THE ONE-SEX BODY ON TRIAL: THE CLASSICAL AND EARLY MODERN EVIDENCE

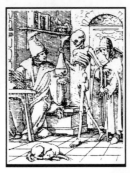

The History of Medicine in Context

Series Editors: Andrew Cunningham and Ole Peter Grell

Department of History and Philosophy of Science
University of Cambridge

Department of History
Open University

Titles in the series include

*Ritual and Conflict: The Social Relations of Childbirth in
Early Modern England*
Adrian Wilson

Medical Consulting by Letter in France, 1665–1789
Robert Weston

Female Patients in Early Modern Britain
Gender, Diagnosis, and Treatment
Wendy D. Churchill

Plague Hospitals
Public Health for the City in Early Modern Venice
Jane L. Stevens Crawshaw

Bad Vibrations: The History of the Idea of Music as Cause of Disease
James Kennaway

'Regimental Practice' by John Buchanan, M.D.:
An Eighteenth-Century Medical Diary and Manual
Edited by Paul Kopperman

The One-Sex Body on Trial: The Classical and Early Modern Evidence

HELEN KING
The Open University, UK

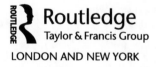

Routledge
Taylor & Francis Group

LONDON AND NEW YORK

First published 2013 by Ashgate Publishing

Published 2016 by Routledge
2 Park Square, Milton Park, Abingdon, Oxfordshire OX14 4RN
711 Third Avenue, New York, NY 10017, USA

First issued in paperback 2016

Routledge is an imprint of the Taylor & Francis Group, an informa business

British Library Cataloguing in Publication Data
A catalogue record for this book is available from the British Library

The Library of Congress has cataloged the printed edition as follows:
King, Helen, 1957-
  The one-sex body on trial : the classical and early modern evidence / by Helen King.
    pages cm. – (The history of medicine in context)
  Includes bibliographical references and index.
  ISBN 978-1-4094-6335-1 (hardcover)
1. Sex differentiation – History. 2. Sex differences – History. I.
Title.
  QP278.K56 2013
  571.8'82 – dc23

                                                                2013011292

ISBN 13: 978-1-138-24762-8 (pbk)
ISBN 13: 978-1-4094-6335-1 (hbk)

Contents

List of Figures

Preface

In the West, making sense of history involves the creation of defining moments, boundaries: befores and afters. We are dominated by a view of time in which there is BC, and AD: or, if you want to see the same division differently, BCE and CE. Within these great swathes of time, we often choose to regard a shorter period as having its own identity, or zeitgeist, and select key images that define what happens before and after our chosen boundary. The history of the body is no exception to this. In the last 25 years, it has been dominated by a particular model in which the 'before' is the 'one-sex' body in which men and women have the same genital organs, only their location – inside or outside – differing. 'After' is the 'two-sex' body, focused on sexual difference. The shift from before to after has been placed in the eighteenth century, so that before becomes 'pre-modern' and after is 'modern'; before is 'them' and after is 'us'. This model was created by Thomas Laqueur in his 1990 book *Making Sex: Body and Gender from the Greeks to Freud.*[1] It has attracted much criticism, yet it has survived, even being enhanced by a 2003 debate in the journal *Isis* following a challenge to it made by Michael Stolberg.[2]

When I first read *Making Sex*, I found the simple two-stage model unhelpful for the texts on which I was then working, the classical Greek treatises on gynaecology found in the Hippocratic corpus, which are not part of Laqueur's 'past'. Here, I was finding neither a 'one-sex' body, nor an interest in the genital organs, but instead an emphasis on differently textured flesh as making women unlike men, a point strongly asserted and used by the ancient writers to suggest that disorders affecting women, throughout their bodies, needed to be interpreted, and therefore treated, very differently from those of men. In the book I published in 1998, *Hippocrates' Woman*, I found that, despite my misgivings about the overall model, much of Laqueur's general approach to the social construction of reality meshed with mine, and I quoted there his comment that 'Experience, in short, is reported and remembered so as to be congruent with dominant paradigms.'[3] But I did not engage directly with his specific views on the ancient world, other than

---

[1]   *Making Sex: Body and Gender from the Greeks to Freud* (Cambridge, MA, 1990).

[2]   Michael Stolberg, 'A Woman Down to her Bones. The Anatomy of Sexual Difference in the Sixteenth and Early Seventeenth Centuries', *Isis*, 94 (2003): 274–99, and subsequent responses and letter to the editor; these will be discussed below, pp. 3–4.

[3]   Laqueur, *Making Sex*, p. 99.

noting in passing that his 'one-sex' model did not work for my material.[4] In 2005, following the *Isis* debate, I was commissioned to write an article on this lack of fit for the ancient Greek world, and on the basis of that I was invited to take part in an exploratory seminar organised by Katy Park at the Radcliffe Institute for Advanced Study, Harvard University, on 'Remaking Sex in Classical, Medieval and Early Modern Medicine'.[5] Here, a group of scholars working on a range of historical periods came together and found that Laqueur's model did not 'work' for any of them. The obvious question this raised was: why did it still survive? In our discussions, we noted the difficulties of challenging a model that is presented as covering such a long span of history, and that appears in a single easily acquired volume; I shall return to the reasons why Laqueur's work was initially so popular, and why it still endures, in the Introduction to the present book.

A few months before the Radcliffe Institute seminar, the survival of Laqueur's model had been vividly illustrated to me when I gave a paper, 'Generating "woman": Jacques Sylvius and Diane de Poitiers', at the 15th Medieval, Renaissance and Baroque Conference at the University of Miami.[6] The theme of the conference was 'When there was no sex or gender?', which I took as an invitation to discuss a 1559 French translation of a treatise on menstruation, and its preface addressed to Diane de Poitiers; this was part of a wider project on Renaissance medicine, another area where Laqueur's model seemed to me to have no value in understanding how the female body was represented. It was clear from the discussion of my paper that nobody could understand why I had not mentioned Laqueur, even once; their first reaction was to ask how what I had said could be made to fit within a 'one-sex' body. While Laqueur's basic model had by that time become irrelevant to my research, it clearly continued to be seen as the starting point by those working in other periods or other humanities disciplines.

This story illustrates the point that the interdisciplinary range and subsequent appeal of Laqueur's work has made it that rare thing: the common property of those working on history and literature, on the early modern period and the modern world. This is despite the many attacks made on it from different directions, some of which will be discussed in detail in the Introduction to this book. Yet it is precisely because of this range and continuing appeal that I believe the present book is necessary. Those coming to *Making Sex* from the many disciplines of the

---

[4]   Helen King, *Hippocrates' Woman: Reading the Female Body in Ancient Greece* (London, 1998), p. 245, citing *Making Sex*, p. 99; see also p. 11.

[5]   The article was 'The Mathematics of Sex: One to Two, or Two to One?', commissioned article for special issue of *Studies in Medieval and Renaissance History: Sexuality and Culture in Medieval and Renaissance Europe*, 3rd series (vol. II, 2005): 47–58.

[6]   Subsequently published as 'Engendrer "la femme": Jacques Dubois et Diane de Poitiers', in Cathy McClive, Jean-François Budin and Nicole Pellegrin (eds), *Femmes en Fleurs: Santé, Sexualité et Génération du Moyen Age aux Lumières* (Université de Saint-Étienne, 2010), 125–38.

arts and humanities are unaware not only of the work on the history of medicine and of the body that has happened subsequent to its publication, but also of the sources Laqueur omits, and the lack of care with which he uses those sources which he does bring into play.

There are other reasons why a book-length examination of Laqueur's work is needed. While he explicitly starts with 'the Greeks', those working in Classical Studies have found his arguments particularly unconvincing. His comments on the classical world in general are very sketchy, and based on a very small sample of evidence; restricted not just to medical texts, but to a subset of these. While he could respond to this criticism by saying that he focused on those ancient authors most cited by the later writers he went on to address in the later parts of his book, this still omits an entire strand of the Western medical tradition. His lack of knowledge of Hippocratic gynaecology, for example, weakens his comments on the sixteenth century, a period in which the Hippocratic insistence on women as entirely different from men was repeated as part of a male claim to be able to treat women's diseases more effectively than could illiterate female healers. This is one aspect of a wider problem with Laqueur: the 'one-sex'/'two-sex' model reduces complexity to simplicity.

Max Weber recommended for comparative study the creation of 'ideal types'; taking and merging features of various real examples, these imaginary constructs could then be used as a basis from which to compare the different examples that can be found in the 'real world'. However, it is central to his methodology that the ideal type itself has never existed. As Julien Freund put it, 'Being unreal, the ideal type has the merit of offering us a conceptual device with which we can measure real development and clarify the most important elements of empirical reality.'[7] In Weber's words, the ideal type 'serves as a harbour until one has learned to navigate safely in the vast sea of empirical facts'.[8] If we were to take them as ideal types, the two stages of Laqueur's model would have some value; but this is not how they have been read. Instead of using them as conceptual, comparative tools to make similarities and differences clearer, the two stages have been reified and the alleged movement from one to the other attached to a specific period, and to other real changes in that period. Ironically, what Laqueur had written about making experience fit the 'dominant paradigms' has also happened in the reception of *Making Sex*.

While further problems concern Laqueur's focus on the genital organs as the locus of sameness or difference – as we shall see in this book, this misrepresents the interest in fluids found in much of Western medicine – I shall be arguing here that the main issue with Laqueur's work is his selective use of 'evidence', and

---

[7] Julien Freund, *The Sociology of Max Weber* (New York, 1969), p. 69. On the ideal type and references to it in Weber, see Richard Swedberg, *The Max Weber Dictionary: Key Words and Central Concepts* (Stanford, CA, 2005), pp. 119–21.

[8] Weber, *The Methodology of the Social Sciences* (eds and tr. Edward A. Shils and Henry A. Finch) (New York, 1959), p. 104.

his lack of close reading of the material he does use. After commenting on some general issues concerning the absence of a 'one-sex' body from the periods on which I work – the classical and the early modern – I shall bring to the debate two stories very different from the canonical medical and scientific works on which he focused. These are the classical stories of Phaethousa, who grew a beard when her husband left her, and Agnodice, the 'first midwife'. I shall show how these have been used over time, and particularly in early modern Europe, to explore issues which are highly relevant to the 'one-sex' body: the possibility of changing sex; whether it is possible to disguise one's sex; and which parts of the body – in addition to the genitalia on which Laqueur's 'one-sex'/'two-sex' model makes us focus – really constitute an individual's sex. In the process of examining these in detail, I shall also focus on the sexual politics of models of the body; for Agnodice in particular, how her story was told and re-told relates to the medical control of the female body, by midwives, medical men, and women seeking to practise medicine. These examples of classical reception will also enable me to say more about the classical world itself, the different interpretations of the two brief key texts helping us to challenge our current readings of the ancient world.

Many people have helped me reflect on these issues over the years, and have encouraged me to continue publishing and thinking about them. I would like to single out Barbara Goff, who encouraged me to start this book, as well as my colleagues Monica Green, Catrien Santing and Manfred Horstmanshoff, all of whom stimulated me to face my problems with Laqueur's model. Above all, I would like to thank Andrew Cunningham, who saw a different book hiding beneath the one I thought I was writing, and persuaded me to rewrite it in its present form. I owe particular debts of gratitude to the Arts and Humanities Research Council, for funding a period of leave in which I could work on it,[9] and to my successive heads of department at the Open University – Phil Perkins and James Robson – and to the Open University Arts Faculty for its support.

Now, nearly a quarter of a century after Laqueur published *Making Sex*, it is time to put the book's central thesis on trial, and to assess more critically the evidence on which it is based, and the use he makes of this evidence. This will enable us to move forward with a better – if more complex – picture of how sexual difference has been made, and remade, over the centuries. By focusing on evidence from the period of his 'one-sex' body, this book aims to explain the unease long felt by scholars about applying his model to the material they know best, and to move the debate forwards in an interdisciplinary way.

---

[9]   AH/I001506/1, 'Following Agnodike and Phaethousa: gender and transformation in the reception of ancient medicine'.

Introduction

Making Sense of *Making Sex*

By far the most influential work on the history of the body, across a range of academic disciplines, remains that of Thomas Laqueur. The son of a pathologist, Laqueur has taught history at the University of California, Berkeley since 1973 and spent a year in medical school from 1980; for his readers, this medical training can be seen as adding authority to his work, with some even confusing the order of events to make him 'a medical student before he became a historian'.[1] First published in 1990, his *Making Sex: Body and Gender from the Greeks to Freud*, presenting a simple two-stage model of change tied to wider social contexts, has now been translated into at least 12 languages.[2] Despite its ubiquity, the model of body history presented in this book is misleading in many ways yet, to date, none of the many challenges made to it has dented its popularity. In this book, I want to put *Making Sex* on trial, presenting evidence from the periods with which I have worked most closely: the classical world and early modern Europe. It is my intention to move the focus away from the canonical texts of the 'great men' of the history of science and medicine used by Laqueur so, after a discussion of the general problems with his model for the period up to around 1700, in the second part of this book I shall investigate two stories originating in the Greco-Roman world that concern the female body and its defining characteristics.[3] These

---

[1]   Lillian Faderman, 'Review', *Signs*, 17 (1992), p. 821: 'Laqueur (who had been a medical student before he became a historian)'. Contrast Thomas Laqueur, 'La Différence: Bodies, Gender, and History', *The Threepenny Review*, 33 (Spring, 1988), p. 12: 'I spent 1980–81 in medical school.' On the opposite trajectory – medical history within the medical curriculum – and the question of who should do medical history, see Frank Huisman and John Harley Warner (eds), *Locating Medical History: The Stories and their Meanings* (Baltimore, MD, 2006). On his medical family, see further *Making Sex*, pp. 16–17 and 243 (great-uncle Ernst Laqueur) and Annick Jaulin, 'La Fabrique du sexe, Thomas Laqueur et Aristote', *Clio: Histoire, femmes et sociétés*, 14 (2001), p. 198. The medical credentials are noticed, and implicitly approved, by readers, for example, 'Laqueur (who did attend a year of med school as preparation for writing this)', in a 2010 review by 'DoctorM' on <http://www.goodreads.com/review/show/90025653> accessed 10 August 2012.

[2]   Laqueur's own CV cites 'French translation with new introduction, Gallimard, 1992; German translation, Campus Verlag, 1992; Italian, Laterza, 1992; Spanish 1994; Swedish, 1995; Portuguese, Lisbon 1997; Brazil 1998; Japanese 1998; Chinese, 1999; Rumanian, 1999; Korean 2000; Hungarian, 2002; Greek 2004' (<http://history.berkeley.edu/sites/default/files/Laqueur_CV.pdf> accessed 12 June 2012).

[3]   This is a more radical shift than that proposed by Donald Beecher, 'Concerning Sex Changes: The Cultural Significance of a Renaissance Medical Polemic', *The Sixteenth*

stories were once widely known, told and re-told by both men and women within the contexts of discussions of sex change, and of the proper roles of women in medicine; areas in which sexual identity was fundamental to the debate.

This book concerns the period which, in Laqueur's model, was that of the 'one-sex' body. His central thesis is that the view of the body that he memorably labelled in this way 'dominated thinking about sexual difference from classical antiquity to the end of the seventeenth century' so that the world before the eighteenth century was thus one 'where at least two genders correspond to but one sex, where the boundaries between male and female are of degree and not of kind'.[4] He traced the 'one-sex body' back to Greco-Roman antiquity, saying that 'For thousands of years it had been a commonplace that women had the same genitals as men except that, as Nemesius, bishop of Emesa in the fourth century, put it: "theirs are inside the body and not outside it".'[5] This imagery is clearly taken from the second-century AD physician, Galen, with whose work Nemesius was very familiar, and who will be discussed at length below. Laqueur's casual 'commonplace ... as Nemesius ... put it' is thus doubly misleading, as it not only glosses over Nemesius' dependence on Galen but also implies many other such rephrasings of the Galenic 'one-sex' body in the period when, in fact, this is a relatively isolated reference. In this 'one-sex' part of Laqueur's model, women and men were believed to have identical organs of generation, only the position of these differing according to the level of heat of the body; the reason why men's genitals were located outside rather than inside was that men's bodies were 'hotter'. In the 'two-sex' model which supposedly replaced this, women and men were understood as fundamentally different, as a result of which their sexual organs could no longer be neatly matched to each other, with each being assumed to have its equivalent in the other's body; instead, according to Laqueur, in the

---

Century Journal, 36 (2005), p. 994, rightly picking up Patricia Parker's point that we need to bring in 'a broader and more complicating textual field' when studying early modern gender; see her 'Gender Ideology, Gender Change: The Case of Marie Germain', *Critical Inquiry*, 19 (1993), p. 339. Where Parker argued for a shift outside the medical literature, Beecher instead moved to other medical literature; but this was itself valuable, as he demonstrated the narrow range of previous scholarship on sixteenth- and seventeenth-century medical discussions of sex change.

    [4]   Laqueur, *Making Sex*, p. 25.

    [5]   Laqueur, *Making Sex*, p. 4 citing Nemesius of Emesa, *On the Nature of Man* (William Tefler, ed., Philadelphia, PA, 1955), p. 369. See now Philip van der Eijk and Robert W. Sharples (eds and tr.), *Nemesius On the Nature of Man* (Liverpool, 2008), p. 155 who translate the key phrase as 'Women have all the same parts as men, but inside and not outside' and Gillian Clark, *Women in Late Antiquity: Pagan and Christian Lifestyles* (Oxford, 1993), p. 72. Katharine Park, 'Cadden, Laqueur, and the "One-Sex Body"', *Medieval Feminist Forum*, 46 (2010), p. 4 (pagination from online version, <http://nrs. harvard.edu/urn-3:HUL.InstRepos:4774909> accessed 10 January 2012) notes that the Latin translation of Nemesius did not circulate in the period before *c.*1500.

eighteenth century, woman ceased to be a colder version of man, and became 'an altogether different creature'.[6]

Laqueur locates the transition between these models of the body in a very specific period, although his critics have found some inconsistency in identifying this; in a review of *Making Sex*, Angus McLaren called the chronology 'maddeningly vague', noting further that, 'Laqueur does not tell us when the shift took place, nor does he tell us why it occurred.'[7] Also picking up the 'why' question, Richard Posner commented on 'Laqueur's inability to come up with an ideological explanation for the change in theory' from 'one-sex' to 'two-sex'.[8] These criticisms are not entirely fair; Laqueur does give various (indeed, maddeningly vague) dates for it and, as we shall see, these do relate to the question of 'why'.

Laqueur asserts that 'Sometime in the eighteenth century, sex as we know it was invented', although elsewhere in his book he has the 'two-sex' model emerging at the end of that century; human sexual nature changed 'in or about the late eighteenth [century]'.[9] In a supportive discussion of Laqueur's work, published in 1997, Tim Hitchcock suggested that these seven years since its publication had already seen the dating of the shift nuanced to cover the period from the 1670s to the 1820s, with an acknowledgement that alternative models of the body continued to exist throughout.[10] In Laqueur's own subsequent comments, the dates have shifted further, but this has still not affected the basic 'one-sex'/'two-sex' model. In 2003, Michael Stolberg challenged the assumptions of both *Making Sex* and Londa Schiebinger's earlier work on eighteenth-century anatomy, on which Laqueur had drawn. Stolberg argued that 'around 1600 many leading physicians, rather than proclaiming a "one-sex model" of female inferiority, insisted on the unique and purposeful features of the female skeleton and the female genital organs and illustrated them visually'.[11] In his response, Laqueur insisted that his model of change remained intact, dismissing apparent

---

6   Laqueur, *Making Sex*, p. 148.

7   Angus McLaren, 'Review', *American Historical Review*, 98 (1993), pp. 832, 833.

8   Richard A. Posner, *Sex and Reason* (Cambridge, MA, 1992), p. 28.

9   Laqueur, *Making Sex*, p. 149, 5 and 6; still quoted as his position by Wendy Churchill, 'The Medical Practice of the Sexed Body: Women, Men and Disease in Britain, *c.*1600–1740', *Social History of Medicine*, 18 (2005), p. 3, who gives the *late* eighteenth century version, and Nadja Durbach, *Spectacle of Deformity. Freak Shows and Modern British Culture* (Berkeley, CA and London, 2010), p. 76. On the various statements Laqueur gave about timing, see Karen Harvey, 'The Century of Sex? Gender, Bodies, and Sexuality in the Long Eighteenth Century', *Historical Journal*, 45 (2002), p. 901.

10   Tim Hitchcock, *English Sexualities, 1700–1800* (New York and Basingstoke), p. 46.

11   Stolberg, 'A Woman Down to her Bones', p. 274. Stolberg assumes that the 'one-sex model' is accompanied by 'female inferiority'; as we shall see, this does not necessarily follow. The piece by Londa Schiebinger which influenced Laqueur was 'Skeletons in the Closet: The First Illustrations of the Female Skeleton in Eighteenth-Century Anatomy', *Representations*, 14 (1986).

divergences from it in the sixteenth to seventeenth centuries, such as that identified by Stolberg, as 'minor revisions', mere 'skirmishes at its metaphysical periphery'.[12] He commented, 'My quarrel with Michael Stolberg is not primarily about whether what I call the one-sex model collapsed 150 years earlier than I claim it did. Over the millennia, what is a century or two?'[13] This is a far more relaxed attitude than that taken in *Making Sex*.

The original choice of a date in the eighteenth century was, however, significant, because it echoed Michel Foucault's chronology for the emergence of the idea of each individual having a single 'true sex'.[14] It also enabled Laqueur to provide this supposed shift between models of the body with a 'why', a social and intellectual context, by tying it to the emergence of 'modernity': 'It is a sign of modernity to ask for a single, consistent biology as the source and foundation of masculinity and femininity.'[15] For him, 'no one was much interested in looking for evidence of two distinct sexes until such differences became politically important';[16] however, we could respond by asking whether, in the history of Western Europe, sexual difference has ever been politically unimportant. Stephanie Libbon published an article in 2007 summarising Laqueur's position on the causative factors of his watershed as follows: '… events surrounding the French Revolution prompted a desire to see difference and therefore a need to create difference. In particular, Laqueur argues that it was the struggle for power between those advocating enfranchisement for women and those opposed to this.'[17] Laqueur further suggests that the paradigm shift occurred because of a greater interest in producing more bodies, as part of the emergence of industrial society, in what he refers to rather vaguely as 'endless micro-confrontations over power in the public and private spheres … in the vast new spaces opened up by the intellectual, economic, and political revolutions of the eighteenth and nineteenth centuries'.[18] In a book

---

[12]   Laqueur, 'Sex in the Flesh', *Isis*, 94 (2003), pp. 301 and 303. *Isis* commissioned responses from both Laqueur and Schiebinger.

[13]   Laqueur, 'Sex in the Flesh', p. 306.

[14]   Park, 'Cadden, Laqueur, and the "One-Sex Body"', p. 2. See Foucault, 'Le vrai sexe', *Arcadie*, 323 (1980); ibid., *Herculine Barbin, dite Alexina B.* (Paris, 1978); English translation *Herculine Barbin: Being the Recently Discovered Memoirs of a Nineteenth-Century French Hermaphrodite*, tr. Richard McDougall (New York, 1980). Further references will be to the English version. For a reassessment of the story told by Foucault, particularly challenging the notion that the 'true sex' is the 'true self', see Geertje Mak, *Doubting Sex. Inscriptions, Bodies and Selves in Nineteenth-Century Hermaphrodite Case Histories* (Manchester and New York, 2012).

[15]   Laqueur, *Making Sex*, p. 61.

[16]   Ibid., p. 10.

[17]   Stephanie E. Libbon, 'Pathologizing the Female Body: Phallocentrism in Western Science', *Journal of International Women's Studies*, 8 (2007), p. 79.

[18]   Laqueur, *Making Sex*, p. 193. Roberta McGrath, *Seeing her Sex: Medical Archives and the Female Body* (Manchester, 2002), pp. 31–2 attributed the rise of the two-sex body

chapter published in 2001 which explicitly endorsed Laqueur's model, Elizabeth Maddock Dillon linked a one-sex to two-sex shift to replacing the collective with the individual as part of 'the move from a monarchical and hierarchical political order to a modern politics of natural rights, equality, and social contract in the Anglo-American world'.[19] Again, this requires the shift to occur in the eighteenth century.

Making a Best-seller

The problems of dating the shift, and the relevance of these in challenging Laqueur's insistence that the rise of the two-sex body was due to specific social and political changes, do not seem to have dented its overall popularity and indeed, in her 2012 book on the legacy of ancient notions of gender, Brooke Holmes notes that the book 'continues to exercise a powerful influence on how contemporary ideas about sex and gender are mapped onto – and authenticated through – the past'.[20] The initial reaction to Laqueur's model, too, was one of great enthusiasm, one reviewer hailing it as 'brilliantly convincing'.[21] Welcoming what he also regarded as Laqueur's 'brilliant' study, Stuart Clark summarised it as focusing on what he called one of the main tenets of the 'binary and analogical thinking' that dominated pre-modern medicine, namely the belief that 'the shape of the female genitals was the exact reverse of the male'.[22] We shall return to this image in the next section of this chapter. In 2003, Londa Schiebinger looked back on Laqueur's book and praised it as 'an arresting and important thesis that has spawned many research projects and observations'.[23] In 2006, *Making Sex* was still being described as one of the 'standard accounts of historical transformation';

---

to a renewed interest in women as 'different' because of the need of an industrialising society to increase the population of workers. On the importance of 'modernity' in the model, see also Heinz-Jürgen Voss, *Making Sex Revisited. Dekonstruktion des Geschlechts aus biologisch-medizinischer Perspektive* (Bielefeld, 2010), pp. 89–90.

[19] Elizabeth Maddock Dillon, 'Nursing Fathers and Brides of Christ: The Feminized Body of the Puritan Convert', in Janet Moore Lindman and Michele Lise Tarter (eds), *A Centre of Wonders: The Body in Early America* (Ithaca, NY, 2001), p. 135.

[20] Brooke Holmes, *Gender: Antiquity and its Legacy* (London, 2012), p. 27. The book as a whole is critical of Laqueur's model, arguing that it fails to understand both sex and gender in the ancient world.

[21] Faderman, 'Review', p. 823. Voss, *Making Sex Revisited*, pp. 18–19 also discusses the reception of Laqueur.

[22] Stuart Clark, *Thinking with Demons: The Idea of Witchcraft in Early Modern Culture* (Oxford, 1997), p. 130. On binary modes of thinking in the ancient world, the classic work remains Geoffrey E.R. Lloyd, *Polarity and Analogy: Two Types of Argumentation in Early Greek Thought* (Cambridge, 1966). For the history of science in the modern period, see Nancy Ley Stepan, 'Race and Gender: The Role of Analogy in Science', *Isis*, 77 (1986).

[23] Londa Schiebinger, 'Skelletestreit', *Isis*, 94 (2003), p. 313.

in 2009 Raphael Cuir stated without any caveats that 'Renaissance human beings had one sex and one body', simply referring to the book in a note.[24]

The remarks of Wendy Sealey Harrison, in a 2006 chapter in which she described the book as 'luminous', illustrate something of why the book has been so successful:

> It dislocates our commonsense understanding of what 'sex' and 'gender' are and how they might be related to one another. Put briefly, what Laqueur argues is that 'sex' is a concept which was invented at a particular point in time in our culture. 'Sex' as a biological entity was 'made' rather than simply discovered, and brought into being for reasons other than the scientific.[25]

This message – of difference between 'then' and 'now', of the primacy of social construction over essentialism, and of the instability of gender – was one that people wanted to hear; Angus McLaren's 1993 review perceptively concluded, 'many readers will want to like this book', and Patricia Simons recently noted that 'Laqueur's daring project suited the times.'[26] One of the oddities of its reception, identified by Janet Adelman, is that 'the authoritative status of Laqueur's thesis is highlighted particularly well by its frequent citation even in places where it is quite tangential to the argument involved'.[27]

---

[24]   Raymond Stephanson, 'Review of Karen Harvey, *Reading Sex in the Eighteenth Century*', *Eighteenth-Century Fiction*, 19 (2006), p. 224; Raphael Cuir, *The Development of the Study of Anatomy from the Renaissance to Cartesianism: da Carpi, Vesalius, Estienne, Bidloo* (Lewiston, Queenston and Lampeter, 2009), p. 80.

[25]   Wendy Sealey Harrison, 'The Shadow and the Substance: The Sex/Gender Debate', in Kathy Davis, Mary Evans and Judith Lorber (eds), *Handbook of Gender and Women's Studies* (London, 2006), pp. 38–9. The point that gender precedes sex was not original to Laqueur; see for example C.S. Lewis' much-quoted comment of 1943 that 'Gender is a reality, and a more fundamental reality than sex', *Perelandra* (London, 1943), p. 200, cited inter alia by Jan Morris, *Conundrum* (London, 1974), p. 25, who prefaced it with 'gender is not physical at all ... it is more truly life and love than any combination of genitals, ovaries and hormones'.

[26]   Angus McLaren, 'Review', p. 833; Patricia Simons, *The Sex of Men in Premodern Europe: A Cultural History* (Cambridge, 2011), p. 155. See also Valerie Traub, 'The Psychomorphology of the Clitoris, or, The Reemergence of the *Tribade* in English Culture', in Valeria Finucci and Kevin Brownlee (eds), *Generation and Degeneration: Tropes of Reproduction in Literature and History from Antiquity to Early Modern Europe* (Durham, NC and London, 2001), p. 157 on how 'Laqueur brilliantly insists upon the force of social construction to impact "biology"'; Traub went on to criticise Laqueur for his 'unifying rubric of explanation' that glosses over variation in either of his two historical periods, noting that in each 'The multiplicity of discourses, their dialogic character, is transformed into a monologic homogeneity' (p. 158).

[27]   Janet Adelman, 'Making Defect Perfection: Shakespeare and the One-Sex Model', in Viviana Comensoli and Anne Russell (eds), *Enacting Gender on the English Renaissance*

From the date of its first publication, *Making Sex* has also been the target of many attacks. While a 1999 review article by the medical historians Mark Jenner and Bernard Taithe noted that *Making Sex* was 'perhaps the most influential work of medical history published in the last two decades', it was from historians of medicine that the very first challenge to Laqueur had come, in the essay review 'Destiny is Anatomy' by Katharine Park and Robert A. Nye; their title is that of Laqueur's Chapter 2 (itself a reference to Freud), and their review was published in *New Republic* in February 1991.[28] Based on their respective specialisms, Park's being early modern medicine and Nye's sexuality in nineteenth-century France, they argued that 'a more complete reading of the sources shows that there was never a one-sex model in Laqueur's sense'.[29] 'Never' is a strong word but, as this book will show, I have found it difficult to identify any historical period in which a 'one-sex' model dominated.

In November 2010, to mark the twentieth anniversary of *Making Sex*, Mineke Bosch and Catrien Santing organised a workshop at the University of Groningen, 'Laqueur Revisited: Between Constructed Bodies and Bodily Materiality', with ten speakers as well as Laqueur himself. The organisers noted that the influence of Laqueur's model has been uneven, varying within different academic disciplines, and one of the questions they posed was 'Why has his book hardly been received in medical history or the history of medicine?'[30] Many aspects of Laqueur's position are ones with which most historians of medicine today would not disagree; centrally, that science constructs rather than discovers, and that what we say about sex will inevitably contain claims about gender.[31] From my own perspective, as a

---

Stage (Urbana/Chicago, IL, 1999), p. 43, cited in Stolberg, 'A Woman Down to her Bones', p. 276, n. 5.

[28] Mark Jenner and Bernard Taithe, 'The Historiographical Body', in John Pickstone and Roger Cooter (eds), *History of Medicine in the Twentieth Century*: Volume 2, *The Body* (New York, 1999), p. 191; Katharine Park and Robert A. Nye, 'Destiny is Anatomy', *New Republic*, 18 February 1991. Freud wrote in his 1912 essay 'On the Universal Tendency to Debasement in the Sphere of Love', James Strachey (ed. and tr.), *The Standard Edition of the Complete Psychological Works* (London, 1957), vol. 11, p. 189; 'the position of the genitals – *inter urinas et faeces* – remains the decisive and unchangeable factor. One might say here, varying a well-known saying of the great Napoleon: "Anatomy is destiny".' Napoleon claimed that 'history is destiny'. Elaine Hoffman Baruch, *Women, Love, and Power: Literary and Psychoanalytic Perspectives* (New York, 1991), pp. 14–15 points out that Freud stated that 'Anatomy is destiny' twice in his work, the second time being in 1924, in a discussion of women's 'penis envy' (Sigmund Freud, *Standard Edition*, vol. 19, p. 178).

[29] Park and Nye, 'Destiny is Anatomy', p. 54.

[30] Conference programme, author's copy; I spoke at this conference on the case of Phaethousa. A similar question about lack of engagement with the model could be posed for Classics; in addition to Holmes, *Gender*, see below, Chapter 1, p. 33 n.12.

[31] Laqueur, *Making Sex*, p. 11. I have commented on the benefits and defects of Laqueur's model in King, 'The Mathematics of Sex'; the present discussion emends and

historian of medicine in the ancient world and also in those periods influenced by the textual traditions of Greco-Roman antiquity, I agree with an assertion found in the preface to *Making Sex*, one which is at odds with Laqueur's subsequent work and its reception; in his words, 'the startling conclusion that a two-sex and a one-sex model [have] *always* been available to those who thought about difference' (my italics).[32] Karen Harvey, for example, has argued that both 'one-sex' and 'two-sex' models coexisted in the long eighteenth century, but featured in different literary genres, with what she classifies as 'erotica' playing with both models; however, she still sets up her argument within Laqueur's picture of a change towards the 'modern' two-sex model, proposing a mixture of old and new images of the body in the period identified as transitional.[33] While Laqueur himself seems to have moved towards a more rigid insistence on the era of the 'one-sex' body being replaced by the age of the 'two-sex' body, his initial statement of the constant availability of both models has generally not been taken up by his users, whether historians or not.

'Men turned outside in'

The main authority for Laqueur's 'one-sex' model is a classical one: Galen. I shall discuss Galen's context in more detail in Chapter 1, when looking at Laqueur's claims for classical Greece and Rome, but it is useful here to reflect on a key Galenic image discussed by Laqueur; the one, I think, which has had the greatest impact on the readers of *Making Sex*. Laqueur's isolation of this image also illustrates something of the problems with his interpretations of pre-modern texts.

In her 2006 chapter supporting Laqueur's model, Wendy Sealey Harrison singled out his use of a poem in which women are 'but men turned outside

---

develops that earlier one.

[32]   Laqueur, *Making Sex*, p. viii. In a letter responding to Mason's review of *Making Sex* in the *London Review of Books*, Laqueur acknowledged that his position had become less rigid, noting that 'Although, for reasons I discuss, a two-sex model based on biological reductionism gained ascendancy after the Enlightenment, both one- and two-sex ways of thinking, contrary to what I thought earlier, have always been, and remain, available'; 'One Sex or Two', *London Review of Books*, 12: 6 December 1990, <http://www.lrb.co.uk/v12/n23/letters#letter4> accessed 1 June 2012.

[33]   Harvey, 'The Century of Sex?'; ibid., *Reading Sex in the Eighteenth Century: Bodies and Gender in English Erotic Culture* (Cambridge, 2004). See below, p. 14–15 for the late seventeenth-century physician Georg Franck von Franckenau, in whose work we can see both models.

in'.[34] She described this as a piece of 'early nineteenth-century doggerel'.[35] This simply repeats Laqueur's own wording; in *Making Sex* he characterised it as 'doggerel verse of the early nineteenth century'.[36] He had previously referred to the same poem in his 1988 article, also as 'doggerel verse of the nineteenth century' (no mention of it as 'early') and as using 'hoary homologies after they have disappeared from learned texts', thus suggesting that popular literature lags behind scientific writing.[37] In fact the source is one of the versions of the popular and much-reprinted guide to pregnancy and childbirth, *Aristotle's Masterpiece*.[38] However, the *Masterpiece*, and hence the poem, is not a nineteenth-century text so, in Laqueur's terms, this cannot simply concern the survival in popular literature of a one-sex model in a two-sex world. Although it was still being reprinted into the early twentieth century, the compilation we know as the *Masterpiece* was first published in 1684, and includes – from the 1702 edition, entitled *Insigne Artificium Aristotelis* – a poem that states

> Thus I the Womens Secrets have survey'd
> And let them see how curiously they're made;
> And that, *tho' they of differente Sexes be,*

---

[34] Harrison, 'The Shadow and the Substance', p. 39. The phrase 'turned the other way out' clearly has had a disproportionate impact on modern readers; for example it is also used in Richard Cleminson and Francisco Vázquez García, 'Breasts, Hair and Hormones: The Anatomy of Gender Difference in Spain, 1880–1940', *Bulletin of Spanish Studies*, 86:5 (2009), p. 630.

[35] Harrison, 'The Shadow and the Substance', p. 39.

[36] Laqueur, *Making Sex*, p. 4.

[37] Laqueur, 'La Différence', p. 13.

[38] Laqueur, *Making Sex*, p. 4; using the Arno Press edition of the 1970s, based on the 1813 edition, thus explaining Laqueur's dating, although elsewhere he seems to think that it 'was continuously reprinted from the middle of the fifteenth century' (*Making Sex*, p. 246, n. 6). On the *Masterpiece* see Roy Porter, '"The Secrets of Generation Display'd": *Aristotle's Masterpiece* in Eighteenth-Century England', in *'Tis Nature's Fault: Unauthorized Sexuality during the Enlightenment* (Cambridge, 1988); Mary Fissell, 'Hairy Women and Naked Truths: Gender and the Politics of Knowledge in *Aristotle's Masterpiece*', *William and Mary Quarterly*, 3rd ser., 60 (2003), and ibid., 'Making a Masterpiece: The Aristotle Texts in Vernacular Medical Culture', in Charles E. Rosenberg (ed.), *Right Living: An Anglo-American Tradition of Self-Help Medicine* (Baltimore, MD, 2003), 59–87; the first version of the *Masterpiece* merges sections of Levinus Lemnius (from a selection published in London, 1664 from his *The Secret Miracles of Nature* (London, 1658; this in turn was a translation of his *De miraculis occulta naturae* (Antwerp, 1564, an expanded version of the 1559 edition)), and Jakob Rueff, *De conceptu et generatione hominis* (Zurich, 1554, translated into English as *The Expert Midwife* in 1637). Fissell, who has identified three different versions of the *Masterpiece* in the seventeenth and eighteenth centuries, is currently working on a monograph on the book and its reception.

Yet in the Whole[39] they are the same as we:
For those that have the strictest Searchers been,
Find Women are but Men turn'd Out-side in:
And Men, if they but cast their Eyes about,
May find they're Women with their In-side out.[40]

It is interesting that, in both his 1988 article and his 1990 book, Laqueur quotes only part of this: the section I have marked in italics here. His choice cuts out the identity of the first-person author as gendered male throughout. It is a man who confidently surveys women's secrets, only to discover that, from one point of view, even men are women; but Laqueur's selection of lines also omits this final, disturbing, truth. The penultimate couplet, which he includes, suggests that there is a single male sex, of which women are a variant, but the final couplet, which he omits, originally served to restore the balance, proposing that neither sex is primary: each is the other, topsy-turvy.[41]

---

[39]   Laqueur uses a later redaction that has 'on the whole' for 'in the whole'. I would suggest that 'in the Whole' in the original is a pun on 'hole', and thus a sexual joke rather than simply expressing 'completely' or 'all things considered'.

[40]   I am quoting here the 1702 edition, *Insigne Artificium Aristotelis: or, Aristotle's Compleat Master-Piece. In two parts. Displaying the secrets of nature in the generation of man*, p. 15; my thanks to Mary Fissell for pointing me to this version. The earliest edition I have located is *Aristotle's Master-piece* (London: J. How, 1690).The poem is not here, nor in the 1694 edition of *Aristotle's Master-piece*, but it also features, for example, in the 1777 *The Works of Aristotle*, p. 14; the 1771 *Aristotle's Compleat Master-piece*, p. 22; the 1799 *The Works of Aristotle*, p. 11; it is the 1791 *The Works of Aristotle*, p. 15 that is quoted in Janet Blackman, 'Popular Theories of Generation: The Evolution of *Aristotle's Works*'; The Study of an Anachronism', in John Woodward and David Richards (eds), *Health Care and Popular Medicine in Nineteenth-Century England* (London, 1977), pp. 69–70, cited by Laqueur, *Making Sex*, p. 246, n. 6. Vern L. Bullough, 'An Early American Sex Manual, or, Aristotle Who?', *Early American Literature*, 7 (1972–73), p. 241 noted that the work contains approximately three to four times as much information on women as on men and argues for its 'erotic' value; the introduction to the 1697 edition contains a warning that 'those that are Filthy and Unclean' may find the book 'an occasion of stirring up their Bestial Appetites'. I have chosen to leave quotations with their original spelling, although mindful of Elaine Hobby's point that 'Not to alter quotations ... gives a false and distancing sense of quaintness' (*Virtue of Necessity. English Women's Writing 1649–88* (Ann Arbor, MI, 1989), 'Note'. I suggest that this is comparable with issues of translation; do we leave in markers of the 'otherness' of the text or erase these so that the text is 'domesticated'? See Lawrence Venuti, *The Translator's Invisibility* (London and New York, 1995), p. 20.

[41]   The final couplet is also omitted by David M. Friedman, *A Mind of its Own: A Cultural History of the Penis* (New York, 2001), p. 69; more accurately than Laqueur, he places the poem 'a century later' than Vesalius. Anthony Fletcher, *Gender, Sex, and Subordination in England, 1500–1800* (New Haven, CT, 1995), p. 37 quotes the final two couplets. Timon Screech, *Sex and the Floating World: Erotic Images in Japan, 1700–1820* (London, 1999), p. 96 reduces the poem to a simple two-line 'rhyme', 'Those

This balanced position is precisely that taken by the classical source which clearly lies behind this passage in the *Masterpiece*: Galen. Laqueur presents the *Masterpiece* as a book that 'transmitted Galenic learning to hundreds of thousands of lay readers'.[42] Although its contents are far more varied in their sources than this comment suggests, it certainly transmitted one key image. In *On the Usefulness of the Parts of the Body*, Galen invited his readers to join him in a thought experiment. In the translation of Margaret Tallmadge May, published in 1968 and so used by Laqueur, Galen wrote:

> All the parts, then, that men have, women have too, the difference between them lying in only one thing, which must be kept in mind throughout the discussion, namely, that in women the parts are within [the body], whereas in men they are outside, in the region called the perineum. Consider first whichever ones you please, *turn outward the woman's, turn inward, so to speak, and fold double the man's, and you will find them the same in both in every respect.*[43]

The section in italics forms the epigraph to Laqueur's Chapter 2, 'Destiny is Anatomy'; but, despite this passage from Galen being so central to his argument, he never quotes it in full.[44] The neutral approach of the *Masterpiece* poem, in which women are men, but men are also women, recalls Galen's 'Consider first *whichever ones* you please' – omitted by Laqueur. Instead, for Laqueur, this becomes a hierarchical relationship in which, in his own words, '*man* is the measure of all things', summarised by Peter Laipson as 'Women were the inverts of men, not vice-versa.'[45] But neither the *Masterpiece* nor Galen added that final negative. Already, Laqueur's 'one-sex' body is not the same as that of his sources.

The 1702 version of the *Masterpiece* featured a further use of inside/outside in the preface 'To the Reader'. Here it appeared with a feminised Nature, stating that Aristotle, in his 'Master piece', has 'made so thorow a Search, that he has (as it were) turn'd Nature's Inside outwards'.[46] This is a very different approach; here

---

whose greatest study it has been / Tell us women are but men turned outside in'. See also Churchill, 'The Medical Practice of the Sexed Body', p. 17 on the late seventeenth- century physician Archibald Pitcairn, who argued that 'a Man is a Woman without a Womb' (*The Whole Works of Dr. Archibald Pitcairn*, tr. George Sewell and J.T. Desaguliers, 2nd edition (London, 1727), p. 235).

[42]   Laqueur, *Making Sex*, p. 151.

[43]   Galen, *De Usu Partium*, 14.6 (ed. Kühn, 4. 158–9), tr. Margaret Tallmadge May, *Galen, On the Usefulness of the Parts of the Body*, 2 vols (Ithaca, NY, 1968), vol. 2, p. 628; Laqueur, *Making Sex*, pp. 25–7.

[44]   Ibid., p. 25.

[45]   Ibid., p. 62; Peter Laipson, 'From Boudoir to Bookstore: Writing the History of Sexuality. A Review Article', *Comparative Studies in Society and History*, 34 (1992), p. 639 summarising Laqueur.

[46]   *Insigne Artificium Aristotelis*, p. i.

Aristotle, and hence the reader, is put in the dominant position as the one who reveals the previously hidden secrets of a passive, feminised Nature. This again contrasts with the poem, in which the world is a more balanced place in which neither sex is superior, despite the dominance of the male 'searcher'.[47]

The earliest versions of *Aristotle's Masterpiece*, in which the poem did not feature, also used inside/outside imagery, but did not restrict themselves to the 'one-sex' model. The 1690 edition, in a chapter on virginity, gave a debate between a one-sex and a two-sex approach concerning whether, with sufficient heat, a female child could turn into a male child *in utero*.[48] This was based on a much earlier author, Severin Pineau, who died in around 1619; he is named here as 'Sever(i)us Plineus' or as 'Pliny', a confusion with the first-century AD Roman author, Pliny the Elder. The *Masterpiece* cited Pineau as a supporter of a 'two-sex model', accurately summarising his views as follows: 'The Genital parts of both Sexes, are so unlike other, in Substance, Composition, Situation, Figure, Action and Use, that nothing is more unequal.'[49] This edition of the *Masterpiece* then turned to the one-sex model, which it attributed to various writers including Galen, from whom it quoted:

> a Man (saith he) is different from a Woman in nothing else but having his Genital Members without his Body: And this is certain, that if Nature having formed a Man, would convert him into a woman; she hath no other task to perform, but to turn his Genital member inward; and a Woman into a Man by the contrary.[50]

---

[47]   The references to men revealing the secrets of a feminised Nature recall the work of Ludmilla Jordanova, *Sexual Visions: Images of Gender in Science and Medicine between the Eighteenth and Twentieth Centuries* (Hemel Hempstead, 1989), Chapter 5, and show that this image was found before the period she describes.

[48]   *Aristotle's Master-piece* (London, 1690).

[49]   Ibid., p. 91; in the 1697 edition, pp. 71–2, 'nothing is more unequal' became 'nothing is more unlike'. Severin Pineau, *De integritatis et corruptionis virginum notis* (Amsterdam, 1663), p. 73, emphasised difference very strongly in a discussion of whether a girl can turn into a boy: *Etenim sunt utriusque sexus partes genitales adeo inter se dissimiles in substantia, magisque in compositione, situ figura, actio et usu, ut dissimilius quicquam vix reperiri posit, et quanto magis inter se similes sunt caeterae omnes totius reliqui corporis partes (exceptis mammis ...) tanto minus genitales partes unius sexus cum alterius partibus convenient, si conferantur ...* 'And indeed, the genital parts of each sex are to such a degree dissimilar to each other in substance, and to a greater extent in composition, location, shape, action and use, so that barely anything can be found that is more different, and much more are all the other remaining parts of the whole body similar to each other (except the breasts), while so much less are the genital parts of the one sex like the parts of the other sex, if they are compared'. On p. 75 Pineau gives the theory that sex change myths arose because midwives tried to cover up the fact that they had assigned the wrong sex at birth; this is also repeated in the *Masterpiece*. As we shall see in Chapter 1, this list of differences comes from sixteenth-century authors.

[50]   *Aristotle's Master-piece* (London, 1690), p. 92.

It is not clear here where the words of Galen end; in fact, before 'And this is certain'. Once again, this is expressed as a balanced model, where sex change can, at least theoretically, operate in either direction. In this model, a female baby could change before birth, with genitals 'issu[ing] forth, and the Child has become a Male, yet retaining some certain Gestures, unbefitting the Masculine Sex, as Female Actions, a shrill Voice, and more feeble than ordinary'.[51] The *Masterpiece* presented the inside/outside model as being essential to generation, and it did not rule out some differences beyond those of location or shape; the organs are 'inverted for the conveniency of Generation, the main reason being that one is more solid than the other'.[52] In the 1697 edition of the *Masterpiece*, the words of Galen were separated out more clearly, by being italicised, while the topsy-turvy nature of the opposition was underlined still further by adding an additional phrase so that the section that forms the direct quotation reads, '*A Man (saith he) is different from a Woman in nothing else, but having his Genital Members without his Body, whereas a Woman has 'em within.*'[53]

If, unlike Laqueur, we study the different versions of the *Masterpiece* rather than ignoring the complexity of this compilation, and if we carry out a close reading of the various editions, we can see that this powerful image of reversal is far more complex than *Making Sex* and its users suggest, and Harrison's uncritical focus on it is misleading. Different versions of the *Masterpiece* made balance more, or less, clear; earlier versions featured a debate between the one- and two-sex models, whereas in 1702 the poem – with its own view of balance – was introduced. Laqueur makes only selective use of the *Masterpiece* verses; he distorts them so that the balance of the original is lost; and he omits the *Masterpiece*'s inclusion of both one- and two-sex models, which in turn derives from sixteenth-century sources that foregrounded a two-sex model, thus supporting sexual difference well before any eighteenth-century 'watershed'.

Making Sex: Appeal and Attacks

This discussion of the *Masterpiece* provides a flavour of the sort of historical and literary work that needs to be carried out on Laqueur's material. If the 'one-sex' model is so misleading, however, why has it been so popular? In addition to images that a modern reader finds surprising or striking, such as the 'outside in' body, and the argument for sexual difference as 'made', I think that we can identify four main aspects explaining the success of *Making Sex*: a clear central thesis, interdisciplinary appeal, a very wide historical range and arresting illustrations.

---

[51]   Ibid., pp. 92–3; in the 1697 edition, pp. 71–2, 'more feeble than ordinary' became 'a more Effeminate temper than ordinary'.

[52]   *Aristotle's Master-piece* (London, 1690), p. 93.

[53]   *Aristotle's Master-piece* (London, 1697), p. 71.

These features combine to make it accessible enough to be very widely used in undergraduate teaching.[54]

First, the book's main attraction lies in what Stephanie Browner's review called its 'simple and compelling argument', which she suggested made the book 'essential reading for all historians'; Dror Wahrman later called it a 'seductively straightforward narrative'.[55] Laqueur's basic two-stage narrative contrasts powerfully with the more complex – and thus more difficult to grasp – approach of those who have produced the most trenchant criticisms of his work, such as Joan Cadden who, for the medieval period (in Laqueur's model, supposedly firmly 'one-sex') instead emphasised 'diversity, eclecticism, and alternatives'.[56] Reviewing the book for the *Journal of the History of Sexuality* in 1993, Sally Shuttleworth commented that in general 'the repetitive prominence accorded to [Laqueur's] overarching theory tends to iron out contextual complexity'.[57] A recent article on the seventeenth-century German physician Georg Franck von Franckenau, framed in terms of Laqueur's model, similarly concluded that

> On the one hand, Franckenau's point about menstruating men seems to reinforce Laqueur's thesis of the one-sex model, since Franckenau shows that men and women shared similar bodily functions. But on the other hand, Franckenau's view of sexual difference is much more complex. He explicitly argues that

---

[54]   Indeed, when I worked at the University of Reading and included this book in reading lists in around 2005, it was one of the few books of its age in the library that was falling apart from use. There is also a Wikipedia entry on 'One sex two sex theory', which summarises the arguments of *Making Sex* without offering any criticisms: <http://en.wikipedia.org/wiki/One_sex_two_sex_theory> (update of 12 January 2012, accessed 20 July 2012).

[55]   Stephanie Browner, 'Review', in *Victorian Studies*, 35 (1992); Dror Wahrman, 'Change and the Corporeal in Seventeenth- and Eighteenth-Century Gender History: Or, Can Cultural History Be Rigorous?', *Gender and History*, 20 (2008), p. 586. See here Sarah Toulalan, 'Introduction' to Sarah Toulalan and Kate Fisher (eds), *Bodies, Sex and Desire from the Renaissance to the Present* (Basingstoke, 2011), p. 1 on how the reception of Laqueur demonstrates the 'tendency to look for "turning points"' in the history of the body. Browner usefully notes that Laqueur seems to have a strong preference for the 'one-sex' model.

[56]   Joan Cadden, *Meanings of Sex Difference in the Middle Ages: Medicine, Science, and Culture* (Cambridge, 1993), p. 4.

[57]   Sally Shuttleworth, 'Review', *Journal of the History of Sexuality*, 3 (1993), p. 634. Shuttleworth is an English Literature specialist. See also the 2004 review by the medievalist Renee Goethe on <http://www.amazon.com/review/R2TN37MTAKKOST> accessed 24 July 2012: 'While Laqueur's model is a nicely simplified version of the past, the question has to arise – when does simplification become distortion? How much detail about the past can be safely ignored in the name of simplicity before you create a useless model?'

female testicles (ovaries) differ from male testicles in many respects, that is, male and female anatomies are significantly different.[58]

This 'on the one hand … on the other hand' approach is more difficult to grasp than a single one-sex/two-sex transition.

Second, Laqueur's book is interdisciplinary, so much so that in her review for the *Journal of Interdisciplinary History* Susan Dwyer Amussen went so far as to hail it as 'a triumph of interdisciplinary scholarship'.[59] It has been read within a wide range of subjects, by specialists on many different historical periods, making it a relatively rare case in which people from very diverse backgrounds can find themselves speaking the same conceptual language. A third, and closely related, point would be its sheer range across the centuries; from the ancient world to modernity, 'from Plato to NATO' or, as the book's subtitle has it, 'from the Greeks to Freud'. This combination of disciplines and chronology makes it very difficult to criticise, an observation taken up in a workshop organised by Katy Park at the Radcliffe Institute in 2006, to which specialists in a wide range of historical periods, including some working on non-Western theories of the body, were invited.[60]

The pattern of attacks on *Making Sex* is normally to say that, while the author accepts the overall validity of Laqueur's model, she wishes to challenge the particular sub-section on which she is an expert; thus the model as a whole manages to survive, despite multiple, and cumulative, challenges.[61] An example

---

[58]   Sari Kivistö, 'G. F. von Franckenau's *Satyra Sexta* (1674) on Male Menstruation and Female Testicles', in Anu Korhonen and Kate Lowe (eds), *The Trouble with Ribs: Women, Men and Gender in Early Modern Europe, COLLeGIUM: Studies Across Disciplines in the Humanities and Social Sciences*, 2 (2007) (<http://hdl.handle.net/10138/25752>). On menstruating men, see below, p. 46.

[59]   Susan Dwyer Amussen, 'Review', *Journal of Interdisciplinary History*, 24 (1994), p. 522.

[60]   I was an invited participant at this event: Radcliffe Exploratory Seminar, 'Remaking Sex in Classical, Medieval and Early Modern Medicine', Radcliffe Institute for Advanced Study, Harvard University, 2006.

[61]   Such challenges include those of Lorraine Daston and Katharine Park, 'The Hermaphrodite and the Orders of Nature: Sexual Ambiguity in Early Modern France', in Louise Fradenburg and Carla Freccero (eds), *Premodern Sexualities* (New York, 1996), pp. 117–36; Katharine Park, 'The Rediscovery of the Clitoris', in David Hillman and Carla Mazzio (eds), *The Body in Parts: Fantasies of Corporeality in Early Modern Europe* (London, 1997), pp. 171–94; Winfried Schleiner, 'Early Modern Controversies About the One-Sex Model', *Renaissance Quarterly*, 53 (2000), pp. 180–91; Jaulin, 'La Fabrique du sexe'; King, 'The Mathematics of Sex'; Katy Park, *Secrets of Women. Gender, Generation and the Origins of Human Dissection* (New York, 2006), pp. 186–8; Amy Lindgren, 'The Wandering Womb and the Peripheral Penis: Gender and the Fertile Body in Late Medieval Infertility Treatises', PhD thesis, University of California, Davis, 2005, p. 10; Park, 'Cadden, Laqueur, and the "One-Sex Body"'. A discussion of the phrasing of challenges features in Churchill, 'The Medical Practice of the Sexed Body', pp. 6–7.

of the phrasing of such an attack features in one of the very first reviews of the book, by Michael Mason; he wrote that 'The first part of the story, up until the Enlightenment, is relatively uncomplicated, and I shall not dwell on it ... I cannot judge if Laqueur's accounts of pre-modern medical ideas on gender are accurate, but I must say that he sometimes seems to have been rushed into errors in the later periods.'[62] In 1992, Richard Posner supported the overall thesis, although moving the date of the watershed even later – 'That something like the one-sex theory was popular, even dominant, until the nineteenth century is powerfully argued and probably true' – but he went on to note that even 'Laqueur's own quotations from Aristotle ... show[s] that Aristotle was a two-sex man.'[63] A more recent example of this phenomenon can be found in Annick Jaulin's blistering attack on Laqueur's elision of Aristotle and Galen, which nevertheless ends with an endorsement of the value of his work for understanding the eighteenth and nineteenth centuries.[64] Howard Hsueh-Hao Chiang's 2007 article on the two-sex model in modern America challenges Laqueur for the modern period, but notes that, overall, 'I am indeed quite confident about Laqueur's historical insight.'[65]

Finally, an important aspect of the success of *Making Sex* is its use of striking visual images, 63 in all; reviewers drew their readers' attention to these.[66] Most memorable, perhaps, is the illustration of the womb, vagina and pudenda from Andreas Vesalius' 1543 *On the Fabric of the Human Body*, in which the human material is cut in such a way that the whole ensemble looks to modern viewers more like a penis (Figure I.1);[67] this mode of representation was used by other authors in the early modern period, as Laqueur himself shows, and the image itself was copied into other treatises. The centrality of the images in *Making Sex* implies that 'seeing' is a simple act, even though in the text Laqueur consistently distinguishes between 'seeing' (reality) and 'seeing-as' (representation). The images are under-referenced, without page numbers from their original locations, and they are separated from the texts that originally accompanied them. I shall further explore the use of images, and the difficulties with Laqueur's interpretation of this Vesalius illustration, in Chapter 2.

---

[62]   Michael Mason, 'Do Women Like Sex? Review of Thomas Laqueur, *Making Sex*', *London Review of Books*, 8 November 1990: pp. 16–17.

[63]   Posner, *Sex and Reason*, p. 28.

[64]   Jaulin, 'La Fabrique du sexe', p. 201.

[65]   Howard Hsueh-Hao Chiang, 'Epistemic Gender, Sex Beyond the Flesh: Science, Medicine, and the Two-Sex Model in Modern America', *eSharp*, Issue 9, *Gender: Power and Authority* (2007) (<http://www.gla.ac.uk/media/media_41212_en.pdf> accessed 1 July 2011), p. 1.

[66]   For example, Faderman, 'Review', p. 821.

[67]   Laqueur, *Making Sex*, Figure 20, p. 82 gives this image but just as Vesalius has chosen to cut the body to make it look like this – and, as the womb, vagina and external genitalia fail to match, possibly chosen to create a composite image – so Laqueur cuts the page to omit the text, showing only the isolated image.

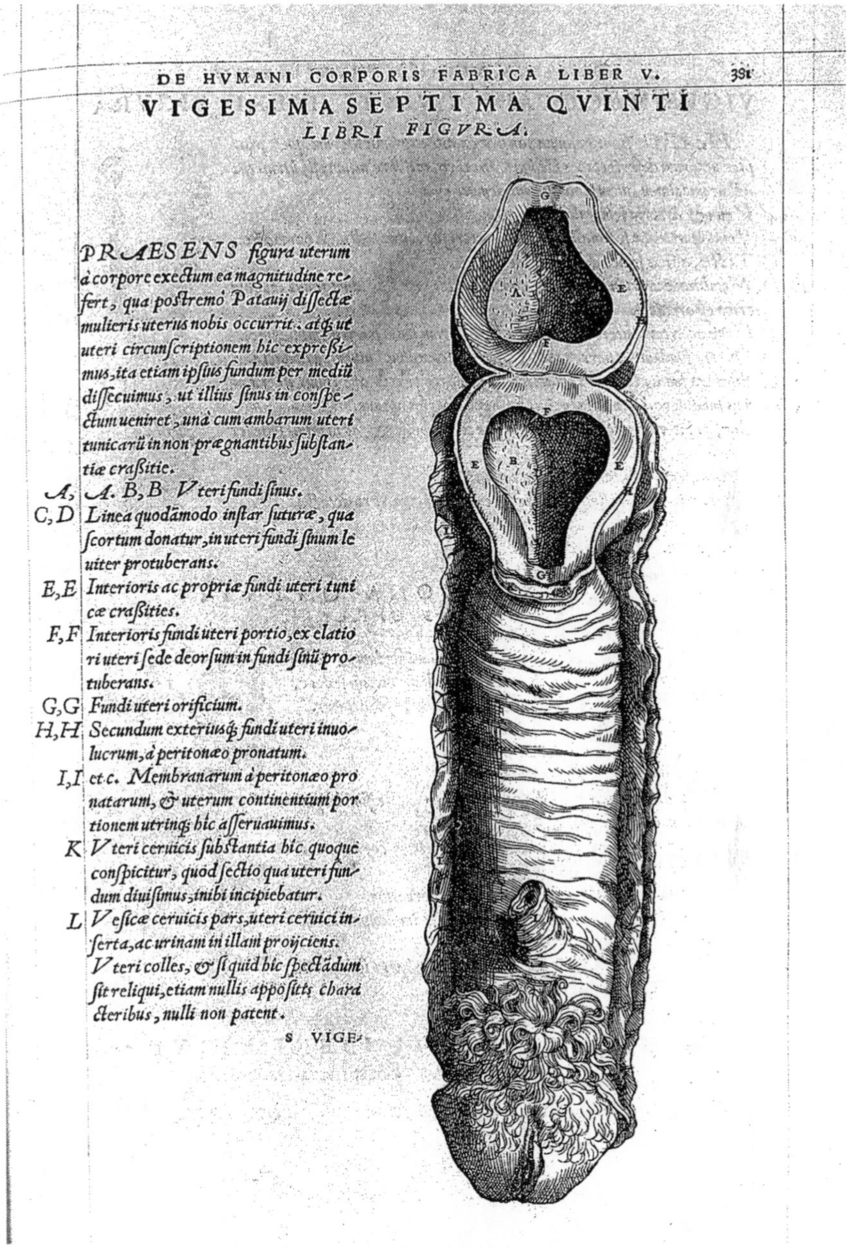

DE HVMANI CORPORIS FABRICA LIBER V. 381

VIGESIMA SEPTIMA QVINTI
LIBRI FIGVRA.

PRAESENS figura uterum
à corpore exectum ea magnitudine refert, qua postremò Patauij dissectæ
mulieris uterus nobis occurrit: atq ut
uteri circunscriptionem hic expressi-
mus, ita etiam ipsius fundum per mediũ
dissecuimus, ut illius sinus in conspe-
ctum ueniret, una cum ambarum uteri
tunicarũ in non prægnantibus substan-
tiæ crassitie.

A, A. B, B Vteri fundi sinus.
C, D Linea quodāmodo instar suturæ, qua
scortum donatur, in uteri fundi sinum le
uiter protuberans.
E, E Interioris ac propriæ fundi uteri tuni
cæ crassities.
F, F Interioris fundi uteri portio, ex elatio
ri uteri sede deorsum in fundi sinũ protuberans.
G, G Fundi uteri orificium.
H, H Secundum exteriusq fundi uteri inuo-
lucrum, à peritonæo pronatum.
I, I et c. Membranarum à peritonæo pro
natarum, & uterum continentium por
tionem utrinq hic asseruauimus.
K Vteri ceruicis substantia hic quoque
conspicitur, quòd sectio qua uteri fundum diuisimus, inibi incipiebatur.
L Vesicæ ceruicis pars, uteri ceruici in-
serta, ac urinam in illam proijciens.
Vteri colles, & si quid hic spectādum
sit reliqui, etiam nullis appositis chara
cteribus, nulli non patent.

S VIGE-

Figure I.1   Andreas Vesalius, *De humani corporis fabrica* (Basle: ex officina Joannis Oporini, 1543), p. 381, Book V, Figure 27.

Beyond Genital Anatomy

In 1993 the medieval historian Joan Cadden succinctly noted in the introduction to her book that 'This analysis differs from that of Thomas Laqueur' and observed that, while some of her material could fit within the 'one-sex' model, nevertheless 'medieval views on the status of the uterus and the opinions of medieval physiognomers about male and female traits suggest evidence of other models not reducible to Laqueur's'.[68] In addition to penis/womb, she identified other key physical distinctions between men and women found in medieval texts; differences in the skull, the brain, the origin of sexual pleasure (in the male, the kidneys: in the female, the navel), body hair and beards.[69]

Cadden's work raises important issues, which this book will explore. Historically, in what parts of the body has sexual identity been thought to reside: in the external genitalia, where Laqueur's inside/outside focus lies, or in non-genital markers of sex? How has this changed over time? Will Fisher has proposed that the beard was more important than the genitalia in defining sex in early modern Europe: Patricia Simons argued against this, pointing out that, as the beard was seen as the result of the presence of semen, it is itself a 'genital' marker, contrary to what we would now expect.[70] What about menstruation as a marker? To us, the beard and the menses may appear very different, one a matter of personal choice, the other of necessity, and one being external and easily visible, with the other resulting from internal processes and not being obvious to the casual observer. However, as we shall see, Western medicine has a long tradition of seeing both as the result of excess bodily fluids. Clearly, we can assume nothing from our own experience. In the following chapters, I want to revisit Laqueur's model by reflecting on the ways in which early modern medical writers posed the questions, 'What constitutes sex?' and 'Is sex change possible?'

While, as I have outlined, a number of attacks have already been mounted on Laqueur's model, in this book I am going to take a different approach. I will take up the generous invitation in his first chapter which, in the reception of his work, has been forgotten; here Laqueur asked his 'readers to decide for themselves, whether the impressions they derive from these pages fit what they themselves know of the vast spans of time that I cover'.[71] Although, like him, I shall begin with the Hippocratic treatises and Galen, my focus after that will be on the period from around 1520 to 1800, when the classical medical authorities – Galen, known as the 'Prince of Physicians', and Hippocrates, the 'Father of Medicine' – still

---

[68] Cadden, *Meanings of Sex Difference*, p. 3. Laqueur is not mentioned any further in this book.

[69] Ibid., pp. 177–83.

[70] Will Fisher, 'The Renaissance Beard: Masculinity in Early Modern England', *Renaissance Quarterly* 54 (2001): pp. 155–87; Simons, *Sex of Men*, pp. 30 and 140.

[71] Laqueur, *Making Sex*, p. 23.

held sway.[72] This dominance survived changes in medical theory and practice; the very range of the theories and practices described in the sixty or so treatises of the Hippocratic corpus meant that new developments continued to find passages of text that meant they too could claim him as their 'Father', or could keep him as a moral exemplar while paying less attention to the medical content of the corpus.[73] In particular, in the sixteenth century, new translations of the Hippocratic corpus introduced a wider range of models of male/female difference than is found in Galen. What I have elsewhere called 'the Hippocratic imperative' demanded that the bodies of men and women were treated in different ways when ill; this was not what Galen had suggested.[74]

Rather than assembling a chronologically organised list of quotations supporting or denying a 'one-sex' body, and then trying to tie this to a major social or cultural shift, I intend here to concentrate on one thread that ran through the period that I am discussing: the lasting power of stories taken from the classical world. The two stories on which I have chosen to focus, unfamiliar to readers today, were very well known in early modern Europe, and highly flexible for their users, so that a simple 'one-sex'/'two-sex' model cannot do justice to them. For both stories, I shall be adopting a methodology different from that of Laqueur; as with the 'outside in' passage discussed earlier in this Introduction, I shall be carrying out close readings of the stories, setting them in their original and later contexts and charting different understandings of the key terms.

The first story is a case history from the Hippocratic corpus, probably dating to the fourth century BC, concerning a woman called Phaethousa, whose body changed when she stopped menstruating. This story helps us consider the question 'Is sex change possible?' But does it concern the ease with which a woman's internal organs can move to the outside, or the inescapable void between woman and man? The text reads as follows:

---

[72]   Helen King, 'The Power of Paternity: The Father of Medicine Meets the Prince of Physicians', in David Cantor (ed.), *Reinventing Hippocrates* (Aldershot, 2001), pp. 21–36.

[73]   Yvonne Knibiehler, 'Les médecins et la "nature feminine" au temps du Code civil', *Annales ESC*, 4 (1976), p. 828 shows that, even within the genre of medical writing, very different models of authority can be used. She usefully distinguished between French 'scientific' medical literature of the late eighteenth and early nineteenth century, in which both Hippocrates and Galen were moved aside in favour of statistics, and French 'moralising' medical literature, where Hippocrates continued to be venerated.

[74]   Monica H. Green, 'Bodily Essences: Bodies as Categories of Difference', in Linda Kalof (ed.), *A Cultural History of the Human Body: The Medieval Age* (New York, 2010), pp. 146–7 suggests that, where the inside/outside image was used in medieval surgery, it had 'therapeutic implications', with treatments for conditions affecting the male genitalia being assumed equally valid for those of women. An increased focus on Hippocrates in the sixteenth century argued instead for totally different treatments; Helen King, *Midwifery, Obstetrics and the Rise of Gynaecology: The Uses of a Sixteenth-Century Compendium* (Aldershot, 2007), p. 33.

In Abdera, Phaethousa the wife of Pytheas, who kept at home, having borne children in the preceding time, when her husband was exiled stopped menstruating for a long time. Afterwards pains and reddening in the joints. When that happened her body was masculinised and grew hairy all over, she grew a beard, her voice became harsh, and though we did everything we could to bring forth menses they did not come, but she died after surviving a short time. The same thing happened to Nanno, Gorgippos' wife, in Thasos. All the physicians I met thought that there was one hope of feminizing her, if normal menstruation occurred. But in her case, too, it was not possible, though we did everything, but she died quickly (*Epidemics* 6.8.32).[75]

Hairiness, in later medical sources from the Greco-Roman world, is the 'mark of a man'.[76] Its presence indicates the greater male body heat that also enables a man to 'concoct' his blood into semen. Women are normally too cold to do this: Phaethousa's missing menstrual blood appears to be turning into her beard and body hair. In early modern writers, too, the beard is 'manhood's ensign'.[77] In the case history of Phaethousa, however, it is a sign not of masculinity, but of sickness. It is not seen as conclusive for her 'true sex', but then neither are her external genitalia, which do not feature here unless we understand 'her body was masculinised' to imply a penis; I shall discuss the options here in more detail in Chapter 3. I shall be arguing that, while her body's surface gives one impression to those around her, it is her womb – hidden, but made evident by her previous childbearing – that convinces the Hippocratic physician recording her case that she is a woman, despite the visible changes to her body. In some Renaissance versions, it is very clear that her 'true sex' remains female, despite the conflicting signals given out by her transformed body: in others, in contrast, she is presented as changing sex, or alongside hermaphrodites.[78] Phaethousa's femininity appears here as a very fragile state, apparently able to be disrupted by the departure of her husband.

---

[75]   [Hippocrates] *Epidemics* 6.8.32; tr. W.D. Smith, Loeb VII, pp. 289–91. References to the Hippocratic corpus and to other Greek and Latin texts from classical antiquity will, where possible, be to this edition with English translation. I initially looked at this story in *Hippocrates' Woman*, pp. 9–10, as an example of the dangers of retrospective diagnosis using modern categories and how this risked losing 'its richness and complexity as a cultural product'. I do not intend to offer any retrodiagnosis here.

[76]   Maud Gleason, 'The Semiotics of Gender', in David Halperin, John J. Winkler and Froma Zeitlin (eds), *Before Sexuality: The Construction of Erotic Experience in the Ancient Greek World* (Princeton, NJ, 1990), p. 400.

[77]   J.B. [Bulwer], *Anthropometamorphosis: Man Transformed; or, the Artificial Changeling* (London, 1650), introductory poem.

[78]   I published a preliminary discussion of these different versions in my 'Barbes, sang et genre: afficher la différence dans le monde antique', in Jérôme Wilgaux and Véronique Dasen (eds), *Langages et métaphores du corps* (Rennes, 2008), pp. 153–68.

The second story, more widely known than that of Phaethousa and re-told up to the nineteenth century, is that of the virgin Agnodice.[79] Known only from the Latin writer Hyginus, it is assumed to be from an ancient Greek original. It is set in an imagined and undated Athens in which 'the ancients had no midwives', and women and slaves are forbidden to practise medicine; women's modesty is such that they prefer to die rather than let a man help them. Agnodice helps us explore the question 'What constitutes sex?', both in her own identity and in the questions she raises about the extent of the difference between men and women as understood by those trying to heal their diseases. Are men and women so different that they need separate branches of medicine, or dedicated personnel to cope with their bodies? The plot is that Agnodice cuts off her hair and dresses as a man to train under 'a certain Herophilus', then treats women patients; first, however, she has to convince them that she is not a man, so she lifts her clothing to prove this. Her success as a physician incurs the jealousy of the male physicians who accuse her of seducing women to gain their custom. Agnodice's own sex is literally put 'on trial'; taken to the Areopagus court, she again lifts her clothes to show she is a woman. But this demonstration in court of her real identity means she is immediately accused of breaking another law, the one preventing women and slaves from practising medicine. Following a protest from the leading women of Athens, this law is then changed so that women of free birth are thereafter allowed to practise medicine.

In this story, Agnodice plays with sexual identity. In an article on early modern views of sex change, Donald Beecher argued that by the end of the sixteenth century there was a 'two-sex' model in which 'sex is grounded in the essences of nature' so that 'gender play becomes a safe and harmless form of self-expression to social ends. A disguise is merely a disguise.'[80] Agnodice's disguise endangers her because it is so successful; her impersonation of a man suggests that it is very easy to pass as the other sex, as she is so convincing that her first patient and her rival male physicians think she is a man. Nevertheless, in this story the external

---

[79] Hyginus, *Fabula* 274. In English translation, Mary Grant (ed. and tr.), *The Myths of Hyginus* (University of Kansas Publications in Humanistic Studies, no. 34. Lawrence, KS, 1960). Now out of print, the translation is available online, for example at <http://www.theoi.com/Text/HyginusFabulae5.html#274> accessed 4 July 2011. M.J. Boyd's brief review in *Classical Review* 13 (1963), p. 350 fairly characterised Grant's translation as 'often loose, not seldom wrong'. Another English translation is now available: R. Scott Smith and Stephen Trzaskoma, *Apollodorus' Library and Hyginus' Fabulae* (Indianapolis, IN, 2007), where this story appears on p. 180. Smith and Trzaskoma call Grant's translation 'derivative' and note that it is in turn based on H.J. Rose's 1927 Latin edition, which has many inaccuracies (p. lv). They use P.K. Marshall's edition of 2002 (*Hyginus: Fabulae. Editio altera*, a revised edition of the 1993 one (Munich, 2002). However, as this was put together from Marshall's notes after his death, it has its own problems; see Wilfrid Major's review in *Bryn Mawr Classical Review*, <http://bmcr.brynmawr.edu/2003/2003-06-37.html> accessed 12 November 2011.

[80] Beecher, 'Concerning Sex Changes', p. 1012.

genitalia immediately and unambiguously demonstrate 'true sex'. However, what precisely does she reveal here: the absence of a penis, or the presence of the female genitalia? This is a question to which I shall return in Chapter 8. In one context, her gesture demonstrates identity (with women): in the other, difference (from men). She is beardless, but apparently nobody suspects from this that she is a woman. Instead, this makes her more attractive as a potential seducer of female patients; her accusers call her 'a smooth-faced [Lat. *glaber*] corruptor of these women'. This contrasts with Phaethousa, who appears as a woman with a beard, rather than an attractive young 'man'. Age is a factor here, and thinking about the self-display of Agnodice, a 'virgin girl' (Lat. *puella virgo*), alongside the changes to the appearance of the mother Phaethousa ('who had previously given birth') also opens a way of discussing the nature of femininity more generally. When does a girl become a woman, and are both equally 'female'? As a girl, Agnodice is able to pass as a man without any difficulty, so much so that her life is threatened by the success of her disguise. Would this be more difficult if she were a mature woman?

Agnodice's visual demonstration of her sexual identity further suggests that the 'outside' is entirely reliable evidence of what is 'inside'. But was this always thought to be the case in the world before dissection?[81] The displayed bodies of both women – displayed in the text itself, in the story of Agnodice, but both laid out for our inspection in the range of later materials that used them – suggest that the variety of signs to be read when deciding an individual's sex was far wider in earlier historical periods. Phaethousa's story shifts the focus from the external genitalia – hidden parts, easily disguised further by clothing – to the rest of the body's surface, to the voice, and to the part on which character and gender is most clearly written: the face. And in versions of Agnodice's story told in the early modern period, factors other than her genitalia came to the fore here too: her face, breasts, hair, skin, voice and intellect. Why? Was this simply due to a reluctance to present her as performing such an apparently lewd gesture, or is there more going on here?

Both stories concern childbirth: Agnodice is presented as 'the first midwife' and Phaethousa has previously given birth more than once, although ceasing to menstruate means she cannot have more children. This interest in birth is not accidental. Just as the womb is the organ that makes a simple male/female genital analogy difficult to sustain – what is its analogue in the male body? – so childbirth is a process for which the one-sex body provides no male equivalent, and I shall be arguing throughout this book that midwifery is a particularly important arena in which to discuss and dispute the extent of the difference between men and women.

---

[81]   Writing on the history of anatomical displays from 1700, Elizabeth Stephens notes the assumption that 'it is in seeing the interior of the body that we see its truth' (*Anatomy as Spectacle: Public Exhibitions of the Body from 1700 to the Present* (Liverpool, 2011), p. 19). This leaves open the question 'At what point in history did it become possible to "see" in this way?' I shall discuss the different possibilities for what Agnodice reveals in Chapter 8.

Laqueur could perhaps dismiss debates about midwifery as one of his 'endless micro-confrontations over power in the public and private spheres' but they will feature throughout this book as a key locus of debate about sex and gender.[82]

Both stories proved flexible enough to be used in often-contradictory ways. Phaethousa could be a victim of circumstances, or an example of the amazing power of the female mind to influence the body. She appeared in discussions of conditions ranging from lovesickness to uterine prolapse, the cause of her transformation being attributed to the fluids of her body, her organs, or her emotions. Where she is a warning, Agnodice can be a role model, but although she may be represented as a heroine, she can become a villain. Two examples will suffice here. For a woman in late seventeenth- or early eighteenth-century London, Agnodice was a heroine: this woman had handbills printed to advertise her skills in healing venereal diseases and skin conditions, and in providing cosmetic services, such as facial makeovers in which she reshaped eyebrows to make the forehead appear higher.[83] Perhaps she was a newcomer to London, trying to find a niche in the market; in any case, she represents herself as having 'Travelled for many Years in Forreign Parts', by no means an unusual claim in these handbills, but interesting in this context because Agnodice travelled to study with her teacher, Herophilus.[84] Searching around for a professional name, she chose to call herself 'Agnodice: The WOMAN Physician'. In the marketplace of early modern medicine, what did this name imply to her, and why would it encourage clients to buy her services?[85]

---

[82]   Laqueur, *Making Sex*, p. 193. I am not using 'sex' and 'gender' in the traditional sense of biological difference versus social roles, as I no longer find it useful to distinguish between biology and society; see also Holmes, *Gender*, pp. 50–51, and Beecher, 'Concerning Sex Changes', p. 993 on the process of 'analogizing from sex to gender, from essential change to artificially fashioned change'.

[83]   In full: 'Agnodice: The Woman Practitioner, dwelling at the Hand and Urinal, next Door to the Blue Ball in Hayden-Yard in the Minories, near Aldgate.' British Library 551.a.32 (199). Kevin P. Siena, 'The "Foul Disease" and Privacy: The Effects of Venereal Disease and Patient Demand on the Medical Marketplace in Early Modern London', *Bulletin of the History of Medicine*, 75 (2001), p. 201 discusses the collections of advertising handbills in the British Library, and this one comes from a collection of 195 items dated to the period 1660–1715.

[84]   On foreign practitioners using handbills, see Siena, 'The "Foul Disease"', p. 204. For Siena, Agnodice is a venereologist and, as he correctly notes, it is to fellow *women* with venereal diseases that 'Agnodice' advertises her skills; see 'The "Foul Disease"', p. 218. But, although this is one of the conditions the handbill mentions, in fact she claims that her practice stretches across women's diseases, including pregnancy testing and infertility remedies, as well as cosmetic treatments.

[85]   The phrase 'the medical marketplace', coined in the 1980s and originally associated with the late Roy Porter, has been criticised as the product of a Thatcherite view of the market economy but, in the context of early modern London, it still seems an appropriate way of characterising the range of competing alternatives on offer, and patient responses to them. See for example Roy Porter, 'William Hunter: A Surgeon and a Gentleman', in

Who was Agnodice for a woman at this time? In contrast, in 1851, the year after the foundation of the Woman's Medical College in Philadelphia – the first all-female medical college – the American physician Augustus Gardner gave a lecture on the history of midwifery in which he argued that women should not be allowed to practise obstetrics, due to 'the past inefficiency and present natural incapacity of females' in this area.[86] Gardner explicitly linked his comments to issues of professional boundaries, saying that there is a proposal 'at the present time' to 'give away the portion of the healing art of which I am treating, if not the whole domain of medicine, to the females'.[87] His dual appeal to both history – the 'past' – and science – what women are 'naturally' able to do – was designed to deflect any such change in the gendering of obstetrics, or of medicine more widely. In his lecture, Gardner compared Agnodice to 'the infamous Restells and Costellos of our day', Madame Restell (Anna Lohman) and Madame Catherine Costello being abortionists in New York and New Jersey respectively.[88] He urged his audience at the New York College of Physicians and Surgeons to 'Conceive, if you can, the books of the world destroyed, schools of medicine abolished, and the practice of midwifery again in the hands of women, even of the intellectual females of the

---

W.F. Bynum and Roy Porter (eds), *William Hunter and the Eighteenth-Century Medical World* (Cambridge, 1985), pp. 7–34: the term 'market-place' appears on pp. 12, 18 and 21. For a perceptive analysis of the emergence and influence of the model, see Andrew Wear, *Knowledge and Practice in English Medicine, 1550–1680* (Cambridge, 2000), pp. 28–9. For an assessment of its relevance in early modern midwifery, see Adrian Wilson, 'Midwifery in the "Medical Marketplace"', in Mark Jenner and Patrick Wallis (eds), *Medicine and the Market in England and its Colonies, c.1450–c.1850* (Basingstoke, 2007), 153–74.

[86]   From the original subtitle of the lecture: 'A History of the Art of Midwifery: A Lecture Delivered at the College of Physicians and Surgeons, November 11th, 1851, Introductory to a Course of Private Instruction on Operative Midwifery; Showing the Past Inefficiency and Present Natural Incapacity of Females in the Practice of Obstetrics by Augustus K. Gardner' (New York, 1852). It was reprinted as the introduction to *The Modern Practice of Midwifery: A Course of Lectures on Obstetrics: Delivered at St Mary's Hospital, London, by Wm Tyler Smith MD* (New York, 1858), from which edition all quotations are taken. The Woman's Medical College of Pennsylvania was founded in Philadelphia in 1850, and was the first medical school in the world to teach only women. See Gulielma Fell Alsop, *History of the Woman's Medical College, Philadelphia, Pennsylvania, 1850–1950* (Philadelphia, PA, 1950); Steven J. Peitzman, *A New and Untried Course: Woman's Medical College and Medical College of Pennsylvania, 1850–1998* (New Brunswick, NJ, 2000).

[87]   Gardner, 'A History of the Art of Midwifery', p. 28.

[88]   Ibid., p. 28. On Madame Restell – Ann Trow Lohman, New York midwife-abortionist – see Clifford Browder, *The Wickedest Woman in New York: Madame Restell, the Abortionist* (Hamden, CT, 1988) and Marvin Olasky, *The Press and Abortion, 1838–1988* (Hillsdale, NJ, 1988), 4–13. On her 'pill war' with her New Jersey counterpart, Madame Catherine Costello, see Olasky, *The Press and Abortion*, p. 15. An advertisement by Restell for her 'Preventive Powders', from the *New York Herald*, is reproduced in Andrea Tone (ed.), *Controlling Reproduction: An American History* (Wilmington, DE, 1997), pp. 101–2.

present day, and after the lapse of fifty or a hundred years, imagine its state!'[89] Agnodice's name, which had once evoked healing, had become an insult.

Before analysing these two stories, this book will begin by setting out the evidence from the classical and early modern periods. In Chapter 1 I shall return to Laqueur's use of Galen, and explore some ancient alternatives to this model, showing that claims for the dominance of the 'one-sex' model fail to account for the complexity of the classical world. Chapter 2 considers in more detail the impact on a modern audience of Vesalius' illustration of the womb, and introduces the general challenges made to a 'one-sex' model, in particular in the sixteenth century. Laqueur concentrates on 'scientific' texts, but beliefs about the body and its sex appear in a wide range of other types of evidence. *Making Sex* does not consider the genres of the evidence used, but in exploring the reception of my two central stories it will be a key feature. The following chapters will therefore provide a close reading of Phaethousa, starting in Chapter 3 with a discussion of the case history genre and of the placement of Phaethousa in relation to bearded ladies and hermaphrodites. Where Agnodice comes from a marginal Latin writer, Phaethousa carries the authority of the 'Father of Medicine', and it is this Hippocratic origin which clearly made her very familiar to generations of medical writers. Yet in many ways she has more in common with sex change stories in later Greek writers. Chapter 4 will explore how her story fared in the period from around 1525 to 1800.

In Chapter 5, I shall turn to Agnodice, again first considering issues of genre. I shall locate the story of Agnodice in its original context, performing a close reading of the text, before identifying the main themes that were picked up by subsequent readers. Agnodice originally featured in a list of inventors/discoverers, and has similar themes to those of ancient novels, but her readers found ways of using the story as evidence of real historical events. In Chapters 6 and 7, I shall look at the different ways in which key features of the story of Agnodice were told in the period from the sixteenth century onwards. Chapter 8 draws out the significance of the 'body in parts', looking at the different parts of the body – and of the mind – identified as significant in readings of both Agnodice and Phaethousa.[90]

---

[89]   Gardner, 'A History of the Art of Midwifery', p. 15. Perhaps only to the modern reader does the dual meaning of the opening, 'Conceive, if you can', seem somewhat ironic when addressed to this all-male audience.

[90]   'Body in parts' is a reference to recent scholarship that focuses on the parts rather than on the body as a whole. See David Hillman and Carla Mazzi (eds), *The Body in Parts: Fantasies of Corporeality in Early Modern Europe* (London and New York, 1997); Mary Beard, 'Did the Romans Have Elbows? or Arms and the Romans', in Pierre Borgeaud (ed.), *Corps Romains* (Grenoble, 2002), 47–59; Florike Egmond and Robert Zwijnenberg (eds), *Bodily Extremities: Preoccupations with the Human Body in Early Modern European Culture* (Aldershot, 2003). In *Generating Bodies and Gendered Selves: The Rhetoric of Reproduction in Early Modern England* (Seattle and London, 2007), p. 43, Eve Keller criticises this approach as glossing over a changing view of the self, from being 'a

Throughout this book, some receptions of the texts will be analysed in detail as case studies: others will be mentioned more briefly. I shall use the many different subsequent readings of my two stories as a place from which to return to the original versions, and shall show how the range of re-imaginings by later readers also help us to reassess what the stories originally meant. The process is circular, with readers in dialogue with each other. At the outset, however, I would like to emphasise here that no reading of either story is 'wrong'. All are valid uses, evidence of the vitality of the classical tradition. The stories of Agnodice and Phaethousa have proved 'good to think with' over a surprisingly long chronological period extending, in some respects, to the present day. History is powerful: classical history, for much of our past, even more so.

I shall end by returning to the issues of sex change, and discussing the difficulties of using Laqueur's model here. His work remains particularly relevant to contemporary discussions of intersex, or what earlier historical periods would have called hermaphroditism. In a one-sex model, a range of body temperatures from hot to cold makes possible a range of gender identities on a spectrum from the very masculine man to the highly feminine woman, a balance between hot and cold leading to a 'perfect' hermaphrodite, with spontaneous sex 'change' from female to male being theoretically possible, under the influence of increased heat: a two-sex model presents an individual with only two possibilities for their 'true sex'. Today, the late nineteenth-century move of locating 'sex' definitively in the tissue of the gonads is no longer thought to close down the discussion.[91] In 1993 Anne Fausto-Sterling, in a proposal she herself later described as 'provocative' but also 'written with tongue firmly in cheek', suggested that a binary model of sex should now be replaced with a five-sex model, including male hermaphrodites, female hermaphrodites and true hermaphrodites; in her 2000 book, *Sexing the Body*, she revisited the question 'Should there be more than two sexes?' and in the same year she published 'The Five Sexes, Revisited'.[92] In a recent study of sex and gender in early modern Europe, Patricia Simons noted that now 'The

---

distributed entity' in the Galenic body to being a separate, and masculine, entity in the early modern period.

[91]   On what she labelled 'the age of gonads', see Alice Domurat Dreger, *Hermaphrodites and the Medical Invention of Sex* (Cambridge, MA and London, 1998). Developing Dreger's work, Anne Fausto-Sterling argued that, in the nineteenth century, hermaphrodites were eventually classified almost out of existence by a new insistence that only people with both ovarian and testicular tissue should count as 'true' hermaphrodites; Anne Fausto-Sterling, *Sexing the Body* (New York, 2000). On the concept of the 'true' hermaphrodite see also Maximilian Schochow, *Die Ordnung der Hermaphroditen-Geschlechter: eine Genealogie des Geschlechtsbegriffs* (Berlin, 2009), esp. pp. 180–84.

[92]   Anne Fausto-Sterling, 'The Five Sexes: Why Male and Female Are Not Enough', *The Sciences*, March/April 1993, pp. 20–24; *Sexing the Body*; 'The Five Sexes, Revisited', *The Sciences*, July/August 2000, pp. 19–23, <http://www.scribd.com/doc/39423403/Anne-Fausto-Sterling-The-Five-Sexes-Revisited> accessed 22 July 2012. Quotation from 'The Five Sexes, Revisited', p. 19.

body is increasingly becoming again a matter of complexity, flux and change, as knowledge grows about the insecurity of sex tests at the Olympics, for instance.'[93] Are we returning to a model of a spectrum of sexes and rejecting the 'two-sex', either/or, biologically reductionist model? And is it a development like this that will finally lead to a rejection of Laqueur's straightforward model of change?

---

[93]   Simons, *Sex of Men*, p. 32. Laqueur, *Making Sex*, p. viii also mentions sex testing at the Olympics.

PART I
Revisiting the Classics

Chapter 1

Making Sex and the Classical World

As we saw in the Introduction, Laqueur's *Making Sex* is a publishing phenomenon. From their reactions, I suspect that what intrigues readers is not the 'two-sex' model, since to them this seems a familiar and 'natural' way of thinking about the body, but instead the 'one-sex' body with its notion that men are women with their 'insides out' – and vice versa.[1] This model reduces the historical and geographical variety of pre-modern Europe into a single image, imposing on it a misleading uniformity, while privileging 'modernity' and giving us, as its representatives, a sense of intellectual superiority.[2] It also suggests that pre-modern Europeans lived with 'the potential instability of their sexuality', as the position of their organs was not fixed once and for all.[3] In Laqueur's version, the 'vice versa' aspect is played down, and instead of being a model of reciprocity, with all organs being shared, differing only in location, it becomes one that favours the male. At one point he argued that the 'one-sex model' 'can be read … as an exercise in preserving the Father, he who stands not only for order but for the existence of civilization itself', going on to say that 'In a public world that was overwhelmingly male, the one-sex model displayed what was already massively evident in culture more generally: *man* is the measure of all things, and woman does not exist as an ontologically distinct category' [Laqueur's italics].[4] The corollary of this is the suggestion that 'the male body has no history'.[5] As we have already seen in discussing the inside/

---

[1] Laqueur does not say that the two-sex model is natural – indeed, for him, 'Two sexes are not the necessary, natural consequence of corporeal difference' (*Making Sex*, p. 243) – but as it is the system with which his readers are familiar, the one-sex model seems surprising and exotic in comparison. For reactions to the book from a range of readers, see the reviews on goodreads.com; for example, 'OMG We are all one sex', <http://www.goodreads.com/review/show/271345368> accessed 10 August 2012.

[2] On 'the uniformity [Laqueur] imposes on his sources and periods' see Rebecca Flemming, *Medicine and the Making of Roman Women. Gender, Nature, and Authority from Celsus to Galen* (Oxford, 2000), p. 121 and Holmes, *Gender*, pp. 50–51.

[3] The phrase is that of Beecher, 'Concerning Sex Changes', p. 1011; he criticises Laqueur for having encouraged a misleading focus on sexual anxiety in early modern Europe, resulting in what he characterises as 'the anxiety-and-indeterminacy school of Renaissance sexuality' (p. 1014).

[4] Laqueur, *Making Sex*, pp. 58 and 62.

[5] Elaine Hobby, '"The Head of this Counterfeit Yard is called Tertigo" or, "It is not Hard Words that Perform the Work": Recovering Early Modern Women's Writing', in Jo Wallwork and Paul Salzman (eds), *Women Writing 1550–1750*, special issue of *Meridian*, 18:1 (2001), p. 19, drawing on the evidence of Jane Sharp in 1671 to criticise Laqueur's

outside model in *Aristotle's Masterpiece*, however, in the late seventeenth century challenges to any view of man as the measure were able to draw on earlier texts, from the sixteenth century and even before.

Yet Laqueur asserts that the 'one-sex' part of his model 'dominated thinking about sexual difference from classical antiquity to the end of the seventeenth century'.[6] In this and the following chapter, I shall begin to reflect in general terms on the claims for this extended heyday of the one-sex body; although, if we were to combine the existing literature critical of Laqueur, we would find it a surprisingly brief phase. For example, Katy Park commented on the medieval period that, 'Before 1500 I could find no convincing expressions of the idea of genital homology at all, even as an alternative to be discarded, except for a few brief passages in the works of several late medieval surgeons'; even in these writers, as Patricia Simons further noted, the reference was 'quickly made in a sentence or so, and was usually noticeable for its isolation'.[7] Park remarked that, while 'Laqueur is correct to point out the power of Galen's one-sex body in sixteenth- and seventeenth-century European culture, ... he wrongly assumes that it spent the intervening centuries percolating along.'[8] However, others working on early modern Europe have raised issues even with this 'sixteenth- and seventeenth-century' timing. Russell West-Pavlov, following Ian Maclean's comments made nearly 30 years earlier, notes that 'By the end of the 1500s, most medical textbooks had rejected the Galenic theory of the parallelism of male and female genitals.'[9] Yet medical textbooks are precisely the sources favoured by Laqueur. Furthermore, Patricia Simons has recently referred to Laqueur's assumption that a 'one-sex' body goes with a 'two-seed' model of conception in which both men and women have testicles and make 'seed', and has argued that 'The death-knell of the two-seed and one-sex idea was already beginning to be tolled as early as the mid- to late sixteenth century.'[10] This leaves very little time for the glory days of the one-sex body; perhaps only from *c*.1500–1550.

---

view 'that the male body has no history, being a stable point of reference against which the woman's was measured and found wanting'. Simons, *Sex of Men* is the most recent example of work demonstrating that the male body does indeed have a history.

[6]   Laqueur, *Making Sex*, p. 25.

[7]   Park, 'Cadden, Laqueur, and the "One-Sex Body"', pp. 4–5; Simons, *Sex of Men*, p. 146. The surgeons alluded to here are Lanfranco of Milan at the end of the thirteenth century, Henri de Mondeville at the start of the fourteenth century, and Guy de Chauliac in 1363; see Simons, *Sex of Men*, pp. 144–5. The model came to them not direct from Galen, but via the intermediary of Avicenna.

[8]   Park, 'Cadden, Laqueur, and the "One-Sex Body"', pp. 4–5.

[9]   Russell West-Pavlov, *Bodies and their Spaces: System, Crisis and Transformation in Early Modern Theatre* (Amsterdam, 2006), p. 48 following Ian Maclean, *The Renaissance Notion of Woman: A Study in the Fortunes of Scholasticism and Medical Science in European Intellectual Life* (Cambridge, 1980), p. 33.

[10]   Simons, *Sex of Men*, p. 148.

But what about the classical world, with which *Making Sex* began, and to which Laqueur attributed the 'one-sex' model? Sally Shuttleworth may have been the first to challenge Laqueur's reading of the classical texts, noting that the ancient Greeks considered women a totally separate race, which sounds more like a 'two-sex' model; while she did not give references, this idea is found in the eighth-century BC poet Hesiod. He described the first woman, Pandora, as a later creation than man, the origin of the 'race of women' (Gk *genos gynaikôn*), with 'the mind of a bitch' and a womb-belly ravenous for food and sex.[11] But Shuttleworth's challenge has not been picked up.[12]

It is striking that, despite his claims to be covering the period 'from the Greeks to Freud', as the subtitle of his book puts it, and his presentation of the 'one-sex' model as 'hoary already in Galen's time', Laqueur's use of the classical material is very restricted; he was clearly reliant on those ancient medical texts available in English translation at the time he was writing.[13] Because he argued from such a limited sample, he did not realise that Galen's remark is just one expression of sex difference in ancient medicine; and, indeed, just one expression within Galen's own work. In this chapter I shall discuss the shortcomings of Laqueur's analysis of classical Greco-Roman medicine, which led him to emphasise genital anatomy at the expense of the physiology of menstruation. Like him, I shall start with Galen, returning to the key passage from *On the Usefulness of the Parts of the Body* already mentioned in the Introduction, before looking at Galen's own sources: Hippocrates, Plato and Aristotle. A 'one-sex' model was only one version of the body, even in the ancient world; Galen's presentation of it is not straightforward, while Laqueur's use of Galen is patchy.

---

[11]   Shuttleworth, 'Review', p. 634; Nicole Loraux, 'Sur la race des femmes et quelques-unes de ses tribus', *Arethusa*, 11 (1978); King, *Hippocrates' Woman*, pp. 25–7.

[12]   Other commentators on Laqueur have uncritically accepted his statements about the ancient world; see for example Maria Eriksson, 'Biologically Similar and Anatomically Different? The One-Sex Model and the Modern Sex/Gender Distinction', *NORA: Nordic Journal of Women's Studies* 6 (1998), p. 32 (online version <http://baer.rewi.hu-berlin.de/w/files/lsbpdf/eriksson.pdf> accessed 12 August 2012), who simply accepts (without giving any references) that 'In the tradition of humoural [*sic*] pathology, dating back to classical antiquity, woman and man were, as stated above, perceived as two versions of the same flesh, of one body.' Within Classics, Flemming, *Medicine and the Making of Roman Women*, pp. 12–16 and 119–21, focuses on the problems of Laqueur's use of Aristotle. Holmes, *Gender*, is also framed as a critique of Laqueur, not simply in terms of his sources, but as misunderstanding the relationship between sex and gender in them.

[13]   Laqueur, *Making Sex*, p. 25; p. 28 moves from Galen to Aristotle, without giving any indication that Aristotle predated Galen by 500 years, a move that may be confusing to readers unfamiliar with these materials.

Location, Location, Location – Galen[14]

Although Laqueur regards the inside/outside model as pre-Galenic, he presents it as having been expressed in a particularly succinct way by Galen before it carried on into the seventeenth century. Before looking at the alternative models of the sexed body in antiquity, we therefore need to explore Laqueur's use of Galen in more detail. Galen is central to the story because Laqueur asserts that 'Across a millennial chasm that saw the fall of Rome and the rise of Christianity, Galen spoke easily, in various vernacular languages, to the artisans and merchants, the midwives and barber surgeons, of Renaissance and Reformation Europe.'[15] It is hard to understand this reference to 'various vernacular languages'; Galen wrote in Greek, but was transmitted mostly in Arabic and subsequently in Latin translations.[16] In Renaissance and Reformation Europe, very little of Galen's work was translated into anything other than Latin. The start and end dates of this 'millennial chasm' are difficult to fathom; the rise of Christianity is conventionally dated to the conversion of Constantine in 312 AD, and the Fall of Rome to 476 AD, although in both cases these are processes over several centuries rather than these culminating 'dates'. If Laqueur meant to identify an entire millennium from *c*.300 AD to 1300 AD as the 'chasm', then *Making Sex* does indeed omit this period almost entirely, even though it implies continuity right across it in the comment that, via Galen, the one-sex body dominates 'from classical antiquity to the end of the seventeenth century'.

Galen's overall model of the body, divided into three regions dominated by the brain, the heart and the liver respectively, was highly influential in Arabic, and then medieval Western, medicine. As we have already seen in the Introduction, he wrote that:

> All the parts, then, that men have, women have too, the difference between them lying in only one thing, which must be kept in mind throughout the discussion, namely, that in women the parts are within [the body], whereas in men they are outside, in the region called the perineum. Consider first whichever ones you

---

[14]   The rules of success in real estate, 'Location, location, location', are popularly associated with the New York property developer William Zeckendorf, although there is disagreement about whether he made the rules, or broke them; Jerome Tuccille, *Trump: The Saga of America's Most Powerful Real Estate Baron* (Washington, DC, 1985), p. 57.

[15]   Laqueur, *Making Sex*, p. 63. The 'chasm' terminology is used by Laqueur in relation to Thomas Kühn's theory of scientific revolutions; *Making Sex*, p. 96. It is also discussed, in terms of its neglect of medieval medicine, in Park, 'Cadden, Laqueur, and the "One-Sex Body"', p. 3.

[16]   Possibly all that Laqueur had in mind here was the *Masterpiece*; see the reference in *Making Sex*, p. 151, discussed above, p. 11.

please, turn outward the woman's, turn inward, so to speak, and fold double the man's, and you will find them the ...same in both in every respect.[17]

What is the status of this passage? It certainly does not represent a summary of anatomical studies; human dissection did not feature in Galen's world. It is clearly a thought experiment, and is introduced as such – 'Consider ...', 'Think ...' – with Galen going on to invite the reader to 'Think first, please, of ...' and 'Think too, please, of the converse ...'.[18] Can we take this apparently isolated passage as evidence that Galen believed in a 'one-sex' body? Patricia Simons suggests instead that, for Galen and also for later surgical writers, the one-sex model was 'an introductory teaching device', 'more an aid to visualization and memorization than the summation of a complex theory of sexual oneness'.[19] One of Laqueur's most trenchant critics, Katy Park, has gone further, alleging that the one-sex body model should be dismissed as merely 'a specific idea contained in a couple of paragraphs of a single book of a single work of Galen'. But this, as I shall now show, is also misleading.[20]

From Laqueur's endnotes it is clear that his comments on Galen are based on just three works: *On the Usefulness of the Parts of the Body*, *On the Natural Faculties* and *On Seed*, the first two of which were available to him in 1990 in relatively recent English translations. *On Seed*, in keeping with its lack of an English translation before 1992, is cited only once.[21] Even within this limited

---

[17]   Galen, *Usefulness of Parts*, 14.6–7, ed. Kühn 4.158–9; translation from May, *Galen, On the Usefulness of the Parts of the Body*, vol. 2, p. 628; Laqueur, *Making Sex*, pp. 25–7.

[18]   In Greek, 'Consider first whichever one you please' is *opotera boulei noêsas protera*. The verb *noeô*, to think, is also used in the other two references; Galen, *Usefulness of Parts*, 14.6, ed. Kühn 4.159. The term 'thought experiment' is applied to this passage by Simons, *Sex of Men*, p. 142.

[19]   Simons, *Sex of Men*, p. 147.

[20]   Park, 'Cadden, Laqueur, and the "One-Sex Body"', p. 5. In what follows, I am revising my more positive evaluation of Park's article made in my 'Sex, Medicine and Disease', in Mark Golden and Peter Toohey (eds), *A Cultural History of Sexuality in the Classical World* (Oxford and New York, 2011), p. 111.

[21]   On the explosion of good editions and translations of Galen from the early 1970s, see John Scarborough, 'Galen *Redivivus*: An Essay Review', *Journal of the History of Medicine and Allied Sciences*, 43 (1988). On Laqueur's emphasis on *Usefulness of the Parts of the Body*, cited in the translation of May, *Galen, On the Usefulness of the Parts of the Body*, see Holmes, *Gender*, p. 39. In the passages Laqueur quotes from May's translation, he makes one significant change; for her glossing of the neck of the womb as the 'cervix' (May, p. 629) he gives 'cervix and vagina' (Laqueur, p. 26). Here I agree with his interpretation; see further Chapter 2 on the terminology of the female body, pp. 58–9. Laqueur cites *On Seed* only once; p. 246, n. 12, in Kühn's Greek/Latin early nineteenth-century edition. It is not clear whether he accessed this through an intermediary secondary source; he could, for example, easily have met it in May, *Galen, On the Usefulness of*

range of Galen's works, Laqueur could have found much more that is relevant
to his theme; in particular, in *On Seed*. Like the bulk of *On the Usefulness of the
Parts of the Body*, this was written between 169 and 175 AD, so we cannot know
whether it is developing the brief comment from *On the Usefulness of the Parts
of the Body*, or *On the Usefulness of the Parts of the Body* is summarising *On
Seed*.[22] There are many points of similarity between the two discussions; both, for
example, use an analogy between the female organs of generation and the eyes of
the mole, which are too weak to come outside.[23] In the second book of *On Seed*,
Galen draws an opposition between the (male) foetus with testicles outside 'and no
uterus anywhere' and the wetter colder (female) foetus with 'testicles and uterus
on the inside'.[24] Here, then, there is not a simple match between organs: there is no
male counterpart to the womb. As we shall see later in this book, the issue of how
to fit the womb into a 'one-sex', inside/outside model would remain a problem into
the nineteenth century, with writers trying to draw up tables of analogies between
the sexual organs of women and men.[25] A few sections later, Galen returned to the
problem, but this time suggesting that the womb is the equivalent of the scrotum:

> If one should think of the female uterus with its double nature as undergoing the
> following two things, falling forward outside the peritoneum, and at the same
> time so reversing itself so that all of it that is outside comes now to be inside,
> and what is inside appears now on the outside, he would in this way produce
> the testicles in the scrotum, the cavity of the uterus having become the scrotum
> and the peritoneum the sheath-like tunic, and the testicles themselves not being
> outside the uterus, as they are now, but inside.[26]

---

the Parts of the Body, p. 629, n. 17. The English translation of *On Seed* by Phillip de
Lacy appeared in the *Corpus Medicorum Graecorum* in 1992. Beecher's 'Concerning Sex
Changes', p. 995 restricts itself to *Usefulness* in assessing Galen's views on the 'one-sex'
model.

[22]   On the dating, see Peter N. Singer (tr.), *Galen: Selected Works* (Oxford, 1977), p. li.

[23]   *On Seed* II 5. 60, *CMG* V. 3, 1, p. 193; *Usefulness of Parts* 14.6, Kühn 4.160.

[24]   See Galen, *On Seed* II 5. 41, *CMG* V 3, 1, p. 189.

[25]   As, for example, James Young Simpson did in his lectures; see King, *Midwifery,
Obstetrics and the Rise of Gynaecology*, pp. 181–2. He commented that 'A considerable
difference of opinion, however, still prevails as to the prototype of the female uterus in the
male system'; James Young Simpson, 'Hermaphroditism', in Robert B. Todd (ed.), *The
Cyclopaedia of Anatomy and Physiology*, vol. 2, DIA–INS (London, 1839), p. 724.

[26]   *On Seed* II 5. 44, *CMG* V 3, 1, p. 189. The 'double nature' is an error based on
analogies with animal wombs; Vesalius later identified it as such, below, Chapter 2, p. 57.
Laqueur, *Making Sex*, p. 90 cites a sixteenth-century attempt (one of many) to identify the
scrotum as the analogous part to the womb, identifying such claims as something a two-sex
world finds 'entirely irrelevant'. Yet even in the supposedly two-sex nineteenth century,
Simpson's work shows that this was still a live issue.

In this convoluted thought experiment, Galen's problem here is that he somehow has to incorporate what he regards as the 'female testicles' (the structures which he believes contain seed, in both men and women, and which in the female body we would now identify with the ovaries) which are normally positioned outside the womb; and they must somehow end up inside the womb/scrotum, presumably pulled into it as it comes out of the body. A few sections later, he says that:

> Thus both the female and the male animal appear to have all their generative parts the same, differing either in position, in that the one set of them is inside the peritoneum, the other outside, or in size, as was noted just now in the case of the prepuce and the testicles.[27]

So although he thinks he has found a way to make the inside/outside model work, it is not just the location, but also the size, that differs; this is already a more nuanced version of the relationship between male and female organs than that found in *On the Usefulness of the Parts of the Body*. Later still in *On Seed* Galen reverted to the simpler version, stating '… they differ in one thing only: the parts are in one case internal, in the other external'.[28]

Rebecca Flemming has drawn attention to a further discussion of male and female by Galen, in his *Doctrines of Hippocrates and Plato*, which as she points out 'clearly contradicts Laqueur's vision of the hegemonic, ancient one-sex model, with its privileging of role over body'.[29] Here Galen discusses how men and women are both similar and different: both are rational animals, but men are stronger, and only women can give birth, because they have 'certain parts of the body prepared for childbearing by their nature'. So, Galen concludes, 'it is correct to say that in one respect women are similar to men, in another they are opposite'.[30]

This is very different to the simple 'one-sex' model that Laqueur presents as Galenic. In another part of *On Seed* Galen further suggested that difference extends far beyond the genitals: 'the male animal differs from the female in its entire body'[31] and:

---

[27]   *On Seed* II 5. 48, *CMG* V. 3, 1, p. 191.

[28]   *On Seed* II 5. 51, *CMG* V. 3, 1, p. 191.

[29]   Flemming, *Medicine and the Making of Roman Women*, pp. 357–8. On the fortunes of this treatise in the sixteenth century, in particular after it was printed in the 1530s, see Vivian Nutton, '*De placitis Hippocratis et Platonis* in the Renaissance', in Paola Manuli and Mario Vegetti (eds), *Le opere psicologiche di Galeno, Atti del Terzo Colloquio Galenico Internazionale, Pavia 10–12 settembre 1986* (Naples, 1988).

[30]   Galen, *Doctrines of Hippocrates and Plato*, 9.3.25–6 (*CMG* V. 4.1, 2 p. 556. 28–37). Book 9 is dated to the same period as *On Seed* and *Usefulness of the Parts* by Singer, *Galen: Selected Works*, p. li. The terminology of similar/different is *homoiôs/enantiôs*.

[31]   Gk *tôi panti sômati*, *CMG* V. 3, 1, p. 180, 20–21.

A person who sees a bull from a distance recognizes it immediately as male, without examining its organs of generation, and it is possible similarly to recognize a male lion and distinguish it from a female lion, a cock from a hen, a buck from a nanny goat, a ram from a ewe. We also distinguish man from woman in this way, not undressing them first so that we may examine the difference in their parts, but viewing them with their clothes on. For they differ in their whole bodies, and of the so-called later parts some are not present in females at all, and some are of the same sort.[32]

A contemporary of Galen, Artemidorus, wrote a guide to the interpretation of dreams. He claimed that 'All things, good and bad, that pertain to the body, if they are seen not in their entirety but in halves, have good and bad fulfilments that are less extreme.'[33] He then describes the wife of Diognetos, who had a dream in which she had a beard, but only on the right side of her face. 'This dream' – and here I think Artemidorus means a woman dreaming of a *full* beard – normally means widowhood, if it is dreamt by a woman who is married, has children and is not pregnant. What the half-beard meant for the wife of Diognetos was a less extreme form of widowhood; she was married, but her husband travelled abroad, leaving her behind to keep house. This recalls the Hippocratic story of Phaethousa, who grew a beard when her husband left.[34] Artemidorus goes on to say that there is no difference between dreams of having a beard and dreams of having a penis, or wearing men's clothes, or having the hair of a man 'or something else virile'; for him, as for Galen, all signs of masculinity are equivalent here. In *On Seed* Galen went on to specify that the sex is clear from the hair (its amount and texture), hips, chest 'and many other differences'. In terms of the story of Agnodice, this 'two-sex' insistence on the very extensive range of signs of sex would suggest that her gesture of revelation should be redundant; there should be no need for her to lift her clothing, as she should be obviously a woman from every other part of her body.

The One-sex World before Galen: Herophilus

In locating earlier expressions of 'one-sex' or 'two-sex' models in the ancient world, there are serious problems regarding the survival of evidence; the work

---

[32]   *On Seed* II 5. 8–12, *CMG* V. 3, 1, pp. 181–3; Gk p. 182, 10–11: *to te gar holon sôma diallattousi.* 'Of the so-called later parts' translates Gk *kai tôn hysterôn onomazomenôn moriôn.* Galen clarifies these as beards, crests, spurs, tusks, horns, body hair, width of hips and chest, 'and many other differences'.

[33]   Artemidorus, *Dream Book*, 4.83; Rudolph Hercher, *Artemidori Daldiani, Onirocriticon Libri V* (Leipzig, 1864), p. 298.1–12; Robert J. White (tr.), *Interpretation of Dreams. Oneirocritica by Artemidorus* (New Jersey, 1975), p. 217.

[34]   The term for 'to keep house' is *oikourein*, Hercher, *Artemidori Daldiani*, p. 298.8. See below, Chapter 4 on *oikouros* in the case history of Phaethousa.

of many ancient medical writers has been lost, and is only known today through isolated quotations and references in treatises by later Greek and Roman writers. Galen, for example, tells us of an early third-century BC version of the two-sex body, by the philosopher Strato, who thought male/female difference extended beyond the genitalia to include the veins and arteries; he himself considered Strato 'very much in error', but as Strato's work does not survive we can say little more.[35] As for the one-sex body, an important figure is another third-century BC Greek medical writer, Herophilus, who wrote one treatise on anatomy and another on midwifery; Agnodice's teacher is named 'Herophilus', so that a story which seems to focus on the genitalia as clear indicators of the 'true sex' appears to have the heroine learning from a supporter of the 'one-sex' model, a point to which I shall return in Chapter 6. As Rebecca Flemming has shown, Herophilus played an important role in spreading a 'one-sex' model, and Galen knew his work well.[36]

Herophilus' aim was to 'demystify the female organs', showing that there were no diseases unique to women; this was a position in a long-standing debate in ancient medicine. The Hippocratic *Diseases of Women* had stated in the fourth century BC that one should not treat a woman as if she had a man's disease because 'the diseases of women and those of men differ very much in their treatment'. The Hippocratic writer also noted that it is hard to know about women's diseases because their embarrassment about them prevents them talking to male physicians; this is very similar to the opening scenario in Agnodice's story.[37] In the second century AD, Soranus summarised the debate up to his own day before insisting that women and men are made of the same material and share the same diseases.[38] Galen's dismissal of Strato notes that he was 'unacquainted with precise dissection'.[39] Herophilus, in contrast, dissected; indeed, in the Greco-Roman world human dissection was only practised during Herophilus' generation in Alexandria, while the city was under Greek rule. Galen, unable for cultural reasons to perform human dissections himself, here supports the dissector over the non-dissector, the material body over theoretical speculation.

In the words of Heinrich von Staden's edition of the surviving fragments of his work, Herophilus was 'fundamentally enslaved' to the idea that both sexes have

---

[35]   *On Seed* II 5. 12–15, *CMG* V. 3, 1, p. 183, 12. Marie-Laurence Desclos and William W. Fortenbaugh (eds), *Strato of Lampsacus: Text, Translation, and Discussion*, Rutgers University Studies in Classical Humanities, XVI (New Brunswick, NJ, 2011), fr. 71, p. 157.

[36]   Flemming, *Medicine and the Making of Roman Women*, p. 121, comparing the relative roles of Aristotle and Herophilus. Galen cites Herophilus many times, for instance in his treatise *On the Dissection of the Uterus*, 4.5 (Diethard Nickel (ed.), Galen, *De uteri dissectione, Corpus Medicorum Graecorum* V 2, 1, Berlin, 1971, p. 42).

[37]   *Diseases of Women*, 1.62 (Emile Littré, *Oeuvres complètes d'Hippocrate*, 10 vols (Paris, 1839–61), 8.126).

[38]   Soranus, *Gynaecology*, 3.1.3–5 and 18–20 (Budé edition); King, *Midwifery, Obstetrics and the Rise of Gynaecology*, pp. 14–15.

[39]   *On Seed* II 5. 13, *CMG* V. 3, 1, p. 182, 11–12.

the same genital organs.[40] For example, he called the ovaries 'the twins' (Greek *didymoi*), the same word that was used for the testicles, and observed that 'they differ only a little from the testicles of the male'; this terminology was still used in Renaissance Latin medical texts.[41] Even here, however, it is worth noting that 'only a little'; this is not a perfect match. Herophilus similarly drew a distinction between the male and the female seed; although women, having testicles, must produce seed, this 'female seed' was unable to play a role in generation because they did not have all the parts to perfect it.[42] From dissection, Herophilus also identified what we now call the Fallopian tubes but, taking the male body as normative, he labelled them 'spermatic ducts', and assumed that they went to the bladder. Galen rectified this assumption, showing that his particular 'one-sex' view of the body was less crude than that of his predecessors.[43]

Aristotle and Deformity

So, although some versions of the body have women as like men, with smaller, weaker, differently located but otherwise identical parts, others stress difference, based on the womb, or on the whole body. In Galen, both models can be found. Two further ancient writers need to be considered here: Aristotle and Hippocrates. Users of Laqueur have been too quick to merge the one-sex model of Galen's *On the Usefulness of the Parts of the Body* with ideas from one of Galen's own sources, the fourth-century BC philosopher Aristotle, whose 'inquiry into nature' included biology and gender.[44] For Aristotle, there was no 'female seed': men contributed seed to generation, and women provided blood. Laqueur presents Aristotle as operating with a commitment to 'the existence of two radically distinct and different sexes' but alongside 'a still more austere version of the one-

---

[40]   Heinrich von Staden, *Herophilus. The Art of Medicine in Early Alexandria* (Cambridge, 1989), p. 168.

[41]   Fr. 61 von Staden.

[42]   Flemming, *Medicine and the Making of Roman Women*, p. 121.

[43]   Von Staden, *Herophilus*, p. 168; Galen, *On the Dissection of the Uterus* 9 (*CMG* V 2.1, p. 48). On Galen and Herophilus, see Anthony Preus, 'Galen's Criticism of Aristotle's Conception Theory', *Journal of the History of Biology*, 10 (1977), p. 81: '[Galen] has learned from the Alexandrian dissectors the existence of the ovaries, which he quite appropriately calls "female testicles"'.

[44]   The 'inquiry into nature' or 'inquiry into the nature of things' is a translation of the Greek *physiologia* and suggests the wide-ranging context of ancient science. Giovanna Ferrari, *L'Esperienza del Passato. Alessandro Benedetti Filologo e Medico Umanistica* (Florence, 1996), p. 137, discussing whether Benedetto (b. 1452) was an Aristotelian or a follower of Galen, suggests that he saw Aristotle as a philosopher, Galen as a physician (Lat. *medicus*).

sex model than [did] Galen'.[45] Specifically, Galen took from Aristotle the notion of women as 'cold', but men as 'hot' and therefore able to concoct (or cook) their blood into semen.[46]

Kathleen Brown's summary of the one-sex model merges the importance of heat with another concept, that of 'deformity'. She writes, 'Lacking the vital heat to develop external genitalia, women's deformed organs remained tucked inside.'[47] But Galen's famous 'Consider ...' in *On the Usefulness of the Parts of the Body* never mentioned deformity in this sense. Aristotle had notoriously commented that 'woman is, as it were, a deformed man' and 'a mutilated man', in terms of the male as the *telos*, the goal or final point towards which humanity strives; however, in Aristotle, in another sense the *telos* of both men and women is to reproduce.[48] In the relevant section of *On the Usefulness of the Parts of the Body*, Galen uses the term *atelesteron*, 'less complete'; women are not as 'complete', not as 'perfect', as men, due to their lack of heat.[49] For us, 'deformed' or 'less perfect' are loaded terms; for Aristotle and Galen, however, they were simply another way of expressing what Rebecca Flemming has called women's 'critical inability', the lack of heat which meant that they could not make semen.[50] The 'deformity' was in the production of fluids, not – as Brown's wording suggests – in the physical form of the organs.

---

[45]   Laqueur, *Making Sex*, p. 28. See Holmes, *Gender*, p. 40 on Laqueur's use of Aristotle as both 'one-sex' and 'two-sex'; she concludes that Aristotle uses one model for the male and female principles, the other for the physicality of bodies.

[46]   Women as too cold to concoct blood into semen: Aristotle, *On the Parts of Animals* 650a8 ff; *On the Generation of Animals* 775a14–20.

[47]   Kathleen Brown, '"Changed ... into the Fashion of Man": The Politics of Sexual Difference in a Seventeenth-Century Anglo-American Settlement', *Journal of the History of Sexuality*, 6 (1995), p. 173.

[48]   The Greek term in Aristotle is *arren pepêrômenon*; Aristotle, *Generation of Animals* 737a26–30. Jaulin, 'La Fabrique du sexe', p. 201 points to the differences between Aristotle and Galen, which Laqueur glosses over, and concludes that 'il est abusif de nommer "unisexe" le modèle antique'. On the Latin translations of Aristotle in the thirteenth century, see Cadden, *Meanings of Sex Difference*, p. 109; on Aristotle's teleology, see Monte Ransome Johnson, *Aristotle on Teleology* (Oxford, 2005), where pp. 174–5 discuss the *telos* as being to reproduce, hence the need for male and female. On Renaissance views on whether the goal is to be a male, see P. Parker, 'Gender Ideology, Gender Change', pp. 338–9 and p. 360 on 'the orthodoxy of irreversibility'.

[49]   *Usefulness of Parts*, K 4.161–2.

[50]   Flemming, *Medicine and the Making of Roman Women*, p. 119: 'It is not so much that the female is inferior as that the inferior is female.' See also Johnson, *Aristotle on Teleology*, on 'the female' as not being equivalent to 'woman' and Nancy Siraisi, 'Vesalius and the Reading of Galen's Teleology', *Renaissance Quarterly*, 50 (1997), p. 4, on Vesalius' modifications of Galen's teleological approach as demonstrated in *On the Usefulness of the Parts*, 'the single work to which the *Fabrica* makes most constant reference'.

Patricia Simons has claimed that the 'deformed male' image was common in fifteenth- and sixteenth-century literature, and it is certainly mentioned in this period, and even before.[51] Karma Lochrie argued that, where the analogy between male and female sexual organs was made in medieval texts, there was always an Aristotelian spin, presenting not a straightforward set of parallels, but a 'failed one-to-one correspondence'; the idea of men and women having the same organs therefore demonstrates not the equivalence of male and female parts, but rather 'the inadequacy of the female anatomy'. What is important in this period is always the superiority of the parts of the male, in addition to 'the location of difference': internal, or external. She quotes the thirteenth-century *Anatomia vivorum*, 'The woman's instrument has an inverted structure, fixed on the inside, where the man's instrument has an [everted] structure extending outwards.'[52] But this does not say that, other than in location, the woman's instrument is the same as that of the man.

By the sixteenth century, however, scholasticism based on Aristotle was being replaced by Galenism; in 1543, in a section on the erroneous medieval belief in a seven-celled uterus, Vesalius commented on the presence at his public dissections of 'the scholastic theologians (who are even more prone than physicians to argue about semen and the genitals ...)'.[53] A seven-celled uterus, of course, is inconsistent with a 'one-sex' model, as the scrotum clearly does not have seven cells. Many medical writers of the sixteenth century were openly arguing against any labelling of women as 'imperfect' or 'lacking'.[54] Instead they saw women as 'perfect' for what they needed to do, namely to provide the raw material for, and bring to birth, a child. This, of course, was precisely Galen's view in *On Seed* and in *On the Usefulness of the Parts of the Body*; clearly engaging with Aristotle's wording, he insisted that 'you ought not to think that our Creator would purposely make half the whole race imperfect and, as it were, mutilated (Gk *ateles kai hoion anapêron*), unless there was to be some great advantage in such a mutilation'.[55]

---

[51]   Simons, *Sex of Men*, p. 130.

[52]   Karma Lochrie, *Margery Kempe and Translations of the Flesh* (Philadelphia, PA, 1991), p. 17.

[53]   Vesalius, *De Humani Corporis Fabrica libri septem* (Basel, 1543), p. 531; translation from William Frank Richardson and John Burd Carman, *On the Fabric of the Human Body: A Translation of De Humani Corporis Fabrica libri septem*, Book V, *The Organs of Nutrition and Generation* (San Francisco, CA, 2007), pp. 171–2. Lat. *a placitis scholasticorum theologorum (quibus frequentior de genitalibus et semine quam medicis disputatio est, quosque quum generationis organa in scholis ostendimus frequentissimos habemos spectatores) declinare veritus, septem sinibus uterum distinctum esse ad iecit*.

[54]   Simons, *Sex of Men*, p. 130. On scholasticism see Maclean, *Renaissance Notion of Woman*, pp. 6–11. On resistance to Aristotle's image of woman as 'deformed', see also Stolberg, 'A Woman Down to her Bones', p. 293.

[55]   *Usefulness of Parts* 14.6, K. 4.162, tr. May, vol. 2, p. 630; Galen, *On Seed* II 5.69 (*CMG* V. 3, 1, p. 184): it is because women are wetter and colder that they are able to provide nourishment for the unborn child.

Clearly reflecting this implied criticism of Aristotle, we read in Thomas Raynalde's *The Birth of Mankind* (itself based on the German apothecary Eucharius Rösslin's 1513 *Rosegarden*, and thus in turn deriving from fifteenth-century sources), that

> ... the woman in her kind and for the office and purpose wherefore she was made, is even as absolute and perfect as man in his kind. Neither is woman to be called (as some do) unperfecter than man (for because that man is more mightier and strong, the woman weaker and more feeble) ... For imperfection is when any particular creature doth lack any property, instrument, or quality which commonly by nature is in all other, or the more part of that kind, comparing it to other of the same kind and not of another kind.[56]

This, then, is not a 'one-sex' model. Men and women are of different 'kinds'; their organs should not be ranked against each other. By the seventeenth century, both male and female writers on midwifery were insisting that there was no reason why women should 'be ashamed of what they have'.[57] Even if men and women had the same parts but in opposite locations due to their different levels of heat, there was not thought to be any value judgement implied here about the relative roles of the sexes in generation.

Hippocrates and Menstruation

Turning now from anatomy to physiology, Hippocrates, as 'father of medicine', was a particularly important source for later writers looking for a classical authority on the body.[58] In the Hippocratic treatise *On Generation/Nature of*

---

[56] For Raynalde, see Elaine Hobby's edition, *The Birth of Mankind, Otherwise Named, The Woman's Book* (Aldershot and Burlington, VT, 2009), pp. 47–8; this passage is discussed in Elaine Hobby, 'Dreams and Plain Dotage: The Value of *The Birth of Mankind*', in Sharon Ruston (ed.), *Literature and Science*: Essays and Studies, The English Association (Cambridge, 2008). On Rösslin's sources, particularly the fifteenth-century physician Michele Savonarola, see Monica H. Green, 'The Sources of Eucharius Rösslin's *Rosegarden for Pregnant Women and Midwives*', *Medical History*, 53 (2009). For the late sixteenth century, see also André du Laurens, *Opera anatomicae* (Lyon, 1593), p. 280 on women as perfect in their kind; p. 285 on rejecting the 'deformed' image.

[57] The wording of Nicholas Culpeper, *A Directory for Midwives or, a Guide for Women, in their Conception, Bearing, and Suckling their Children* (London, 1651), p. 26, echoed by Jane Sharp, *The Midwives Book* (London, 1671), p. 32: 'we cannot be without ours no more than they can want [that is, lack] theirs'.

[58] While some writers, including Laqueur, still use the name 'Hippocrates', it is standard now to refer to 'the Hippocratic writers', thus acknowledging that there is no agreement on any one text of those in the collection of treatises we know as 'the Hippocratic corpus' that can be firmly attributed to the historical Hippocrates. See further Wesley D. Smith, *The Hippocratic Tradition* (Ithaca, NY, 1979); revised edition, 2002, <http://www.

the Child, the English translation of which, published in 1981, was available to and used by Laqueur, sex is determined by a mixture of the 'seeds' contributed by the man and the woman, and there is a spectrum from the manly male to the feminine woman.[59] The presence of two seeds is similar to Galen, but contrasts with Aristotle, for whom there is no female seed, but only male semen imposing 'form' on a woman's blood.[60]

Laqueur did not, however, use another group of Hippocratic treatises, which even today are not available in full in English translation, and which show us once again that the 'two-sex' body is not a creation of some eighteenth-century watershed between the early modern and modern worlds. These are the late fifth- or early fourth-century BC *Diseases of Women* treatises: the Greek title, *Gynaikeia*, can mean 'diseases of women', 'remedies for women', 'female genitalia', or 'menstruation'. Here, not only is women's contribution to generation simply the 'raw material' of menstrual blood, but also men and women are entirely different and, as I have already noted, it is stated that 'the diseases of women and those of men differ very much in their treatment'.[61] The lack of female 'seed' is matched by a lack of interest in seeing the organs of men and women as analogous; what is important here is not the genitalia, but the difference located in every part of the female body, in particular in the soft and spongy nature of female flesh, which absorbs more fluid from the diet and thus makes menstruation necessary. Women are like unprocessed fleece, men like a closely woven garment, and if someone were to put fleece and garment in the same damp place for the same length of time,

---

biusante.parisdescartes.fr/medicina/Hippo2.pdf>. On the shift from anatomy to physiology, from structures to fluids, see the comments on Laqueur in Simons, *Sex of Men*, p. 141 and the papers in Manfred Horstmanshoff, Helen King and Claus Zittel (eds), *Blood, Sweat and Tears: The Changing Concepts of Physiology from Antiquity into Early Modern Europe*, *Intersections* 25 (Leiden, 2012).

[59] Iain M. Lonie, *The Hippocratic Treatises 'On Generation,' 'On the Nature of the Child,' 'Diseases IV'* (Berlin and New York, 1981).

[60] For Galen, women must produce semen in order to explain the resemblance between a child and its mother. Since men do not produce menstrual blood, resemblance cannot pass from blood; therefore it must pass through semen, and so women must produce semen. See *On Seed*, Book 2.1.57–74. Ruth Gilbert, *Early Modern Hermaphrodites: Sex and Other Stories* (Basingstoke, 2002), p. 38 opposes to Aristotle a 'Hippocratic/Galenic position' on generation, but this demonstrates her reliance on Laqueur who, as I shall show, used only a limited group of Hippocratic treatises. Beecher, 'Concerning Sex Changes', p. 991 uses the term 'Aristotelean-Galenic' for the 'one-sex' model; as this chapter has shown, the position of these ancient writers is, however, far from being identical.

[61] *Diseases of Women* 1.62 (Littré 8.126), a statement described as 'the founding act of Greek gynaecology'; see Paola Manuli, 'Donne mascoline, femmine sterili, vergini perpetue. La ginecologia greca tra Ippocrate e Sorano', in Silvia Campese, Paola Manuli and Giulia Sissa, *Madre Materia. Sociologia e biologia della donna greca* (Turin, 1983), p. 154; King, *Hippocrates' Woman*, p. 12; von Staden, *Herophilus*, p. 297.

it is the fleece that would draw up more moisture.[62] The full versions of these texts re-entered the Western medical tradition in the sixteenth century, following the Latin translation of the entire Hippocratic corpus by Marco Fabio Calvi in 1525, including the books on the diseases of women from which only a few chapters had previously been known.[63] By showing that Hippocrates had thought women's diseases sufficiently important to devote entire treatises to them, Calvi's edition paved the way for Hippocrates as 'Father of Gynaecology'. Men who were already well established as experts on women's diseases gained further support from this new/ancient ally.[64] As Maurice de la Corde, the first to write a commentary on the first volume of the Hippocratic treatise *Diseases of Women*, put it, only 'our divine Hippocrates, with sure reasoning and purpose, has embraced the complexity of the diseases which affect woman throughout the whole course of her life'.[65] This was not an entirely new image of Hippocrates; a Latin translation of parts of *Diseases of Women*, produced in the late fifth or early sixth century AD, had prefaced the text with praise of Hippocrates, 'Herald of truth and master who does not lie', who 'also provided human health to the female race, and talked about their cures because of women's weakness'.[66] Women are weak, needing male medical attention, or they are complex, needing a theoretically based medicine that takes into account the many ways in which a virgin's internal structure differs from that of a childbearing woman, and the body of a widow has needs different from those of a married woman. In the sixteenth century, praising Hippocrates as the ultimate authority for men to treat the diseases of women also, conveniently, supported the corollary of this; the restriction of women's role to helping in childbirth.

What sixteenth-century and later writers took from the *Gynaikeia* model of sexual difference was an even greater interest in menstruation. As a visible sign of what was happening inside the female body, this was fundamental to being a woman; women's flesh accumulated excess blood and needed to evacuate it regularly to maintain health, so as Wendy Churchill put it for the seventeenth

---

[62]   *Diseases of Women* 1.1 (Littré 8.10–14); King, *Hippocrates' Woman*, pp. 28–9.

[63]   King, *Midwifery, Obstetrics and the Rise of Gynaecology*, pp. 18–19. Calvi owned the fourteenth-century manuscript of the Hippocratic texts, *Vaticanus graecus* 277, known as 'R', which derives from the manuscript tradition associated with *Marcianus Venetus* 276 or 'M'; see Volker Langholf, *Medical Theories in Hippocrates: Early Texts and the 'Epidemics'*, Untersuchungen zur antiken Literatur und Geschichte, vol. 34 (Berlin, 1990), pp. 9–10.

[64]   King, *Midwifery, Obstetrics, and the Rise of Gynaecology*, esp. pp. 18–20.

[65]   Maurice de la Corde, *Hippocratis Coi, Medicorum principis, liber prior de morbis mulierum* (Paris, 1585), pp. 8–9; discussed by King, *Midwifery, Obstetrics and the Rise of Gynaecology*, pp. 33–4.

[66]   Translated by Laurence Totelin, 'Old Recipes, New Practice? The Latin Adaptations of the Hippocratic Gynaecological Treatises', *Social History of Medicine*, 24 (2011), p. 86, based on Innocenzo Mazzini and Giuseppe Flammini, *De conceptu: Estratti di un'antica traduzione latina del Περὶ γυναικείων pseudoippocratico* (Bologna, 1983).

century, 'Depending upon the circumstances, menstruation could be regarded as a cause, a symptom, or a cure.'[67]

Not being aware of the *Gynaikeia* tradition, Laqueur plays down the pre-modern importance of menstruation in defining what it is to be female, replacing this with his focus on inside/outside organs. For example, he argued that menstruation was not seen as particularly 'female' in the seventeenth century, and described menstrual blood as merely 'a local variant in this generic corporeal economy of fluids and organs', writing that, in a 'one-sex' model, 'what matters is losing blood in relation to the fluid balance of the body, not the sex of the subject or the orifice from which it is lost'.[68] Here he was clearly aware of the interest of medical writers – indeed, up to the early twentieth century – in phenomena such as male menstruation and menstrual diversion, a variant of which features in the story of Phaethousa; it is when her menses stop that her beard grows.[69] In the Hippocratic treatise *Aphorisms*, highly influential in the education of physicians in the medieval, early modern and modern worlds, we are told for example that 'A nosebleed is a good thing if the menstrual period is suppressed' and even that 'Vomiting blood ceases when menstruation commences.'[70] At the beginning of the first century AD the Roman writer Celsus described what to do in women 'If blood bursts forth from the nose at a time when it should do from the genitals'.[71]

But in ancient medicine, none of this made menstruation a 'local variant' in the body of fluids. Instead, it lay at the very centre of what it is to be a woman; in the words of the writer of the Hippocratic text *On Generation/On the Nature of the Child* – in a passage Laqueur did not pick up – it was 'simply a fact of her original constitution', so that 'if the menses do not flow, the bodies of women become sick'.[72] For the medical writer Soranus, writing in the early Roman Empire,

---

[67]   Churchill, 'The Medical Practice of the Sexed Body', p. 13.

[68]   Laqueur, *Making Sex*, pp. 35, 37 and 105.

[69]   Laqueur, 'Sex in the Flesh', p. 305. Male menstruation has been widely discussed. See for example Gianna Pomata, 'Menstruating Men: Similarity and Difference of the Sexes in Early Modern Medicine', in Valeria Finucci and Kevin Brownlee (eds), *Generation and Degeneration: Tropes of Reproduction in Literature and History from Antiquity to Early Modern Europe* (Durham, NC and London, 2001), pp. 109–52; on the medieval myth that Jewish men have been condemned to menstruate since Christ's crucifixion, see J. Beusterien, 'Jewish Male Menstruation in Seventeenth-Century Spain', *Bulletin of the History of Medicine*, 73 (1999) and Irven M. Resnick, 'Medieval Roots of the Myth of Jewish Male Menses', *Harvard Theological Review*, 93 (2000).

[70]   *Aphorisms* 5.32–3. On the *Aphorisms* passages and the place of the text in medical education, see King, *Hippocrates' Woman*, pp. 58–9. Laqueur, *Making Sex*, pp. 36–7 mentions these aphorisms.

[71]   Celsus, *De medicina*, 4.27.1. M.H. Green, 'Bodily Essences', pp. 152–3 also demonstrates that male menstruation beliefs can be accompanied by a model of 'absolute' distinctions between male and female.

[72]   *Nature of the Child* 15 (Littré 7. 494); *Generation* 4 (Littré 7. 474); Lonie, *The Hippocratic Treatises*, p. 8.

evacuating blood is 'the first function' of the womb.[73] There was no sense that one could miss a period. In Hippocratic descriptions of amenorrhoea, the blood is described as 'hidden'; the verb is *kryptomai*, as in 'cryptic'.[74] In this pre-ovulation version of the body, then, rather than a missed period, one has a hidden period. Nor was this simply a pre-modern view of the female body; in eighteenth-century France, for example, menstruation continued to be seen as essential in order to maintain women's health.[75]

In *Making Sex*, Laqueur discussed Jacques Moreau, who published his *Histoire naturelle de la femme* in 1803. Located on the other side of Laqueur's watershed, Moreau knew his Hippocrates *and* his Galen, and referred to both. His concern to distinguish the 'four ages of woman' (birth to puberty, youth, maturity, decline) and the hygienic regime appropriate to each, is comparable to the study of woman as virgin, married woman, pregnant woman and old woman in Renaissance gynaecological texts, while his synoptic table (vol. 1, p. 32) recalls those of sixteenth-century commentaries on the Hippocratic treatise, *Diseases of Virgins*.[76] Laqueur summarised Moreau's position as being that 'A woman is a woman ... everywhere and in all things, moral and physical, not just in one set of organs.'[77] Moreau argues, for example, that one cannot compare male and female sexual pleasure in terms of one being 'stronger' or 'weaker' than the other, as they are simply different: 'il est autre'.[78] 'La femme ... est femme par toutes ses parties,

---

[73]   Soranus, *Gynaecology* 3.2, Budé p. 5: *prôton ergon hysteras ê katharsis* (purging is the first function of the womb).

[74]   King, *Hippocrates' Woman*, p. 146, citing *Diseases of Women* 1.2 (Littré 8. 14); *Diseases of Women* 1.3 (Littré 8. 22) etc. The *Index Hippocraticus*, Fasc. II, p. 459 cites a total of 15 uses of the verb in a menstrual context.

[75]   See for example Lisa Smith, 'Imagining Women's Fertility before Technology', *Journal of Medical Humanities*, 31 (2010), p. 75.

[76]   Jacques L. Moreau, *Histoire naturelle de la femme*, 2 vols (Paris, 1803), vol. 1, p. 16; Helen King, *The Disease of Virgins: Green Sickness, Chlorosis and the Problems of Puberty* (London: Routledge, 2003), pp. 52–3.

[77]   Laqueur, *Making Sex*, p. 149 and p. 281 n. 3, citing Moreau, *Histoire naturelle de la femme*, referring simply to '1, chap. 2'. In his initial summary of the views of the ancients on female difference (vol. 1, pp. 62 ff.), Moreau does not mention Hippocrates, but later in his argument, when discussing the difference between male and female muscles, he notes 'L'éducation, les habitudes, peuvent y ajouter, augmenter, peut-être la délicatesse des parties, comme Hippocrate était forcé de l'avouer, sans qu'il soit possible d'en rien conclure pour rejeter l'idée d'une différence radicale, innée, qui a lieu dans tous les pays et chez tous les peuples' (p. 111). Moreau did not see the absence of an analogue for the womb as a problem, writing that 'Galien, confondant les sexes, même, dans les parties où leur caractère se manifeste davantage, n'admet d'autres différences entre les pièces diverses de l'appareil mâle et les parties de l'appareil féminin, que celles qui dérivent du développement et de la situation; l'addition de *l'utérus* dans la femme ne lui parait pas même une objection ...' (Moreau, *Histoire naturelle de la femme*, pp. 66–7).

[78]   Moreau, *Histoire naturelle de la femme*, p. 186.

sous tous les points de vue.'[79] But to a reader familiar with Hippocratic medicine, none of this is new. There too, women themselves are 'the Other', with the audience of the texts being reminded that women should not be treated medically as if they are men, because in fact 'the healing of women differs greatly from that of men'.[80] There too, women's difference extends beyond the organs of generation to every part of the flesh: men are firm and hard, women are wet and spongy. In terms of the texture of their bodies as a whole, men are like woven cloth, women are like fleece.[81] At least in the *Gynaikeia* treatises, the Hippocratic woman cannot be understood by reference to the organs of the male body.

Even if we restrict our analysis to medical treatises alone, it is clear that, in the classical world more broadly, the range of models of the body was much greater than Laqueur allows. Although in Herophilus' dissections, a belief in the sexes as analogous led to the identification of the ovaries as 'female testicles', the 'one-sex' model was far from being dominant. It could feature more as a thought experiment than as a statement of how things are. Expressions of the all-embracing difference between men and women are found in Galen as well as in the Hippocratic *Gynaikeia* writings. If the male is the goal, the female must be inadequate: but if reproduction is the goal, both sexes are equally necessary. So 'one-sex' statements that identified women as 'deformed' men could become 'two-sex' claims for each sex having its own specific, and divinely ordained, role in the process of generation. In many ancient medical texts, what mattered was not so much genital anatomy, as the centrality of menstruation in the economy of the female body.

---

[79]   Ibid., p. 210.
[80]   *Diseases of Women* 1.62 (Littré 8. 126); King, *Hippocrates' Woman*, pp. 27–36.
[81]   *Diseases of Women* 1.1 (Littré 8. 10–12); King, *Hippocrates' Woman*, pp. 28–9.

Chapter 2
Picturing the Womb: Vesalius and the Sixteenth Century

In the previous chapter, we saw that, even within the canonical texts used by Laqueur, various models of sex centred on difference existed in the ancient world, with Galen himself focusing sometimes on similarity, sometimes on difference. While Laqueur thought the emergence of the 'two-sex' model in the eighteenth – or late eighteenth – century (or at some point after 1670) was what needed to be explained, those working on earlier periods have found more interesting what they identify as an increased interest in a 'one-sex' model in the early sixteenth century. In her 2010 article on Laqueur and medieval images of the body, Katy Park's closing question was 'What needs explaining, then, is not, as Laqueur claims, "why did the attractions of this [one-sex] model fade at all?" (61), but why did they appear?'[1] Monica Green has recently proposed an answer to this question, suggesting that the one-sex model had been mentioned in passing by medieval surgeons, who were learning more about the male genitalia from new ways of treating inguinal hernia, as 'a way to make up for their relative lack of information on female pelvic anatomy'.[2] Like Herophilus in the third century BC, they were transferring knowledge of the male onto the female, and postulating a 'one-sex' body made it a valid move to apply discoveries from the visible outside of the male body to the invisible insides of women.

The respective roles of male and female in generation were particularly fascinating for pre-modern European culture; as Monica Azzolini noted, 'reproduction was a hidden process, and while the results were in front of everybody to observe, the mechanisms were wrapped in mystery'.[3] In this context, an analogy between the penis and the neck of the womb was an obvious one to make, since clearly the former must fit into the latter, as in Leonardo da Vinci's famous imagined scene of coitus. Not discussed by Laqueur, this was drawn in the years between 1490 and 1493, before Leonardo had performed any human dissections.

In the sketchier female figure on the left, the penis goes right through the cervix to deposit its seed, drops of which are visible; Leonardo represents the

---

[1]   Park, 'Cadden, Laqueur, and the "One-Sex Body"', p. 5.

[2]   M.H. Green, 'Bodily Essences', p. 147.

[3]   Monica Azzolini, 'Exploring Generation: A Context to Leonardo's Anatomies of the Female and Male Body', in Alessandro Nova and Domenico Laurenza (eds), *Leonardo da Vinci's Anatomical World: Language, Context and 'Disegno'* (Florence, 2011), p. 83.

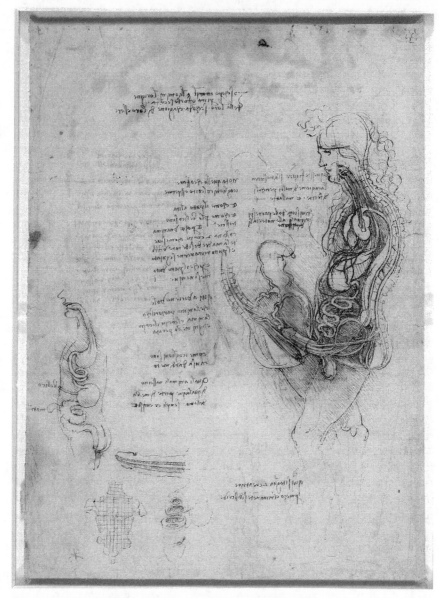

Figure 2.1   Leonardo da Vinci, Coition of a Hemisectal Man
              and Woman, Windsor, Royal Library 19097v

womb as having many chambers, perhaps a reference to the medieval seven-celled womb, and he may be suggesting that the womb is actively drawing the male seed up into its cavities.[4] As I noted in the previous chapter, this seven-celled womb is not part of a 'one-sex' model. Leonardo's notes include a line going to the diaphragm, stating this is where the spiritual parts (in the chest) are separated from material parts (in the abdomen); this is based on Plato's division of the body into three sections (the other division being at the neck), which was in turn used by Galen. The penis, shown in detail elsewhere on this page, has two channels, one for seed and one for urine; this was not the only position taken in medicine in the late fifteenth century, as other writers followed Avicenna and had three different channels.[5] Leonardo also portrays channels going from the womb to the breasts; these too are part of the heritage of ancient medicine, allowing menstrual blood to be further concocted into breast milk.[6] Monica Azzolini has suggested that, in this drawing, Leonardo may have been giving a visual version of the text of Mondino's *Anatomia*.[7] This suggestion warns us against using visual images, even those that may to us appear 'obvious', out of context; despite its appearance, this image is not based on dissection, and may be illustrating an (absent) text.

This chapter will explore the transmission of Galen's comments about an inside/outside model of the body in the sixteenth century, when Hippocratic 'two-sex' models were coming back into play; the publication in 1525 of Marco Fabio Calvi's Latin translations of the Hippocratic *Gynaikeia/Diseases of Women* treatises, with their emphasis on treating women not as if they were men, but on their own terms, reinforced what was already a growing interest in women's diseases, even though these texts argued against a 'one-sex' model of analogy. I shall first discuss in some detail what Laqueur saw as a visual expression of the 'one-sex' body, Vesalius' image of the womb and vagina; here I shall be arguing that the key image is one that has a very specific context. How would a viewer contemporary with Vesalius' image have read it? Vesalius' *Fabrica* (1543) appeared within an environment in which women's 'secrets' still remained the ultimate challenge, with their revelation being the Holy Grail for anatomy, but also at the same time as learned men – and women – in Europe were first reading the account of Agnodice's self-display in court; her story first appeared in a printed book in 1535. I shall then focus on those working in the decades around the 1590s to 1620s when, as the rest of this book will go on to show, the 'one-sex' and 'two-sex' models were in dialogue and were using the classical stories of Agnodice and Phaethousa as a way of exploring the nature of sex.

---

[4] Simons, *Sex of Men*, pp. 135–6; Carmen C. Bambach, 'Leonardo's Drawing of Female Anatomy and his "Fascciculu Medjcine Latino"', in Alessandro Nova and Domenico Laurenza (eds), *Leonardo da Vinci's Anatomical World: Language, Context and 'Disegno'* (Florence, 2011), pp. 123–4 on the very different, spherical, womb in his later drawings.

[5] Azzolini, 'Exploring Generation', pp. 89–90.

[6] Ibid., p. 80.

[7] Ibid., p. 91, n. 38.

The Vagina as Penis?

I noted in the Introduction that one of the reasons for the popularity of *Making Sex* is the use of visual images. Here I want to concentrate on the most powerful of them all: the womb in Vesalius' Figure 27 (Introduction, Figure I.1).[8] In general, Vesalius trod a fine line between challenging Galen – famously accusing him of being 'deceived by his apes' because he did not dissect humans – and showing a high level of appropriate deference, engaging with the original Greek text with what Nancy Siraisi has characterised as 'intensity', above all with *On the Usefulness of the Parts of the Body*, but also with *Doctrines of Hippocrates and Plato*.[9] Roger French has described the *Fabrica* as 'a focused critique of Galen's writings, especially *De Usu Partium*' but, as Andrew Cunningham has demonstrated, Vesalius wanted to emulate Galen, not to bury him.[10]

Vesalius' magisterial account of the body, *De humani corporis fabrica* ('On the Fabric of the Human Body'), was published in 1543, nearly two decades after Calvi's Latin translation of the Hippocratic *Diseases of Women* appeared; a second, revised, edition was published in 1555 and notes for a third edition have recently been identified.[11] It was not until 1585 that Maurice de la Corde's commentary on these treatises engaged with the differences between the Hippocratic and the Galenic models of the female body, but already by the 1550s writers were hailing Hippocrates as the expert on women.[12] On the famous title page of the *Fabrica*, Vesalius presents himself as merging the established anatomical roles of lecturer, dissector and demonstrator as he opens up a female cadaver, and what he reveals

---

[8]   Laqueur, *Making Sex*, p. 82, Figure 20; Vesalius, *De humani corporis fabrica*, Book 5, Figure 27; 2nd edition (Basel, 1555), p. 584.

[9]   'Deceived by his apes', *at vero suis deceptum simiis*, features in the Preface to *Fabrica*. On Vesalius' engagement with Galen, see Siraisi, 'Vesalius and the Reading of Galen's Teleology', p. 2 and V. Nutton, '*De placitis Hippocratis et Platonis* in the Renaissance', pp. 305–6.

[10]   Roger French, *Dissection and Vivisection in the European Renaissance* (Aldershot, 1999), p. 175; Andrew Cunningham, *The Anatomist Anatomis'd: An Experimental Discipline in Enlightenment Europe* (Aldershot and Burlington, VT, 2010), p. 29 on Vesalius as 'trying to emulate Galen' in his emphasis on dissection; cf. Cunningham, *The Anatomical Renaissance: The Resurrection of the Anatomical Projects of the Ancients* (Aldershot, 1997), p. 115: 'Vesalius as vivisectionist was simply Galen restored to life' and p. 116, on Vesalius even in 1540 as 'not just following what Galen said one should do in anatomy, but trying to *be* Galen in the present'.

[11]   Unless otherwise stated, references here are to the 1543 edition. On the third edition, see <http://www.myscience.cc/wire/new_material_from_founder_of_modern_human_anatomy_comes_to_warwick-2012-warwick> accessed 30 July 2012 and Vivian Nutton, 'Vesalius Revised: His Annotations to the 1555 *Fabrica*', *Medical History*, 56 (2012): 415–43.

[12]   On de la Corde, see King, *Disease of Virgins*, p. 44; ibid., *Midwifery, Obstetrics and the Rise of Gynaecology*, pp. 11 and 19.

is the womb.[13] Some medical works of a similar period showed a woman pulling back or lifting up flaps of her own skin to reveal her internal organs of generation, recalling Agnodice lifting her clothes, but on Vesalius' title page the female cadaver is passive, giving up her agency to the dissector.[14]

For Laqueur, Figure 27 is clear evidence of the 'one-sex' model in action. He described Vesalius' earlier version of the image, published in 1538, as 'the vagina as penis', phrasing echoed by Londa Schiebinger in the 2003 article in which she supported Laqueur against Michael Stolberg's critique.[15] But this was a very different image, showing ligaments and 'female testicles', none of which feature in Figure 27, where the focus is explicitly on the womb. Whatever we may see here now, this image is labelled not as 'the vagina' but as 'the womb cut out of the body' and it has a very specific purpose, being described in the caption as showing the size of the parts in a woman who is not pregnant: 'This figure concerns, with respect to its size, the womb cut out of the body, in the manner of the womb of the last woman we dissected at Padua' is followed by a reference to the 'thickness' of the tunics or layers of the womb here 'in women who are not pregnant'.[16] In Laqueur's version the image appears as a freestanding one,

---

[13]   On the three roles, G. Ferrari, *L'Esperienza del Passato*, p. 124; on the significance of Vesalius being shown dissecting a woman, Katy Park, 'Dissecting the Female Body: From Women's Secrets to the Secrets of Nature', in Jane Donawerth and Adele Seeff (eds), *Crossing Boundaries: Attending to Early Modern Women* (Newark, NJ and London, 2000), pp. 29–47 and ibid., *Secrets of Women*; on the title page, Andrea Carlino, *Books of the Body: Anatomical Ritual and Renaissance Learning* (Chicago, IL, 1999), pp. 42–53; Sachiko Kusukawa, *Picturing the Book of Nature: Image, Text and Argument in Sixteenth-Century Human Anatomy and Medical Botany* (Chicago, IL, 2012), pp. 200–10; Giovanna Ferrari, 'Public Anatomy Lessons and the Carnival: The Anatomy Theatre of Bologna', *Past and Present*, 117 (1987), p. 62 suggests that the anatomy theatre shown in the title page is the temporary structure used at Bologna for Vesalius' 1540 lectures there. On these lectures, see further below, pp. 60–2.

[14]   I disagree here with Jonathan Sawday's interpretation in *The Body Emblazoned: Dissection and the Human Body in Renaissance Culture* (London and New York, 1995), pp. 112–3, where he suggests that she is 'looking directly' into Vesalius' face and so 'is by no means simply a passive object for our contemplation. She too is watching the process of dissection which is mirrored in the face of her dissector.' I owe this reference to Laura Robson.

[15]   Laqueur, *Making Sex*, p. 82 with Figure 18; Stolberg, 'A Woman Down to her Bones'; Schiebinger, 'Skelletestreit', p. 310 on 'Vesalius's remarkable image of the female genitalia portrayed as a male penis'. The image is on <http://www.zol.be/internet/vesalius/Tabulae/Tabulae1/body_tabulae1.html> accessed 15 May 2012 and in Laqueur, *Making Sex*, p. 80, Figure 18. On the debate, see further above, pp. 3–4.

[16]   *Fabrica*, 1543, p. 381 (this should be numbered 481, but the pagination is incorrect from pp. 313–91). Lat. *Praesens figura uterum a corpora exectum ea magnitudine refert, qua postremo Patavii dissectae mulieris uterus nobis occurrit* (the translation of Richardson and Carman, p. 44, 'This figure shows a uterus cut away from the body: it is the same size as the uterus of the woman who was the subject of our last dissection at

but it originally had a caption and accompanying labels which, as in all Vesalius' figures, are tied not only to small letters on the image, but also to references in the inner margin of the main body of the text. In the 1543 edition the captions were to the left of this image, and in the 1555 edition they appeared on the following page.[17] I mentioned above the possibility that Leonardo's section of a couple having intercourse may have illustrated a text that is not mentioned on that page; in some medieval manuscripts, such as the late thirteenth-century Ashmole 399, the text and images 'transmit related but separate bodies of knowledge'.[18] For Vesalius, in contrast, captions and illustration are intricately connected. Yet Laqueur chose to omit both caption and labels when he reproduced Figure 27. Elaine Hobby has pointed out the same need to read this particular image in conjunction with its caption in the 1560 edition of *The Birth of Mankind*, which repeated this picture from the *Fabrica*; here, as in the Vesalian original, the accompanying text again clearly showed that the focus was not on what Hobby calls 'the monstrous vagina', but instead on the womb.[19] While Laqueur hails

---

Padua' misses Vesalius' emphasis on size as the *purpose* of the illustration). Vesalius goes on to explain that he has shown the womb opened so that the thickness or density of the cavity and tunics of the womb in a non-pregnant woman can be clearly seen; *sinus ... una cum ambarum uteri tunicarum in non praegnantibus substantiae crassitie.*

[17]   On the general issues of keying the image to the text, and the implications for the reader, see Nancy G. Siraisi, 'Vesalius and Human Diversity in *De humani corporis fabrica*', *Journal of the Warburg and Courtauld Institutes*, 57 (1994), p. 64; Vivian Nutton, 'Representation and Memory in Renaissance Anatomical Illustration', in Fabrizio Meroi and Claudio Pogliano (eds), *Immagini per conoscere: dal Rinascimento alla Rivoluzione scientifica* (Florence, 2001), pp. 61–80; French, *Dissection and Vivisection*, p. 175; Kusukawa, *Picturing the Book of Nature*, p. 188.

[18]   Karl Whittington, 'The Cruciform Womb: Process, Symbol and Salvation in Bodleian Library MS. Ashmole 399', *Different Visions: A Journal of New Perspectives on Medieval Art*, 1 (2008), p. 4.

[19]   Hobby, *The Birth of Mankind*, p. xxix. Compare Figure 9, 1560 *Birth of Mankind*, taken from the copy of Vesalius's Figure 27 in Thomas Geminus, *Compendiosa totius Anatomie delineatio* (London, 1553), no page number; <http://alfama.sim.ucm.es/dioscorides/consulta_libro.asp?ref=X532785400&idioma=0> image 110. 'And the ninth figure showeth the matrix cut forth of the body, being of that bigness as it was seen taken forth of a woman at the last anatomy which I did see at the University of Padua in Italy. And moreover we have so divided and cut asunder the bottom of the matrix by the middle, that the concavity and hollow bought [= sheepfold] within the same matrix might be perceived, and the thick substance also of both the coats of the matrix in women, when they be not with child' (Hobby, *The Birth of Mankind*, pp. 77, 94–8). In the 1545 edition this image also appeared, but here as Figure 5: 'This fifth figure is portrayed after the quick [that is, from the life] both in length and breadth, according to the length and breadth of a woman which was cut open for the same purpose by physicians. But here ye must understand that here the found or body of the womb or matrice is divided in the midst, the forepart of the which is turned up, for because that ye may the better perceive the cavity of the matrice' (Hobby, *The Birth of Mankind*, p. 225). The 'found' is the Latin *fundus* or base.

this image as 'not incredible or "wrong". Its proportions are roughly those of "accurate" nineteenth-century engravings … and illustrations from a modern text', medical practitioners today regard the vagina as too long and too wide for the uterus, the cervix as nowhere near thick enough, and they point out that the labia minora and majora are confused. They query whether the vagina could be dissected out in the way in which it is shown here – from the outside – and note that the section through the heart-shaped womb is simply incorrect, while the external genitalia with the strangely-positioned pubic hair are unbelievable.[20]

How would Figure 27 have been seen in the sixteenth century? Do its caption, its discussion within Vesalius' text, and its labelling by those who copied and used it in the following 20 years or so suggest that it expressed for them a 'one-sex' body or a more Hippocratic 'otherness' and difference? Today, when we illustrate the womb in medical works or elsewhere, we often show it with the Fallopian tubes, and we omit the external genitalia; for us, womb-and-tubes form the 'organ'. But in Vesalius' image, there are of course no signs whatsoever of the tubes because these were 'discovered' by Vesalius' pupil Gabriele Falloppio only in 1561, so in Vesalius even their points of entry into the womb do not appear.[21] He never discusses the Galenic 'inside out' passage, either in the caption to Figure 27, or elsewhere in his text where, like other sixteenth-century writers, he mixes one-sex and two-sex points. In his image of 'the womb cut out of the body', there is no sign of the 'female testicles'; yet, if this were really a 'one-sex' image, they should appear, since Galen described them in his comments about the womb 'reversing itself so that all of it that is outside comes now to be inside'.[22]

Galen's comment is given visual representation in an illustration of the womb in a treatise first published 20 years before Vesalius' *Fabrica*, Berengario da Carpi's *Isagoge breves*, based on Mondino and Galen (Figure 2.2). In his text, Berengario duly described men's and women's organs as respectively 'complete and outside', and 'diminished and inside', with the neck of the womb 'like a penis'.[23] In the

---

[20]   Laqueur, *Making Sex*, p. 85. My thanks to the audience at the conference, 'Vital Traditions', Princeton, 19–20 April 2013 for their comments on this image, and above all to Henry Schneiderman, M.D. and Vivian Nutton.

[21]   Gabriele Falloppio, *Observationes anatomicae* (Venice, 1561), 196v on the *uteri tuba*; Robert Herrlinger and Edith Feiner, 'Why Did Vesalius Not Discover the Fallopian Tubes?', *Medical History*, 8 (1964), p. 338 notes that Vesalius' Figure 27 shows no points of entry into the womb for the tubes.

[22]   Above, p. 36.

[23]   Berengario da Carpi, *Isagogae breves* (Bologna, 1522), p. 22r–v, *Matrix tota cum suis Testiculis et uasis seminariis est similis membris generationis uirorum sed membre uirorum sunt completa extra propter suum calorem expulsa: foeminae uero sunt diminuta intra retenta propter suum diminutum calorem … collum matricis est quasi virga*. Laqueur, *Making Sex*, p. 80, Figure 17 reproduces two of the Berengario images but interprets them as showing 'the correspondences between male and female organs'; in fact, they are simply showing the female organs.

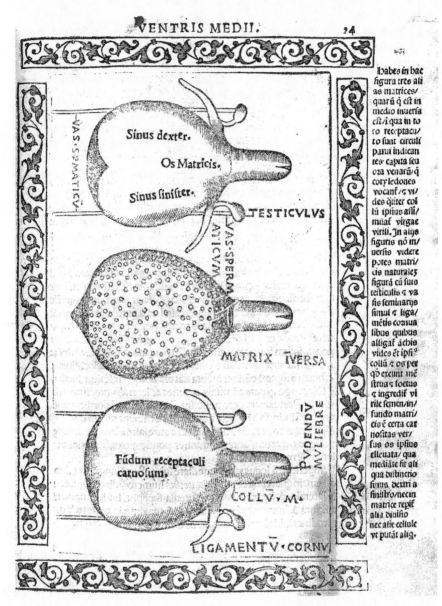

Figure 2.2   Jacopo Berengario da Carpi, *Isagogae breves* (Bologna: Benedictus Hectoris, 1522)

outer images of this illustration, the woman's 'testicles' are visible; but the central image is labelled 'matrix inversa', the womb inverted. The woman's 'testicles' are no longer visible here because, following Galen, Berengario is imagining the womb turned inside out so that they go inside it, in the manner of the male ones retained in the scrotum.

In contrast, however, Vesalius' Figure 27 is divorced from this model. It is consistent with this separation from the Galenic inside-out model that Vesalius is adamant that Galen had *never* seen a human uterus, only those of cows, goats and sheep; there is thus no reason why he should want to represent Galen's views of this organ in Figure 27, as 'not even in his dreams did Galen ever see a woman's womb'.[24] On similar grounds, he also criticises Galen's comments on the 'double nature' of the womb (above, p. 36): in fact, he insists, it 'is not double and elongated like an intestine; this is its form in the dog and the pig and, in short, in animals that almost always produce several foetuses together'.[25] However, although it is clearly not a medieval seven-celled womb, it is still seen as a heart-shaped structure, which is perhaps a relic of the 'double nature'. Berengario da Carpi's outer two illustrations of the womb (above, Figure 2.2) also have this shape, and Berengario commented that 'It has a single cavity or cell, which somewhere near its fundus is divided into two parts, as if there were two uteruses terminated at one neck.'[26]

In terms of a 'one-sex' idea of shared organs in different locations, Vesalius certainly draws analogies between various parts of the male and female organs of generation; for example, like Galen in *On Seed* he links the appearance of the womb to that of the scrotum, and he comments that the mouth of the womb resembles the opening in the glans of the penis.[27] He considers that 'Nature has given the substance of the neck of the uterus something in common with the male penis, or more specifically with the substance that forms the two bodies and the glans of the penis as described earlier.'[28] The neck of the uterus here is not our

---

[24]   *Fabrica*, p. 532: margin, *Galenum humanum uterum nunquam inspexisse*; text, Galen *ne per somnium quidem muliebrem uterum unquam inspexisse*. In the accompanying text, Vesalius cites the Galenic treatises *Usefulness of Parts*, *On Seed* and *Dissection of the Uterus*.

[25]   *Fabrica*, p. 537 (tr. modified from Richardson and Carman, p. 185); Lat. *Non enim geminus cernitur, et intestini instar oblongus, qualis cani et sui, et illis denique animalibus obtigit, quae plures simul foetus semper propemodum enituntur.*

[26]   Berengario da Carpi, *Isagogae breves*, p. 22v *Unicam cauitatem seu cellulam habet: quae tunc aliqualiter circa eius fundum in binas partiri: ac si essent duae matrices ad unum collum terminatae*; tr. L.R. Lind, *A Short Introduction to Anatomy* (Chicago, IL, 1959), p. 82.

[27]   *Fabrica*, pp. 531 (where the marginal note refers the reader back to Figure 27) and 532.

[28]   *Fabrica*, p. 535 (tr. Richardson and Carman, p. 180); Lat. *Cervicis porro uteri substantiae aliquid commune cum virili pene Natura elargitur, eam dico qua duo penis corpora et glandem praecipue formari diximus.* On the significance of 'Nature' in Vesalius, see Siraisi, 'Vesalius and the Reading of Galen's Teleology', pp. 14–28.

'neck', the cervix, but rather what we think of as the vagina; in the words of Karl Whittington, writing on a late thirteenth-century English manuscript illustration of the womb, it is both entrance, and chamber.[29] For Berengario (Figure 2.2), although a line from *collum*, neck, points at the cervix, the label extends the full length of the vagina to the external genitalia (*pudendum muliebre*).

Laqueur attributes to the other side of his eighteenth century watershed the naming of female parts, saying that it was only then that 'Organs that had not been distinguished by a name of their own – the vagina, for example – were given one.'[30] The naming of 'parts' is a difficult matter, the dividing line between them being a matter of choice.[31] 'Vagina' – which is simply the Latin for 'sheath' – in fact appeared before the eighteenth century; Laqueur himself notes that Realdo Colombo had earlier used it in a metaphorical sense, noting that the penis is placed 'as it were' into a vagina, or sheath.[32] According to the *Oxford English Dictionary*, the first use of 'vagina' in English texts was in Thomas Gibson's 1682 *Anatomy of Humane Bodies*. But Gibson's use was just as metaphorical as Colombo's, and he included other similarly metaphorical names: 'It has its name *Vagina* or Sheath, because it receives the Penis like a Sheath. It is called also the *door of the Womb*, and its *greater Neck* ...'. Outside the specific chapter on the vagina Gibson continued to use 'neck of the womb'; the 1703 edition shifted from this terminology to 'the vagina *of the womb*' to set it apart from other 'sheaths' in the body.[33]

Laqueur distances us unnecessarily from the past in suggesting that the vagina previously had no name in English; it had many, but – as in the label 'the vagina of the womb' – they linked it to other parts, simply because that was how the vagina was seen. In Raynalde's *The Birth of Mankind*, for example, the vagina is the 'womb passage' and the cervix the 'womb gate' or 'womb port'.[34] In Vesalius, the label 'the neck of the uterus' (Latin *uteri cervix*) translates Galen's 'neck of the

---

[29]   Whittington, 'The Cruciform Womb', p. 7.

[30]   Laqueur, *Making Sex*, p. 149, repeated by Eriksson, 'Biologically Similar and Anatomically Different?' p. 32: 'A specific terminology for the female anatomy was not developed until the 18th century'. This myth persists; for example, Katherine Crawford, *European Sexualities, 1400–1800* (Cambridge: 2007), pp. 106–108, who claims that 'Female parts were not distinct enough to merit separate names.'

[31]   As T.S. Eliot reminded us about the naming of cats.

[32]   Laqueur, *Making Sex*, p. 96.

[33]   In the first edition, *The Anatomy of Humane Bodies Epitomized* (London, 1682) mostly the term 'the neck of the womb' was used for the vagina (for example, p. 15), but there is a separate chapter on 'the vagina and its contents'; Book 1, Chapter 28, pp. 152–4. On the name, see p. 152. In the sixth edition (London, 1703), in addition to the separate Chapter 28, pp. 191 ff., other references in the text have moved from referring to 'the neck of the womb' to calling it 'the vagina of the womb' (cp. p. 20 of the 1703 edition to p. 15 of the 1682 edition).

[34]   Hobby, *The Birth of Mankind*, pp. 32, 34, 37.

wombs', in Greek, *ho auchên tôn mêtrôn*; literally 'the neck/gullet of the wombs' as, like many Hippocratic writers, Galen used the plural term for womb, as part of his belief that it was 'double'. In *On the Usefulness of the Parts of the Body* Galen described the ability of this neck to straighten and to stretch during intercourse; 'Nature made the neck of the wombs quite hard, so that while it is stretched and at the same time expanded during the entrance of the male seed, it will be sufficiently straightened and dilated both to be able to give an unblocked road for the semen and to close the orifice afterwards.'[35] Vesalius, similarly, discussed the flexibility of this part, observing that 'When we pull up the uterus in the course of dissection the neck stretches out to an astonishing length.'[36] Thus our vagina and womb were here seen as a single organ, womb-with-neck, and, in Vesalius' Figure 27, as in the Berengario image, these are also joined to the external genitalia.

So, even if we see it that way, this is not a vagina-as-penis: as the label makes clear, for a sixteenth-century audience, this is the womb and its constituent parts.[37] Understanding it in this way helps us to understand what I think is the key point about this image: the emptiness of the womb. Vesalius tells us that the woman whose womb is represented here also features in a second image, of her torso; Katy Park has further identified her as the woman on the iconic title page of his book. Giovanna Ferrari has drawn attention to Alessandro Benedetti's 1502 description of the ideal cadaver for dissection, namely someone 'who had been hanged, especially if they were middle-aged, neither fat nor thin, and of larger

---

[35]   Galen, *Usefulness of Parts*, 14.3, K 4.148; translation modified from May, p. 624.

[36]   Lat. *nam nobis uterum inter dissecandum attollentibus, in miram longitudinem cervix porrigitur*; Vesalius, *Fabrica*, p. 533 (tr. Richardson and Carman, p. 176). I disagree with May who, in her translation of *Usefulness of Parts*, p. 614, n. 7, insisted that 'Galen really means the cervix when he speaks of the neck of the uterus', citing Galen's treatise *On Anatomical Procedures*, Book 12, Chapter 2; see W.L.H. Duckworth, *Galen On Anatomical Procedures: The Later Books* (Cambridge, 1962), p. 112. In *On Anatomical Procedures* there is a reference to 'the neck and cervix of the uterus' as the part 'between the vagina, the female pudenda, and the uterine cavity'. As Book 12 is lost in Greek and Latin, this is based on the Arabic translation, and may therefore significantly modify the original text. The many references to *uteri cervix* in *Fabrica* include descriptions of how it sometimes collapses in on itself, and sometimes expands (p. 378, caption to Figure 24).

[37]   This issue of not identifying 'organs' in the same way across time also applies to the male body; while we regard the penis as an organ, in early modern works it was likely to be represented only as an ensemble with the testicles, and presented merely as a conduit for the seed which they produced. It was the ability to produce and project seed that made 'a man'. Simons, *Sex of Men*, p. 10: 'From ancient Greece to well past the Renaissance, the standard visual signifier of male sex was the ensemble of testicles, penile shaft, foreskin and glans'; p. 134: 'Testicles ... were considered the true seat of virility.' See also Helen King, 'Inside and Outside, Cavities and Containers: The Organs of Generation in Seventeenth-Century English Medicine', in Patricia A. Baker, Han Nijdam, Karine van 't Land (eds), *Medicine and Space: Body, Surroundings and Borders in Antiquity and the Middle Ages*; *Visualising the Middle Ages* 4 (Leiden, 2011), pp. 37–60.

overall stature than average, "so that there is material that is in greater abundance and more evident for the spectators"'.[38] Vesalius' woman fits this description; she was 'unusually large' (Lat. *rarae magnitudinis*), middle-aged, and had given birth many times and, having been condemned to be hanged for a crime that is nowhere identified, she had tried to avoid her sentence by claiming that she was pregnant.[39] Rather than 'womb-as-penis' or 'vagina-as-penis', this then is 'the empty womb and its neck'. His exposure of her womb on the title page image and in Figure 27 emphasises that women's word cannot be trusted as evidence of their pregnancy – or lack of it.

Agreeing and Disagreeing: Galen in the Sixteenth Century

Although Vesalius does not repeat the Galenic inside/outside passage, he was clearly familiar with it. Three years before the publication of the *Fabrica*, Vesalius was already being cast as the new voice in medicine when he was invited to demonstrate anatomy at Bologna University. Only 25, he was performing alongside the much older Curtius, who although he was 65 saw himself as representing what was then the 'modern' view of the body: supporting careful analysis of Galen's

---

[38]   G. Ferrari, 'Public Anatomy Lessons and the Carnival', p. 59, citing Alessandro Benedetti, *Anatomice: sive, de historia corporis humani libri quinque* (Venice, 1502), Book 1, folio Civ; there were also editions published in Cologne and Paris in 1527, and in Strasburg in 1528 (G. Ferrari, 'Public Anatomy Lessons and the Carnival', p. 57, n. 30).

[39]   Park, *Secrets of Women*, pp. 207 and 211; Vesalius, *Fabrica*, p. 539 explains the origins of this cadaver and its use for Figures 24 (*Fabrica*, p. 377) and 27 (*Fabrica*, p. 381); *Quae autem postremo nobis obtigit, et qua in vigesimaquarta et vigesimaseptima figuris exprimendis usi sumus, suspendii metu se gravidam falso finxerat*: Richardson and Carman, p. 189; 'The last one we obtained, which was the subject of our Figures 24 and 27, had falsely claimed to be pregnant from fear of being hanged.' Midwives were used to check her story, and discounted it; the woman went to her punishment. On p. 533 Vesalius again refers specifically to Figure 27 and notes – as in the caption – that this is the size of the womb in women who are not pregnant: *Vigesima septima tamen praesentis libri figura, eam uteri magnitudinem exprimit, quae frequenter in non praegnantibus, et praecipue in huius anni consectione Patavii occurrit*; the translation of Richardson, p. 177 changes the emphasis on size and adds 'often seen', thus implying more about eye-witness evidence than does the Latin. I would translate as 'For all that, Figure 27 of the present volume shows the size of the womb, as happens often in women who are not pregnant, and especially in a dissection at Padua in this very year.' In the 1555 edition, p. 663 develops the comment on 1543, p. 539 above, giving instead *Quae autem postremo nobis obtigit, rarae magnitudinis, mediaeque aetatis mulier, suspendii metu se gravidam falso finxerat*. Laqueur, *Making Sex*, p. 82 calls the woman who was the basis of the three illustrations 'a young woman'; it is not clear what his authority is for this assertion.

original Greek text against Mondino's version of it.[40] Curtius began each day with an exposition of Mondino's views on the body, contrasting these with Galen, and Vesalius would then go on to challenge Curtius from the evidence of a real cadaver. Regardless of the part on which Curtius had lectured, Vesalius' demonstrations concentrated on the muscles. Notes taken by the student Baldasar Heseler record Curtius picking up Galen's remarks on reversal in *On the Usefulness of Parts of the Body* and in *On Seed*, teaching in his 20 January 1540 lecture that

> Galen says that the organs of procreation are the same in the male and in the female, only that in the female all is reversed to the male, in whom that which is inside in the female is outside. And again in the male all is contrary to the female. For if you turn the scrotum, the testicles and the penis inside out you will also have all the genital organs of the female, like they are in the male. (Yet the penis of the male is more solid, the neck of the uterus of the female more excavated and concave and much more extendable in time of coitus and parturition.) Vice versa, if you turn inside out the genital organs of the female, you will have all the organs of the male. Thus, they differ only by being reversed.[41]

It is not clear here how we should read the material in brackets. Was Curtius both summarising Galen, and inserting into his summary a challenge to him?[42] Or are these Vesalius' words, as he interrupts the older man? The editor of Heseler's notes, Ruben Eriksson, suggests that the bracketed material is Heseler's own; at the end of each day of lecture and demonstration, he would write up his rough notes, sometimes adding a comment.[43] While some such remarks are clearly Heseler reflecting on how what he has just seen reminds him of an earlier experience, and one definitely records Vesalius' comments at the time, others – particularly those, like this one, which start with the Latin *tamen* (yet/however) – express

---

[40]   On the way in which 'medieval predecessors were far more likely to be criticised for failure to understand ancient authority than for slavish dependence on it', see Siraisi, 'Vesalius and the Reading of Galen's Teleology', p. 1; Cunningham, *Anatomical Renaissance*, pp. 102–16. On the Bologna dissections see also French, *Dissection and Vivisection*, pp. 165–8.

[41]   Ruben Eriksson (tr.), *Andreas Vesalius' First Public Anatomy at Bologna, 1540: An Eyewitness Report* (Uppsala and Stockholm, 1959), Curtius' fifteenth lecture, 20 January 1540, pp. 180–81. The Latin of the central passage is: *Si enim conuertas scrotum, testiculos et penem uirorum, tunc habebis quoque omnia membra spermatica in mulieribus, sicut in uiris sunt. (Tamen coles in uiris est magis solidus, collum autem matricis in mulieribus magis excauatum concauum et magis extensibile multum tempore coitus et partus.). Coles* here is for *caulis*, a term for the penis. My thanks to Laura Robson for discussing the Heseler notes with me.

[42]   This would recall the *quaestio* format, on which see below, pp. 64–5.

[43]   Eriksson, *Andreas Vesalius' First Public Anatomy*, p. 42: 'Heseler himself often indicated his own additions to Curtius' lectures and Vesalius' explications during the demonstrations by ().' See also Eriksson, pp. 17–19 on Heseler's note-taking practices.

disagreement with Curtius.[44] In one bracketed section, the words 'my good Curtius' are included, which could mean that here Heseler is giving Vesalius' own response to Curtius' claims.[45] In this particular passage, the comments that Heseler inserts into his notes on Curtius' lecture concern the highly 'extendable' neck of the womb (= vagina); as we know that this was something Vesalius wrote about in 1543, this could also point to him as the source of the disagreement with Curtius here. But, as we have just seen, Galen too discussed the way in which the 'neck of the womb' could stretch.

Whatever the source of Heseler's bracketed comments on the differences that undercut a 'one-sex' model, they contrast with Laqueur's version of Galen, in which 'only' the inside/outside location distinguished men from women. Laqueur claimed that 'The notion, so powerful after the eighteenth century, that there was something concrete and specific inside, outside, and throughout the body that defined male as opposed to female, and provided the foundation for the attraction of opposites, was absent in the Renaissance.'[46] But in Heseler's record of Vesalius' work at Bologna, again we see not only that a simple inside/outside difference was already being challenged in the mid-sixteenth century – supposedly the period when Laqueur's 'one-sex' model dominated – but also that there were plenty of challenges to it even within the work of Galen himself.

How did the works of Galen and the Hippocratic treatises speak across Laqueur's 'millennial chasm' to other sixteenth-century writers? In terms of how well they were known in Western Europe, the different treatises of Galen had different fates; Vesalius was able to engage with, and challenge, *On the Usefulness of the Parts of the Body*, but it had not been translated in full from Greek into Latin until the fourteenth century, and had only been printed in 1528. Before it appeared in print, manuscripts of the Latin translation of 1317 were used for example by Mondino and Gentile da Foligno in the fourteenth century, and it was engaged with in more detail by Gabriele de Zerbi in 1502.[47] A version of the inside/outside imagery and the homology between the sexual parts of men and women was also

---

[44]   Eriksson, *Andreas Vesalius' First Public Anatomy*, p. 149: Heseler uses the brackets to reflect on what he saw at the dissection of a thief in Leipzig; p. 155: Heseler uses the brackets to note that 'our anatomist Andreas [Vesalius] said however …'; p. 198: the brackets record the amusement of 'all the Italians' present, at a comment that the penis does not always become erect when it should, especially in old people.

[45]   Eriksson, *Andreas Vesalius' First Public Anatomy*, p. 181. Heseler also refers to Curtius as 'the good Curtius' in another bracketed comment where he adds 'See how Curtius has lied', *Vide quomodo Curtius mentitus sit.*

[46]   Laqueur, *Making Sex*, p. 133. It is not clear when Laqueur dates the Renaissance; on occasion he uses it for Jane Sharp, who wrote in 1671, so he appears to be using it for the period up to the eighteenth century; ibid., pp. 65 and 67–8.

[47]   French, *Dissection and Vivisection*, p. 82 (Gabriele da Zerbi); p. 67 (Mondino); p. 59 (Gentile da Foligno); Park, 'Cadden, Laqueur, and the "One-Sex Body"'; M.H. Green, 'Bodily Essences', pp. 146–7.

known to Renaissance medical writers as a result of its appearance in Avicenna's eleventh-century *Canon*, based on Galen and translated into Latin in the twelfth century; here, 'the membrane of the uterus is like the scrotum and the penis is like the neck of the uterus and the two eggs are in women as in men'. The Latin term for 'eggs' is *ova* – a further reference to the idea that both men and women have 'testicles' in which their seed is stored. But, while the penis is 'complete [Lat. *completum*] and stretches outside' the womb is 'diminished and retained inside and is like an inverted male instrument'.[48] While the inside/outside imagery is clear, this is not just a simple homology; the organs are respectively diminished, or complete.

Ten years before *Making Sex* appeared, Ian Maclean published *The Renaissance Notion of Woman*. Laqueur refers to this important study only once in his text, and three times in his notes. Maclean showed that the analogies of the 'one-sex' body were rejected after 1600 by most medical writers; the difficulties of maintaining them, in the face of anatomical discoveries such as those of the clitoris and the Fallopian tubes, from the 1560s onwards, were simply too great.[49] We have already seen both acceptance and challenge (possibly both deriving from Galen) within the notes Heseler took from Curtius' lectures in 1540. In the final quarter of the sixteenth century, the 'one-sex' model was still being repeated by the Spanish Juan Huarte, whose 1575 *Examen de ingenios* appeared in English translation in 1594. Huarte, interestingly, appealed to anatomical knowledge not to overturn the 'one-sex' body, but instead to support it. He stated that man differs from woman

> in nought els (saith *Galen*) than only in hauing his genitall members without his body. For *if we make anotomie of a woman*, we shall find that she hath within her two stones, two vessels for seed; and her belly of the same frame as a mans member, without that any one part is therin wanting. And this is so very true, that if when nature hath finished to forme a man in all perfection, she would conuert him into a woman, there needeth nought els to be done, saue only to turne his instruments of generation inwards. And if she haue shaped a woman, and would make a man of her, by taking forth her belly [i.e. womb] and her cods, it would quickly be performed (my italics).[50]

---

48   Avicenna, *Canon* (Venice, 1507), 3.21.1.1, fol. 360.

49   Maclean, *Renaissance Notion of Woman*, p. 33. Beecher, 'Concerning Sex Changes', supports this dating from sex change stories in particular.

50   Juan Huarte, *Examen de ingenios, para les sciencias* (Baeça, 1575); *The Examination of Mens Wits in whicch [sic], by Discouering the Varietie of Natures, is Shewed for what Profession Each One is Apt, and How Far he shall Profit Therein. By Iohn Huarte. Translated out of the Spanish tongue by M. Camillo Camili. Englished out of his Italian, by R.C. Esquire* (London, 1594), p. 269. On Huarte see Or Hasson, 'On Sex-Differences and Science in Huarte de San Juan's *Examination of Men's Wits*', *Iberoamerica Global*, 2 (2009): 194–212; <http://iberoamericaglobal.huji.ac.il/Num5/Art_15.pdf> accessed 28 August 2012.

Here, the belly (womb) is 'of the same frame', or structure, as the penis, in every part. In the English translation, this passage was accompanied by a marginal note stating that 'This is no chapter for maids to read in sight of others.'

For Huarte, the reversal could still go either way, at least *in utero*: 'Contrariwise, nature hath sundrie times made a male with his genetories outward, and cold growing on, they haue turned in ward, and it became female.' But he also suggested that it could occur later in life to women, 'should a beard grow on her chin, and her floures [menses] surcease, and she become as perfect a man, as nature could produce'; in its first two points, although not the third, precisely what happened to Phaethousa of Abdera in the Hippocratic case history.[51] He proposed that there are three levels of coldness and of heat, and the factors of understanding, demeanour, voice, flesh, complexion, hair, and attractiveness allow an observer to determine whether a woman is cold in the first, second or third degree.[52]

Huarte shows that anatomy – 'if we make anotomie of a woman' – could be invoked by those supporting a range of models of the body. But as Laqueur believes that anatomical knowledge was not the prime mover here, playing only a secondary role to other changes that made two sexes necessary – changes he locates in the eighteenth century – it is perhaps not surprising that he makes little use of Maclean, retaining his watershed over a century later. From my own research into this period, I would add that, although the 'one-sex' model and its attribution to Galen continued to feature, as in Huarte, the late sixteenth-century pattern of discussing generation was commonly to include a short summary of Galen on the inside/outside body but to follow this with a discussion of the 'two-sex' alternative. Some further examples will demonstrate how this worked.

'You will never make a penis'

One of the sixteenth-century writers singled out by Maclean as giving 'a very coherent account' of the dispute over whether the organs of generation were parallel in men and in women is the French physician and rector of Montpellier University, André du Laurens. In 1593, in his *Opera Anatomicae* (*Anatomical Works*, appearing in a later version as *Historia Anatomica Humani Corporis*, 'An Anatomical Account of the Human Body'), du Laurens summarised the accepted wisdom of his day as regards male/female difference, and asked 'Whether the reproductive organs of a woman differ only in their location, contrary to the ancients and Galen.'[53] This was framed as a debate, or *quaestio disputata*, in

---

[51]   *The Examination of Mens Wits*, pp. 269 and 271.

[52]   Ibid., pp. 272–3; I am rendering Huarte's 'wit' as understanding here, and 'manners' as demeanour.

[53]   Maclean, *The Renaissance Notion of Woman*, p. 33; du Laurens, *Opera Anatomicae*, pp. 261–5, *Controversiae, Quaestio* VII: *An mulierum genitalia solo situ a virorum genitalibus distinguantur, contra veteres & Galenum*. In the later *Historia Anatomica*

which a proposal was made and then the arguments on both sides assembled, with a view to reconciling apparent contradictions between ancient authorities; a feature of education inherited from the Middle Ages, the basic form survived well into the seventeenth century.[54] Donald Beecher has correctly pointed out that sixteenth-century writers 'typically began by reciting the established beliefs and thereby accommodating the ancients, but they are to be watched for the dissent embedded in their statements of putative conciliation'.[55] Following this pattern, du Laurens' response began with the 'one-sex' model: 'The ancient belief in the books of illustrious men, confirmed by the writings of generally all anatomists, is that the parts of generation of women do not differ from those of men in the parts relating to seed, except in their location,' and he added that most writers 'today' share these beliefs.[56] It is noteworthy that he described the parts in terms of 'seed', supporting Patricia Simons' arguments for a model focused more on the fluid of semen, than on the organs, in this period.[57] Du Laurens then went on to list similarities between the organs; for example, the central raised line on the scrotum is like that along the base of the womb. He noted that 'Generally all the anatomists proclaimed' that it was only in location, not in shape (Lat. *forma*), that the spermatic organs differed.[58] But, as the title of the section had suggested – *contrary* to – in the second section of the *quaestio* du Laurens then challenged this 'one-sex' position, the marginal note stating 'The ancient view is rejected.'[59] Here he discussed the Hippocratic case history of Phaethousa as evidence of a two-sex model, ending this section by identifying her as a clear case of a woman retaining all her female organs of generation, including her womb, despite her outwardly masculine appearance.[60] Observation, *autopsia*, should be trusted,

---

Humani Corporis (Paris, 1600), this became *Quaestio* VIII, pp. 358–60. Laqueur's response to Stolberg, 'Sex in the Flesh', addressed du Laurens specifically, but focusing on the 'one-sex' model rather than on the second part of the *quaestio* in which du Laurens challenges it.

[54] Brian Lawn, *The Rise and Decline of the Scholastic 'Quaestio Disputata' with Special Emphasis on its Use in the Teaching of Medicine and Science* (Leiden, 1993); Azzolini, 'Exploring Generation', pp. 83–6.

[55] Beecher, 'Concerning Sex Changes', p. 995.

[56] Du Laurens, *Opera anatomicae*, p. 261: *Vetus est opinio clarissimorum virorum monumentis & omnium fere Anatomicorum scriptis confirmata, non differre mulierum genitalia a virorum spermaticis partibus, nisi solo sito.*

[57] Simons, *Sex of Men*.

[58] Du Laurens, *Opera anatomicae*, p. 262: *id Anatomici fere omnes clamabant ... Non distinguebantur ergo forma, sed solo situ spermatica organa.*

[59] Lat. *Opinio vetus improbatur*, du Laurens, *Opera anatomicae*, p. 263 and ibid., *Historia Anatomica*, p. 359.

[60] Du Laurens, *Opera anatomicae*, p. 265.

and this shows that women's organs differ from those of men in number, shape, size, substance and structure.[61]

Challenges like this one were common, often based on observation and expressed in terms of 'difference'. The 1599 fugitive sheet *The Anatomie of the Inward parts of Woman, very necessary to be knowne to physitians, surgians, and all other that desire to know themselues* opened by stating that 'here we will declare the situation and manner of such partes as are in a woman, different from the parts in a man'; 'situation' or location was not everything, as 'manner' featured too.[62] In 1604 Caspar Bauhin followed Galen in presenting a strong inside/outside division; however, he added to this some other binary oppositions not given in the key passage of Galen, namely spacious/narrow and thin/thick.[63] Caspar Bartholin, one of Bauhin's pupils in Basle, published his Latin work on anatomy, *Institutes Anatomicae*, in 1611. He too repeated these denials that location was the only difference, appealed to the evidence of dissection, and ridiculed the different lists of analogies between the female and male organs that had so far been proposed. In the English translation of 1663 he insisted that

> the generative Parts in Women differ from those in Men, not only in Situation, but in their universal Fabrick, in respect of Number, Surface, Magnitude, Cavity, Figure, Office, and Use, as is sufficiently manifest to a skilful Anatomist, and to any one that will compare what follows to what went before. And the falsity of their Opinion is sufficiently apparent, by means of the sundry Conjectures which they bring. For some liken the Womb to the Cod of a Man, and some to the Nut of the Yard. Some will have the Neck of the Womb to answer the Mans Yard, and others will have the Clitoris.[64]

---

[61]   Ibid., p. 263: *Differunt utriusque sexus genitalia non situ modo, sed etiam numero, forma et structura* and p. 264.

[62]   *The Anatomie of the Inward parts of Woman, very necessary to be knowne to physitians, surgians, and all other that desire to know themselues* (London, 1599).

[63]   Caspar Bauhin, *Institutiones Anatomicae Corporis Virilis et Muliebris Historiam Exhibentes* (Berne, 1604), p. 77; ibid., *Theatrum Anatomicum* (Frankfurt am Main, 1605), pp. 210–11. The vocabulary is that of *intus/extra*; women's organs are 'hidden inside' (*intus sunt conditae*) while those of men are located outside (*extra ad perinaeum sitae*).

[64]   See *Bartholinus Anatomy*, tr. Nicholas Culpeper and Abdiah Cole (London, 1663), p. 62. The 1611 *Anatomicae institutiones corporis humanis* was revised by Caspar Bartholin's son Thomas in 1641 to take account of William Harvey's work, before this English translation based on the revised version was issued. See Nancy Siraisi, *History, Medicine, and the Traditions of Renaissance Learning* (Ann Arbor, MI, 2007), pp. 34 and 275. On Bartholin see Ole P. Grell, 'Caspar Bartholin and the Education of the Pious Physician', in Ole P. Grell and Andrew Cunningham (eds), *Medicine and the Reformation* (London, 1993), pp. 78–100. In the 1626 edition, *Anatomicae institutiones corporis humanis* (Strasburg, p. 114), this passage reads in full: *Neq. n. existimandum est cum Galeno, Archangelo, Fallopio & aliis, haec muliebria dicta membra à virilibus non differre nisi solo situ. Quae opinion nata est ex iis, qui putarunt, foeminam esse tantum*

In terms of parallels between the male and female generative parts, the discovery of the clitoris in 1560 (Realdo Colombo) / 1561 (Gabriele Falloppio) had further complicated attempts to draw up a satisfactory list.[65] Bartholin included in the main text the Galenic comment on location, but the summary in the margin of the book undercut it, stating simply 'The similitude of the yard and of the Womb, ridiculous'. Nor was this a view that emerged only at the beginning of the (very) 'long eighteenth century'. In its Latin original, it was equally dismissive: *Similitudo penis cum utero inepta est.*[66] While Russell West-Pavlov recently called this marginal note 'succinct and scathing', and Kaara Peterson described it as 'One of the more memorable dismissals of isomorphism', both ignore its presence in the 1611 Latin edition and instead cite only the 1663 version, thus concluding that, in West-Pavlov's words, 'By the *end* of the [seventeenth] century, the differences between male and female had crystallized fully' (my italics).[67] In fact, something very similar had also been stated in 1593 by du Laurens, who may be Bartholin's source here: he wrote that any claim that the vagina and the penis were the same in form was 'absolutely absurd', *absurdissimum*. 'However you perform an inversion of the vagina, you will never make a penis from it.'[68] This is a clear and explicit attack on Galen.

Du Laurens and Bauhin were the two main Latin sources for the 1615 *Microcosmographia: A Description of the Body of Man*, by Helkiah Crooke, who observed that 'It was the opinion of Galen ... that women had all those parts belonging to Generation which men have.'[69] But to state something as 'the opinion

---

virum imperfectum ... Caeterum muliebres partes non tantum situ a virilibus differre, sed universa structura, ßßquoad numerum, superficiem, magnitudinem, cavitatem, figuram, officium et usum, satis manifestum est perito Anatomico, et cuivis, qui sequentia haec cum praecedentibus conferre velit. Et satis apparet opinionis eorum falsitas, ex multiplici, quam afferunt, conjectura. Quidam n. uterum scroto virili assimilant, quidam glandi penis. Peni virili aliqui uteri collum respondere volunt, aliqui clitorida. Quae omnia propria fragilitate cum concidant ad explicationem partium accedimus. Similitudo penis cum utero inepta est.

[65] Simons, *Sex of Men*, pp. 147–8.

[66] See *Bartholinus Anatomy*, p. 62; Bartholin, *Anatomicae institutiones corporis humanis*, p. 114. The Latin *ineptus* has the sense of 'foolish' or 'silly'.

[67] West-Pavlov, *Bodies and their Spaces*, p. 49; Kaara L. Peterson, *Popular Medicine, Hysterical Disease, and Social Controversy in Shakespeare* (Aldershot, 2010), p. 34.

[68] Du Laurens, *Opera anatomicae*, p. 263: *Iam vero dum cervicem uteri inversam mentulae virilis formam referre volunt, absurdissimum ... Quocunque igitur modo uteri cervicem invertas, numquam ex eo penem efformabis.* He justified this dismissal by listing the differences – for example, the vagina has only one channel, the penis has two – and also dismisses Falloppio's equation of the clitoris and the penis. Simons, *Making Sex*, p. 148 notes du Laurens' rejection of the reversal model.

[69] Helkiah Crooke, *Microcosmographia: A Description of the Body of Man* (London, 1615), p. 216. Crooke's version of du Laurens is at times a direct translation from the Latin, at other times a simplification, as titles and chapter numbers of the ancient texts du Laurens used are omitted. As Jennifer Jordan, '"That ere with Age, his strength is utterly decay'd":

of Galen' is not to agree with it, and Crooke, like his sources, did not believe that
one should stop at Galen's 'opinion'. Crooke cut out du Laurens' comment that the
ancients and writers 'today' think that men and women differ only in the location
of their organs of generation; perhaps, from his standpoint over 20 years later,
and working within an English rather than a French context, that was simply no
longer true, and if this interpretation is correct then it would further support the
argument that the 'one-sex' body, already moribund in 1593, was dead by 1615.[70]
But he followed du Laurens in stating that there are parts in men that simply do
not exist in women, and others where the number of the parts differs between
the sexes; while 'Howsoever ... the neck of the womb [i.e. the vagina] shall be
inverted, yet will it never make the virile member' because the latter is made of
three hollow bodies (the opinion, as mentioned above, of Avicenna), the former
only of one.[71] Still following du Laurens, Crooke added that those arguing for the
clitoris – which he elsewhere calls the 'womans yard' – as the female analogue
for the penis were also mistaken, because the clitoris is small, not linked to the
bladder, and has no passage from which it can emit seed.[72] Crooke's other source,
Bauhin, was more conservative in his views on the clitoris; Crooke's 'womans
yard' simply translates Bauhin's *penis muliebris*, Bauhin stating that the clitoris is
'properly called the woman's penis, because it corresponds to the virile member'.
However, even Bauhin gave some examples of differences between these two
organs: in length, channels and muscles.[73]

In Jane Sharp's *The Midwives Book* of 1671, the first book by an English
midwife, we again see a reflection of the pattern of the *quaestio*. Sharp drew on
a number of published male authors, including Crooke, but, as Elaine Hobby and

---

Understanding the Male Body in Early Modern Manhood', in Sarah Toulalan and Kate Fisher
(eds), *Bodies, Sex and Desire from the Renaissance to the Present* (Basingstoke, 2011),
pp. 28–9 points out, Crooke also issued a smaller version of this in 1616, designed to be
portable and to focus the reader's attention on the illustrations: *Somatographia anthropine.
Or, A description of the body of man By artificiall figures representing the members, and
fit termes expressing the same. Set forth either to pleasure or to profite those who are
addicted to this study* (London, 1616). This contained simply the illustrations and the tables
explaining them. Jordan comments that the womb is 'distinctly phallic in appearance', but
like the other illustrations, this is taken from Vesalius, and the interpretation of the womb as
phallic tells us more about ourselves than about the early modern body.

[70]   I would like to modify Gianna Pomata's comment, in her edition of Oliva Sabuco
de Nantes Barrera's *The True Medicine* of 1587 (Toronto, 2010), p. 57 that 'Some late
Renaissance anatomists abandoned the Galenic homology of the male and female genitalia';
this was a wider movement rather than the choice of 'some'.

[71]   Crooke, *Microcosmographia*, pp. 249–50.

[72]   Ibid., p. 238 ('womans yard') and pp. 249–50; noted by Crawford, *European Sexualities*,
p. 109. However, Crawford gives too much credit here to Crooke, who is merely (and openly, by
interspersing his section with 'saith Laurentius'/'saith he') following du Laurens.

[73]   Bauhin, *Institutiones Anatomicae*, p. 86: *proprie virga muliebris, quod virili
membro respondeat*, and pp. 258–9.

Eve Keller have shown, she gave these sources her own spin.[74] In the first part of her book she repeated the inside/outside model, saying that 'Galen saith that women have all the parts of Generation that Men have, but Mens are outwardly, womens inwardly. The womb is like to a mans Cod, turned the inside outward.'[75] However, at the start of Book 2 of *The Midwives Book* she follows Crooke in challenging this view, writing that 'the parts of men and women are different in number, and likeness, substance, and proportion; the Cod of a man turned inside outward is like the womb, yet the difference is so great that *they can never be the same*' (my italics).[76] Furthermore, Sharp disputes Galen's conclusions more widely, following Vesalius in noting that they were based on dissecting apes rather than human beings; on ancient Greek knowledge of the body, she comments that 'the inside of men or women they saw not, and so were ignorant of the difference between them'.[77] This 'difference', rather than the 'inside/outside' model, is for Sharp the best way of regarding men and women. Eve Keller commented on Sharp's reading, 'The Galenic model, then, is less a biological "reality," than a hermeneutic: it offers a way of reading the body, but is not constitutive of the body itself.'[78] Sharp copies Crooke, Crooke copies Bauhin and du Laurens; none of them seems to have any investment in the model, and they explicitly mark it as what 'Galen says' rather than as the truth.

In the sixteenth and seventeenth centuries, then, alongside the repetition of what 'Galen says' which Patricia Parker called 'the rhetoric of insistence', there was considerable unease with the one-sex model.[79] Laqueur accepted that this unease existed, but for him this was about authors who 'seemed incapable of transcending the ancient images [they] explicitly rejected'.[80] I would instead suggest that the coexistence of both models in one text reflects the *quaestio* form; giving both sides of an argument is the normal format. However, even within this form, the objections to the 'one-sex' model were being made more forcibly than Laqueur suggests; it was silly, ridiculous, absurd. Medieval writers had used the

---

[74] Elaine Hobby, '"Secrets of the Female Sex": Jane Sharp, the Reproductive Female Body, and Early Modern Midwifery Manuals', *Women's Writing*, 8 (2001), pp. 201–12; ibid., '"The Head of this Counterfeit Yard"'; ibid., 'Yarhound, Horrion, and the Horse-Headed Tartar: Editing Jane Sharp, *The Midwives Book* (1671)', in Katherine Binhammer and Jeanne Wood (eds), *Women and Literary History: 'For There She Was'* (Newark, DE and London, 2003), p. 33; Eve Keller, 'Mrs Jane Sharp: Midwifery and the Critique of Medical Knowledge in Seventeenth-Century England', *Women's Writing*, 2 (1995), pp. 101–11.

[75] Jane Sharp, *The Midwives Book* (London, 1671), ed. Elaine Hobby, p. 37.

[76] Ibid., p. 67. On Sharp's undercutting of Galen here, see Keller, 'Mrs Jane Sharp', p. 106.

[77] Sharp, *The Midwives Book*, ed. Hobby, pp. 56–7.

[78] Keller, 'Mrs Jane Sharp', p. 106.

[79] P. Parker, 'Gender Ideology, Gender Change', p. 340.

[80] Laqueur, *Making Sex*, p. 92 on Bartholin.

'one-sex' model to emphasise male superiority, but also as a way of speculating about the unseen insides of women's bodies. Sixteenth- and seventeenth-century writers stressed that each sex has its purpose; they were not only more familiar with the female body, as a result of dissection, but also had a greater knowledge of a Hippocratic model of difference, which encouraged them to regard women as so unlike men that they required a separate branch of medicine to make sense of their bodies. Vesalius's infamous Figure 27 concerns the emptiness of the womb, and the unity of what we would see as the womb and the vagina as a single organ with its extendable 'neck'; it challenges our assumption about the lines between parts of the body.

In this and the previous chapter I have emphasised the importance of close reading within their cultural context not only of texts, but also of images. The material used has largely come from the great men of the canon, those also used by Laqueur. But, as I noted in the Introduction, there are other ways of thinking about making sex in the period before the eighteenth century. While Laqueur's method is to weave together statements from mostly medical or other scientific sources, in the rest of this book my method will be very different: I am taking two stories that were the common property of medical writers and lay people, men and women, across a long time period. I have already commented on Vesalius' investigations into the female body, and his revelation of its secrets, happening at the same time as the story of Agnodice became known. The story seems to have peaked in popularity in the period around the 1590s to 1620s, when that of Phaethousa was also particularly frequently told; as we have seen in this chapter, it was a time when the dialogue between 'one-sex' and 'two-sex' models was particularly vigorous. By showing the power of classical tales, the two stories thus raise many questions that are important to the history of medicine more broadly. For example, on what authority does medical knowledge depend? What is the relationship between texts and observation? What is the status of evidence, and of the different groups and individuals who claim expertise?[81] I shall show how the texts could provide continuity, even though they were being read in different ways in order to accommodate them into new explanatory frameworks. Because her popularity peaked before that of Agnodice – in the sixteenth century – it is with Phaethousa that I shall start. Her absence of menstruation and growth of a beard were thought by some readers to be part of a 'one-sex' shift from female to male, but by others to be evidence that such change is impossible. At a simple level, approaching the story in terms of Laqueur's model challenges the date of his historical rupture; if, however, we think outside the model altogether, we are better able to understand the richness of early modern readings of this classical Greek story.

---

[81]   Discussing Thomas/Thomasine Hall in Virginia in 1629, Kathleen Brown notes that 'We can thus analyze each group's articulation of sexual difference by comparing it to their investigatory method, their claims (often implicit) to expertise, and their authority in the community'; '"Changed … into the Fashion of Man"', p. 173.

PART II
Phaethousa

Chapter 3

Phaethousa: Gender and Genre

Drawing on a range of evidence from Latin and vernacular medical writers, the previous chapters have challenged Laqueur's claim that there was no notion of 'something concrete and specific inside, outside, and throughout the body that defined male as opposed to female' in the Renaissance, or indeed in the classical world.[1] In the sixteenth century, while Galen's striking inside/outside thought experiment was frequently mentioned in terms of women's reproductive organs being 'just like' (Lat. *sicut*) those of a man, differing only by being reversed, we have seen that in fact medical writers often challenged it from experience or from other authorities – including other passages of Galen himself. The tone of these challenges became increasingly scathing not in the eighteenth century, as Laqueur would have it, but at the end of the sixteenth, when Hippocratic notions of the extent of male/female difference came to the fore. So, for du Laurens in 1593, observation showed that women's organs differed from those of men in number, shape, size, substance and structure, while it was 'absolutely absurd' to claim that the vagina and the penis had the same shape. However you turn the vagina inside out, you will never make it into a penis.[2] In 1611, for Caspar Bartholin, 'The likeness of the penis and the womb is foolish.'[3] For Jane Sharp, merging the views of the established authorities in 1671, 'the difference is so great that they can never be the same'.[4] All these writers also repeated versions of the Galenic inside/outside image, but without investing in it.

In this and the following chapter, I shall be producing a different kind of evidence against Laqueur's claims for the history of the body. I shall be concentrating on the various alternative readings of Phaethousa, in order to show how different models of the female body engaged with a single Hippocratic story. In a 'one-sex' model, as the genital organs only differed in terms of location, and were placed where they were because of different levels of heat in the body, then logically they should be able to change their location if the level of heat altered. Did this represent a 'woman' becoming a 'man', however, or simply the late emergence of the 'true

---

[1] Laqueur, *Making Sex*, p. 133. His phrasing is noteworthy; defining 'male'. Here I shall be concentrating on 'defining female'.

[2] Du Laurens, *Opera Anatomicae*, pp. 263–4; note that Jane Sharp's 'number, and likeness, substance, and proportion' (Sharp, *The Midwives Book*, ed. Hobby, p. 67) clearly comes from du Laurens, via Crooke.

[3] *Bartholinus Anatomy*, p. 62; Bartholin, *Anatomicae institutiones corporis humanis*, p. 114.

[4] Sharp, *The Midwives Book*, ed. Hobby, p. 67.

sex'? Phaethousa provided evidence for both 'one-sex' and 'two-sex' readers, and I shall be demonstrating that there was a shift in reading her story in the second half of the sixteenth century; from seeing Phaethousa as one example of an ever-lengthening list of 'sex change' or hermaphrodite cases (an outcome reached only by omitting the original ending of the story – her death), some writers instead used her in a 'two-sex' way, as evidence of the impossibility of such a change. In 1596, for example, Schenck von Grafenberg included her death and noted that, for a woman, growing a beard endangered her health and her life.[5] For him, bearded women should be seen not as sex change cases, but as women at risk of death. This shift not only in telling, but also in interpreting, Phaethousa supports the demise of any one-sex model in the sixteenth – not Laqueur's eighteenth – century. After introducing some of the contexts in which Phaethousa was later told, in the rest of this chapter I shall turn to the classical original of Phaethousa, and what it says to Laqueur's model; in its original context, was this ever a 'one-sex' story?

Beards, Menopause and the Virago

Readings of Phaethousa alongside cases of sex change and of hermaphroditism can be found on both sides of Laqueur's watershed, in the sixteenth as much as in the nineteenth century. Phaethousa combines clear signs of being a woman – in particular, the capacity to menstruate and to bear children – alongside markers of masculinity. In the sixteenth century, her story could be told as the first of a sequence of classical 'sex change' stories, which I shall discuss in the next chapter. Stories which resonate with hers come not only from the medical literature but also from accounts of displaying the body for entertainment, where the 'bearded lady' has been a regular fixture, particularly in the mid-nineteenth century, when 'the beard movement' was significant in British culture, with the full beard for men moving 'from the social margins inhabited by artists and Chartists into the respectable mainstream'.[6] For Victorian writers, beards were beneficial to health, filtering the air and keeping the throat warm, but also as a visible sign of their wearers' manly qualities.[7] So how could a woman survive without one? The author

---

[5] Johannes Schenck von Grafenburg, *Observationes Medicae Rarae, Novae, Admirabiles et Monstrosae* (Frankfurt: Becker, 1596); in the 1600 edition this is Book 4, pp. 10–11: *mortua est*, 'she died'. Schenck von Grafenburg uses Amatus Lusitanus – on whom see below, pp. 114–16 – for the Maria Pacheca sex change story, in Book 4, observatio 5 (on which see Beecher, 'Concerning Sex Changes', pp. 997–8), but when he tells the Phaethousa story he stresses the risks to women of growing beards (*non sine valetudinis et vitae periculo*) and includes her death.

[6] Christopher Oldstone-Moore, 'The Beard Movement in Victorian Britain', *Victorian Studies*, 48 (2005), p. 7. Oldstone-Moore draws attention to the 'beard manifesto' pamphlets issued in the 1850s.

[7] On health arguments see Oldstone-Moore, 'The Beard Movement', pp. 21–2.

of *An Apology for the Beard* responded: 'By the protection of the same Providence that made her without', going on to argue that there was more internal fat in a woman to protect her throat.[8] As beards became more important to manhood in this period, so bearded women became a focus of fascinated and horrified interest. In 1853, Henry Morley and William Henry Mills wrote a short piece entitled 'Why Shave?' in Dickens' *Household Words*; this was followed up by a 44-page pamphlet by Morley in which he noted 'The beard is not an excellent thing in women, but there have been numerous remarkable instances.'[9] At about the same time, James Ward observed 'No woman would like a man without a Beard, as no man would like a woman with one.'[10]

It was at the height of this 'beard movement', in 1857, that the bearded Julia Pastrana was first exhibited in London; as Rebecca Stern has shown, she was also embalmed and displayed after her death, allowing audiences to gaze at her without any of the potential embarrassment felt at being in her living presence.[11] While some people argued that women like her were really men in female clothing, physicians were brought in to certify that they were women.[12] But a further possibility existed: were these individuals hermaphrodites?

In 1903, when Cesare Taruffi published his medical study of hermaphrodites, *Hermaphrodismus und Zeugungsunfähigkeit. Eine systematische Darstellung der Missbildungen der menschlichen Geschlectsorgane*, his bibliography listed 1891 items.[13] One of the cases he mentioned (his Observation 84) was that of Virginia Mauri, born in Rome in 1859, who menstruated at the age of 16, had

---

[8] 'Artium Magister', *An Apology for the Beard* (London, 1862), p. 7.

[9] Henry Morley and William Henry Mills, 'Why Shave?', *Household Words*, 13 (August 1853); H[enry] M[orley], *Why Shave? Or, Beards v. Barbery* (London, 188? [precise date not given]), p. 18 on women.

[10] James Ward, *An Essay Written in Defence of the Beard* (n.d., probably 1854; London, 1954).

[11] Rebecca Stern, 'Our Bear Women, Ourselves. Affiliating with Julia Pastrana', in Marlene Tromp (ed.), *Victorian Freaks. The Social Context of Freakery in Britain* (Columbus, OH, 2008), pp. 214–5. Stern has listed the many parallels between Pastrana and the character Marian Halcombe in Wilkie Collins' *Woman in White*, which was serialised in 1859–60. For example, we are told that Halcombe's 'complexion was almost swarthy, and the dark down on her upper lip was almost a moustache', and that while she had a 'perfectly shaped figure' the viewer is 'almost repelled by the masculine form and masculine look of the features in which the perfectly shaped figure ended' ('Our Bear Women, Ourselves', pp. 226–7).

[12] Erin N. Burrows, 'By the Hair of her Chin: A Critical Biography of Bearded Lady Jane Barnell' (MA thesis, Sarah Lawrence College, 2009), p. 27.

[13] Cesare Taruffi, *Hermaphrodismus und Zeugungsunfähigkeit. Eine systematische Darstellung der Missbildungen der menschlichen Geschlectsorgane* (Berlin, 1903). I am using the term 'hermaphrodite' in preference to the modern 'intersex' because this was the term used in the periods I am studying; it clarifies the element of 'both' rather than 'between', being composed of the two deities Hermes and Aphrodite.

sexual relationships with men and suffered miscarriages. This apparent capacity to conceive would in many cases be definitive in making her a woman, even though she did not bring any of these supposed conceptions to birth. Furthermore, a Dr Ravaglia 'observed her menstruation'. However, these female signs were challenged because she also had a penis 5.5 cm in length.[14] The illustration of Mauri commonly reproduced shows her heavily bearded, reclining on cushions, her legs spread to show her vulva and penis, naked except for stockings, women's boots tied with ribbons, a double strand of pearls around her neck, and pearl earrings.[15] Like the nineteenth-century 'freak shows' and the cartes-de-visite of 'bearded ladies', this is deliberately posed to shock, contrasting the evidence of the beard (and in this case, also the penis) with the femininity of the subject. On cartes-de-visite and in the circus, 'bearded ladies' were displayed very much as normative women, here elegantly dressed, sometimes with a low neckline drawing attention to the bust, and seen doing needlework or at other feminine occupations, or even with their children.[16] Even the terminology of 'ladies' suggests this alarming normality.

Cartes-de-visite and their successors, the cabinet cards, were, as Christopher Smit notes, intended 'to communicate, almost instantly, a sense of grandeur and dignity'; he adds that the photographer and the subject worked together in a 'collaborative aesthetic' to achieve this.[17] Full eye contact was made with the viewer, establishing a link with him or her, as in the unidentified bearded lady shown in Smit's Figure 12.3, who poses in her wedding dress, holding the viewer's gaze.[18] In this tradition, in Figure 3.1, Delina Rossa is seated next to a flower arrangement, her lace neckline and necklace drawing attention to her bust.

These bearded ladies may still challenge or disturb our notions of sex and gender, but – unlike Phaethousa – in the nineteenth century they were not seen as 'ill'. Instead, they were part of a spectrum of possibilities that still existed, even though Laqueur would see this as a 'two-sex' age in which men and women were entirely different.

---

[14]   Ibid., p. 548.

[15]   Ibid., p. 336, illustration p. 335.

[16]   Durbach, *Spectacle of Deformity*, p. 105; 'Madame Clofullia' was shown with her child. 'Miss Maud Temple, Britain's Bearded Beauty' could be seen in Glasgow in 1909; on the poster advertising her appearance, she was shown riding side-saddle, with the images around this central figure show her cycling, playing golf, at the piano and sewing. <http://www.vintagevenus.com.au/vintage/reprints/info/C269.htm> accessed 18 June 2013.

[17]   Christopher R. Smit, 'A Collaborative Aesthetic: Levinas's Idea of Responsibility and the Photographs of Charles Eisenmann and the Late Nineteenth-Century Freak-Performer', in Marlene Tromp (ed.), *Victorian Freaks. The Social Context of Freakery in Britain* (Columbus, OH, 2008), p. 294.

[18]   Ibid., p. 298.

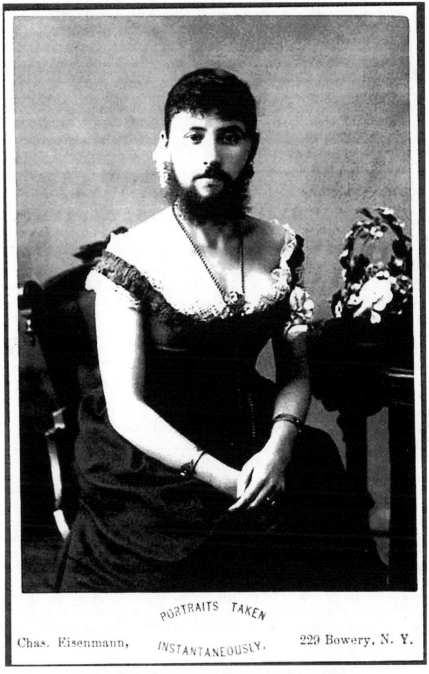

Figure 3.1   Delina Rossa, <http://www.sideshowworld.com/81-
SSPAlbumcover/Beard/BL-35.jpg>

Taruffi's study of hermaphroditism included a section on 'Change of sex'. Here, his Observation 1 was not a case, but rather the 'one-sex' model phrased in the past tense, namely that

> Aristotle and Galen thought that the genitals of the man differ from those of the woman only in location, so that the exterior organs of one sex are completely similar to those of the other, but situated inside, so the transformation of a woman into a man, which at times appears to happen, was attributed to the appearance outside of organs which previously existed inside.[19]

There was no discussion or critique given of this 'one-sex' body statement; it merely introduced the following sequence of named cases extending from Hippocrates to the nineteenth century. His Observation 2 was the case of Phaethousa, named here as Phartus; *De Phartus Pistae uxore*. The brief comment noted the existence of Nanno, stating that there were in fact two separate examples in this passage of Hippocrates of women who 'took on a masculine appearance after the cessation of menstruation'.[20] For Taruffi, again, these women were not 'ill'. In 1908, when Neugebauer repeated this section from Taruffi, he made a slight alteration so that any ambiguity in Taruffi's timing of this event within the female life cycle was removed: he gave 'Hippocrates describes two women, who took on a masculine appearance *at the age of menopause*' (my italics).[21]

Is this a valid reading of the original story, or is it changing it into something else? I have already given the relevant Hippocratic text in full in the Introduction, in Smith's translation, but here I repeat it in my own modified translation, and with the Greek terms I shall be exploring in this and the following chapter italicised:

> In Abdera, Phaethousa the wife of Pytheas, a stay-at-home wife (*oikouros*), having been highly fertile (*epitokos*) in the preceding time (*tou emprosthen chronou*), because her husband was exiled/fled (*phygontos*), stopped menstruating for a long time (*chronon polun*). Afterwards pains (*ponoi*) and reddening in the joints. When that happened her body was masculinised (*to te sôma êndrôthê*) and grew

---

[19] 'Aristoteles und Galenus meinten, die Geschlechtsteile des Mannes unterscheiden sich von denen des Weibes nur durch die Lage, so dass die äusseren des einen Geschlechts denen anderen vollkommen ähnlich seien, aber innerlich lägen, daher wurde die Verwandlung einer Frau in einen Mann, die bisweilen vorzukommen scheint, dem äusseren Auftreten der vorher im Inneren vorhandenen Organe zugeschrieben.' Taruffi, *Hermaphrodismus*, p. 364.

[20] Taruffi, *Hermaphrodismus*, p. 364, 'Er bringt zwei Beobachtungen von Frauen, die nach dem Aufhören der Menstruation ein männliches Aussehen annahmen.' The next group of cases in Taruffi are sex change stories from Pliny, Aulus Gellius, Phlegon (on whom see below, Chapter 4) and St Augustine.

[21] Franz Ludwig von Neugebauer, *Hermaphroditismus beim Menschen* (Leipzig, 1908), p. 250, 'Hippocrates beschreibt zwei Frauen, die im klimakterischen Alter ein männliches Assehen annahmen.'

hairy all over, she grew a beard, her voice became harsh, and although we did everything we could to bring forth menses (*ta gynaikeia*) they did not come, but she died after surviving for not long after. The same thing happened to Nanno, Gorgippos' wife, in Thasos. It seemed to all the physicians I met/talked to that there was one hope (*elpis*) of feminising her, if normal menstruation (*ta kata physin*) occurred. But in her case too it was not possible, though we did everything, but she died, and not slowly (*Epidemics* 6.8.32).[22]

Phaethousa had given birth 'in the preceding time', 'beforehand', and she fails to menstruate 'for a long time'. Earlier in this volume of the *Epidemics*, a list is given of the many things a physician should consider, including 'The time of the disease, the things that follow on it, the periods [of time], and of the periods the longer ones and whether they are increasing ...'. One category concerns what is appropriate to the patient's age: 'Of an age with one's age, or earlier or later than is proper for the age ... Or earlier or later than appropriate' and goes on to mention 'excess and defective growth of hair, thickness, toughness, diminution'.[23] In the context of *Epidemics* 6, Phaethousa's absence of menses is evidently seen as inappropriate to her age, as is her hair growth; modern attempts to see this as menopause, explaining 'growing a beard' in terms of hormonal change, are thus anachronistic.[24] Sixteenth-century translators of the story appreciated this, making it clear that both women had stopped menstruating *before* the natural time; for example, du Laurens says that Phaethousa 'perdit ses purgations avant le temps'.[25]

---

[22]   A range of manuscripts of *Epidemics* 6 survives, the earliest known version of the whole book in its original Greek being the manuscript Marcianus graecus 269 (= M), which dates to the tenth century AD; see Daniela Manetti and Amneris Roselli, *Ippocrate. Epidemie Libro Sesto* (Florence, 1982), p. lxx. Latin translations circulated in the Middle Ages; Pearl Kibre listed 21 manuscripts and two different versions, one from the ninth- or tenth-century Florence manuscript Laur. Plut. 73, 12, and we know that Galen was familiar with this case history in the second century AD because he wrote a commentary on it. There are three main variants in the manuscript tradition; Phaethousa is 'the woman who kept at home'/'the housekeeper' (*oikouros*) or 'the servant' (*hê kouros*); her husband is 'in flight'/'in exile' (*phugôn*) or 'keeping guard' (*phulattôn*); and her voice becomes not only rough (*trêcheê*) but also harsh, *kai sklêron*; for rough 'and harsh', Manetti and Roselli, *Ippocrate*, p. 195 note that 'the reading, which is received from the indirect tradition, is certainly authentic'.

[23]   *Epid.* 6.8.11 (Loeb VII, p. 283).

[24]   The much-reprinted collection, George M. Gould and Walter L. Pyle, *Anomalies and Curiosities of Medicine* (Philadelphia, PA, 1896), is probably responsible for contemporary claims about this; p. 228: 'Hippocrates mentions a female who grew a beard shortly after menstruation had ceased. It is a well-recognized fact that after the menopause women become more hirsute.'

[25]   *Controverses anatomiques*, Book 7, ch. 8 of du Laurens, *Les Oeuvres*, pp. 224r–225r cited in Donald A. Beecher and Massimo Ciavolella (tr. and ed.), *Jacques Ferrand, A Treatise on Lovesickness* (Syracuse, NY, 1990), p. 381, n. 17.

Neugebauer's 1908 study of hermaphroditism also includes the slightly fuller version of the story given by Johann Wier, in which 'her body was entirely male' (*wurde ganz männlich*); this will be discussed in more detail in Chapter 4.[26]

For Taruffi, then, 'change of sex' was an appropriate category to include in a study of the hermaphrodite, but on his interpretation Phaethousa and Nanno were not changing sex, nor even suffering from an illness; they were going through a normal stage of life. In an earlier account of these women that appeared in 1839 in one of his first publications, an account of hermaphroditism for the second volume of Robert Bentley Todd's *Cyclopaedia of Anatomy and Physiology*, James Young Simpson also referred to Phaethousa and Nanno as being somewhere on the hermaphrodite spectrum, and like Taruffi he did not class them as true hermaphrodites.[27] For him, however, this was not menopause, but evidence of the existence of the virago. He wrote that

> Women, both young and aged, with this tendency to the male character, are repeatedly alluded to by the Roman authors under the name of viragines, and Hippocrates has left us the description of two well-marked instances.

The virago is a category that extends across Laqueur's one- and two-sex worlds, and in the seventeenth century, too, Phaethousa had been labelled in this way. In *The Sick Woman's Private Looking-Glass*, John Sadler included 'Phaetusa' in his section on menstrual suppression, referring to the story in passing as if expecting his readers to know it, but also changing it so that she is the one who is exiled.[28] He described external causes of this condition – too much heat using up the surplus blood, or too much cold thickening it so that is unable to flow out – and then went on to internal causes. These originate, he says, either in the womb or in the blood, and Phaethousa's condition comes from the blood. Rather than the suppression causing her masculinisation, he may be suggesting that she was already masculine and that this is why she did not menstruate; he describes 'Viragoes and virill women, who through their heat and strength of nature, digest and consume all their last nourishment, as Hippocrates writes of Phaetusa, who being exiled by her husband Pythea, her terms were suppressed, her voice changed, and had a beard, with a countenance like a man.' While 'virago' did not always have negative nuances in this period, Sadler says that such women are

---

[26]   Quoted as: 'Der Leib der Phaetusa, Frau des Pytheus, wurde ganz männlich, die Stimme wurde männlich, Bartwuchs trat ein, dasselbe geschah in Thasos mit Mamysia, der Frau des Gorgippus.' Neugebauer, *Hermaphroditismus*, p. 250.

[27]   Simpson, 'Hermaphroditism'; a work with over 90 contributors, this was initially published in parts and then collected into five volumes. The section in which Simpson's piece appears came out in summer 1839; see Morrice McCrae, *Simpson. The Turbulent Life of a Medical Pioneer* (Edinburgh, 2011), p. 47. Simpson's footnote is to the edition of Anuce Foës.

[28]   John Sadler, *The Sick Woman's Private Looking-Glass* (London, 1636), p. 17.

'women-eaters' not 'women-breeders, because they consume one of the principles of generation, which gives a being to the world, viz. the menstrual blood'.[29] One possible reading of this is that Sadler's Pytheas wanted to be rid of his masculine wife: another would be that she reacted to her exile by rejecting her womanly role. As we shall see in Chapter 4, although it shares an interest in body heat and in menstruation as the direct cause of the symptoms, this is very far from the highly fertile Phaethousa of the Hippocratic text. And, unlike in a 'one-sex' model, the effect of the heat here is not to cause a change of sex.

Keeping Company with Hermaphrodites

Like the bearded woman, the hermaphrodite mixes features of both sexes; but, until the nineteenth-century emphasis on gonads, in the hermaphrodite the focus was placed on the external genitalia. While popular representations from the sixteenth to the nineteenth century put both the bearded woman and the hermaphrodite on display, early modern and later scientific literature tried to deconstruct the category of 'hermaphrodite' to classify it out of existence.

Hermaphrodites featured widely in classical Greek and Roman art and myth, sometimes as ideals, sometimes as monstrous.[30] While I know of no classical Greek parallels for the 'freak show', there was a 'monster market' in Rome during the period of the early Roman Empire, where slaves with a range of unusual physical traits were in demand.[31] In the Renaissance, human oddities were as much sought after for the collections of curiosities of the courts of Europe as were any other items seen as in some way 'extraordinary'.[32] By the seventeenth century, hermaphrodites were not only private possessions, but were put on public display as curiosities for close inspection, as well as being the object of scientific discussion; Alexander Pope wrote of his pleasure in seeing a hermaphrodite displayed for a shilling in

---

[29] Ibid., p. 17. *OED* suggests that a positive use is for a 'man-like, vigorous, and heroic woman'; it cites Richard Montagu, The *Acts & Monuments of the Church before Christ Incarnate* (London, 1642), p. 361: 'Shee so ruled as Queene eight yeers and better: a man-like virago of a stout and noble spirit.'

[30] On ancient hermaphrodites, see Marie Delcourt, *Hermaphrodite: mythes et rites de la bisexualité dans l'antiquité classique* (Paris, 1958, tr. as *Hermaphrodite: Myths and Rites of the Bisexual Figure in Classical Antiquity*, London, 1961); Luc Brisson, *Le Sexe incertain. Androgynie et hermaphrodisme dans l'Antiquité gréco-romaine* (Paris, 1997, tr. as *Sexual Ambivalence: Androgyny and Hermaphroditism in Graeco-Roman Antiquity*, Berkeley, CA, 2002).

[31] See Plutarch, *Moralia* 520c, discussed by Carlin A. Barton, *The Sorrows of the Ancient Romans: The Gladiator and the Monster* (Princeton, NJ, 1995), pp. 86–8.

[32] For example, Merry Wiesner-Hanks, *The Marvellous Hairy Girls* (New Haven, CT and London, 2009). See also Paul Semonin, 'Monsters in the Marketplace: The Exhibition of Human Oddities in Early Modern England', in Rosemarie Garland Thomson (ed.) *Freakery. Cultural Spectacles of the Extraordinary Body* (New York, 2006), 69–81.

1714.[33] Sex change stories can be seen as a diachronic form of hermaphroditism; where they require movement between the sexes, discussions of hermaphrodites seem to accept the possibility of being fixed as neither man nor woman, or as both man and woman. However, this distinction should not be overstated and, rather than their uncertain sex being seen as a stable identity, hermaphrodites' stories could emphasise change over their lifetimes.[34]

Hermaphrodites were not, however, a focus for ancient medical writers; there is no Hippocratic case history of one, while Galen appears to have found it hard to believe in them, and talked about 'the so-called hermaphrodites that artists fashion'.[35] His contemporary Aulus Gellius drew attention to Pliny's comment that *androgynoi*, 'men-women', once seen by the Romans as prodigies (signs of divine disfavour), had by the first century AD come to be regarded *in deliciis*; the Loeb translation is 'as instruments of pleasure', but this could simply mean 'as pets', the sense being delight in their company, or perhaps specifically sexual delight.[36] Ancient writers themselves thus perceived a shift in how hermaphrodites had been interpreted over time.

For the early modern period, scholars still regard the section in Ambroise Paré's 1575 treatise on monsters as the most influential text on the hermaphrodite. Donald Beecher, however, has argued that Paré does not represent the norm, but rather the dying stages of the 'one-sex' interpretation of sex change; if change between the sexes no longer seemed possible, then anyone showing the characteristics of both must be reinterpreted as holding the categories together rather than being in transit between them.[37] The problem with this interpretation is that ancient authors had written about both stable hermaphrodites and changes in sex so, once again, there may be no need to adopt Laqueur's model and then insert a transitional period here. Paré attributed the cause of hermaphroditism to equal amounts of 'seed' being provided by both parents; this recalls the Hippocratic *On Generation/ Nature of the Child*, used by Laqueur and mentioned above.[38] But this, his 'perfect hermaphrodite' or 'male and female hermaphrodite', with two sets of organs, both

---

[33]   Alexander Pope, 'To a Lady in the Name of her Brother', in *The Correspondence of Alexander Pope* (ed. George Sherburn), 5 vols (Oxford, 1956), I, p. 277, cited by Gilbert, *Early Modern Hermaphrodites*, p. 158. On this encounter, see further below, pp. 85–6.

[34]   Gilbert, *Early Modern Hermaphrodites*, pp. 144–58.

[35]   *On Seed* II 3.17, *CMG* V 3, 1, p. 171.

[36]   Leofranc Holford-Strevens, *Aulus Gellius. An Antonine Scholar and his Achievement*, revised edition (Oxford, 2003), p. 103 n. 30. Pliny's reference to *in deliciis* is at *Natural History* 7.3.34, before the description of the various cases at 7.4.36.

[37]   Beecher, 'Concerning Sex Changes', p. 999.

[38]   Ambroise Paré, *Les œuvres d'Ambroise Paré, conseiller et premier chirurgien du Roy* (Paris, 1575), p. 811 (English, *On Monsters and Marvels*, tr. Janis L. Pallister, Chicago, IL and London, 1983, p. 26). The English is abbreviated from the 1575 French edition, the latter including a section on same-sex female behaviour. There is also a fairly loose seventeenth-century English version, *The Workes of that Famous Chirurgion Ambrose*

of them capable of use, was only one of four possibilities, the others being the male hermaphrodite, capable of impregnating a woman; the female hermaphrodite, who produces female seed and menses and, although she has a penis, cannot achieve erection; and hermaphrodites who are 'neither one nor the other' sex, because they have no functioning sexual organs.[39] Another French physician, Jacques Duval, included hermaphrodites in his 1612 midwifery text, following Paré in arguing that a hermaphrodite resulted from the perfect balance of the contributions of seed from both parents.[40] However, this category of the 'perfect hermaphrodite' was often doubted; could anyone really function in both the male and the female role in generation?[41] In all these iterations, in addition to organs, what mattered were the fluids of the body and their power, or lack of power, to generate.

In the ancient world, Phaethousa did not appear in the company of hermaphrodites. But in the early modern period, she became the first of a developing 'cumulative list' of both ancient and contemporary examples of sex change stories.[42] These included ancient stories, which I shall discuss in Chapter 4, alongside sixteenth-century ones such as Marie who became Germain, when male genitalia emerged as she jumped over a ditch – a story told by Paré in 1575 and inserted into Montaigne's *Essays* in 1588 – and Marie le Marcis, whose sexual identity was debated by Jacques Duval and Jean Riolan in 1601. In Paré's terms, Duval saw Marie le Marcis as a 'male hermaphrodite', with a functioning penis that emerged only late in his life and only when he was aroused: Riolan regarded her as a woman with an enlarged clitoris or a womb extending outside her body.[43] These stories of change most commonly involved a girl on the cusp of full sexual maturity from whose body a penis and testicles suddenly emerged but, as we shall

---

Parey translated out of Latine and compared with the French, tr. Thomas Johnson (London, 1634).

[39] Paré, *Les œuvres*, p. 811; Pallister, pp. 26–7. Jenny C. Mann, 'How to Look at a Hermaphrodite in Early Modern England', *Studies in English Literature*, 46 (2006) argues for a genre difference here; while physicians became increasingly interested in the detail of the hermaphrodite genitalia, sixteenth-century poets kept the hermaphrodite's sexuality blurred, neither one thing nor the other.

[40] Jacques Duval, *Des hermaphrodits, accouchemens des femmes, et traitement qui est requis pour les relever en santé, et bien élever leurs enfants* (Rouen, 1612), p. 328.

[41] For example, François Gayot de Pitaval, *Causes celebres et interessantes avec les jugements qui les ont décidées*, vol. IV (Paris, 1734), pp. 453–4.

[42] Beecher, 'Concerning Sex Changes', p. 992; Beecher also proposes that the first person to add a contemporary story to the inherited list of ancient examples was Raffaele Maffei, who in 1511 described the case of a girl who changed sex on her wedding day in the time of Pope Alexander VI (1492–1503) (p. 997).

[43] Ibid., p. 1008; for a careful reading of Marie Germain, see P. Parker, 'Gender Ideology, Gender Change', pp. 341–4, which takes this account as part of Montaigne's discussion of male impotence. Laqueur, *Making Sex*, pp. 126–9 uses these stories.

see in the next chapter, there were also stories of this happening when a woman was already married.[44]

While Paré's classification had already reduced the number of those seen as fully hermaphrodite, eighteenth-century writers often went further still, assigning all to one sex. This too picked up on even earlier ways of looking at bodies of uncertain sex; Albucasis, basing his work on the sixth-century AD Paul of Aegina, had argued that their condition was due to excess, and that 'the superfluous growths must be cut away so that every trace is destroyed'.[45] Writing as the result of the display in London in June 1740 of an Angolan hermaphrodite, James Parsons argued that all so-called hermaphrodites were really *female*. He addressed the ancient view that somebody could have the features of both sexes if the seed provided by both parents was entirely equal in quality and quantity, but rejected it, instead claiming that it was 'an extraordinary Elongation in the Clitorides of Females' that had led to the myth of the hermaphrodite.[46] But in his 1771 lectures, Thomas Young asserted the reverse: 'I am of the opinion that such as go under this name are all *male*'. What appeared to be an enlarged clitoris should more properly be identified as a penis; this recalled discussions a century earlier in which 'not over-expert Midwifes [*sic*]' were blamed for classifying as female a child who was really male, but who had only a small penis.[47]

Other than midwives, who decided an individual's sex, particularly when that individual was raised as a girl but then developed a penis? When he wrote the introduction to the English translation of the memoirs of Herculine Barbin, who was born as a woman in 1838 and committed suicide in 1868 after being compelled to re-identify as a man due to her testicular tissue, Foucault painted a picture of a pre-modern Europe in which it was up to the individual to decide for him/herself, followed by a less generous Europe in which tissue was decisive.[48] But there are stories from early modern Europe that suggest, firstly, that not everyone of uncertain sex possessed agency and, secondly, that not everyone with agency

---

[44]   On sex change stories in this period see for example Gilbert, *Early Modern Hermaphrodites*; Beecher, 'Concerning Sex Changes', p. 992 on the search for alternative explanations, other than a shift in the location of the organs to the outside; he argues that the familiar tales were 'recycled' to become stories of hermaphrodites rather than any 'change'.

[45]   Martin S. Spink and G.L. Lewis, *Albucasis, On Surgery and Instruments. A Definitive Edition of the Arabic Text with English Translation and Commentary* (London, 1973), p. 454 (section 2.70, based on Paul of Aegina, 6.69).

[46]   James Parsons, *A Mechanical and Critical Enquiry into the Nature of Hermaphrodites* (London, 1741), pp. 7–9, 31. Gilbert, *Early Modern Hermaphrodites*, p. 33. On the Angolan person, see ibid., p. 154.

[47]   Royal College of Surgeons, Edinburgh, Ms lectures of Thomas Young, 1771, vol. 2; R. C., I. D., M. S. and T. B., *The Compleat Midwife's Practice Enlarged ... The second edition corrected* (London, 1663), p. 274.

[48]   Foucault, *Herculine Barbin*, p. vii. One of the characteristics Herculine shared with Phaethousa was excessive body hair.

chose to be simply one sex or the other. It is not clear whether those on display gained financially from it, but a disturbing case can be found in lecture notes taken from the man-midwife Thomas Young's classes. In order to cast further doubt on the existence of hermaphrodites, Young described how the body could be manipulated to create one. He had seen a person who 'had been manufactured when young, in order to make more money of him by making him resemble both sexes'; the testes had been removed, the scrotum divided to create 'labia', and a small 'vagina' formed by making a hole just large enough to admit a little finger.[49] This deliberate surgical creation of 'hermaphrodites' reverses the widely criticised modern practice of reducing intersex people to one sex. Young's manufactured hermaphrodite comes across to us as a victim of other people's financial ambitions, but in his 1988 book *Freak Show* Robert Bogdan has argued that those displayed in such shows in the nineteenth century – including hermaphrodites and bearded ladies – were active agents, making a living. David Gerber has criticised Bogdan for suggesting that such people were in control, and has instead linked issues of consent to slavery and prostitution, seeing these performers as tragic figures.[50]

But, whether for financial or other motives, some people may not have wanted to be confined to one sex. People of doubtful sex could manipulate audiences, just as those audiences manipulated them; in the latter case, sometimes literally, as in the case of Marie le Marcis, where Jacques Duval manipulated the hidden penis to make it ejaculate, thus proving that he was a man, or with the hermaphrodite seen by Pope, already mentioned.[51] This person was the child of 'a Kentish Parson and his Spouse', the advertising handbills announcing the display of 'her personal curiosities'.[52] Pope was accompanied by a priest and a physician who, like him, both inspected and touched the person's genitals; he writes of 'the surest method of believing, seeing and feeling'.[53] But the evidence was not found conclusive; the priest decided this was a man, while the physician concluded that this was a woman, and attributed the presence of something like a penis to the maternal

---

[49]   Royal College of Surgeons, Edinburgh, Ms lectures of Thomas Young, 1771, vol. 2, p. 8.

[50]   Robert Bogdan, *Freak Show: Presenting Human Oddities for Amusement and Profit* (Chicago, IL, 1988) and 'The Social Construction of Freaks', in Rosemarie Garland Thomson (ed.) *Freakery. Cultural Spectacles of the Extraordinary Body* (New York, 2006), pp. 23–37; David A. Gerber, 'The "Careers" of People Exhibited in Freak Shows: The Problem of Volition and Valorization', in Thomson (ed.) *Freakery*, pp. 38–54; for a detailed biography of one of the most famous bearded ladies, born hirsute and sold as a child to a circus, see Burrows, *By the Hair of her Chin*; Burrows stresses the agency of her central character, Jane Barnell.

[51]   Joseph Harris, '"La force du tact": Representing the Taboo Body in Jacques Duval's *Traité des hermaphrodits* (1612)', *French Studies,* 57 (2003), p. 312.

[52]   A. Pope, 'To a Lady in the Name of her Brother', pp. 277–8.

[53]   Ibid., p. 279.

imagination; 'nothing being more common than for a child to be mark'd with that thing which the mother longed for'.[54]

Could the person's own desire be used as a marker of the true sex here? To the women who paid their shilling the person Pope saw said that 'he has the Inclination of a Gentleman' but 'she tells the Gentlemen she has the Tendre of a Lady'.[55] Geertje Mak has recently uncovered another example of two different physicians giving contradictory accounts of the nineteenth-century hermaphrodite Katharina/Karl Hohmann's own desires, and here the primary source could again be taken to suggest that the story offered by the hermaphrodite depended on the amount of money paid to hear it.[56] Gottlieb Göttlich travelled around Europe in the 1830s, making money by being viewed by a succession of curious physicians and surgeons in London, Liverpool, Dublin, Glasgow, Edinburgh and Aberdeen, as well as in continental Europe; he carried with him the certificates they presented to him, stating what they had found. They open with the 1833 decision of the Heidelberg authorities that 'attentive examination' has shown that Marie Rosine Göttlich is 'a man with genitals of uncommon conformation' and that he should take the name of Gottlieb Göttlich and dress as a man.[57] Sexual preference was not seen as any help in determining Göttlich's sex, as the certificates he carried with him state that 'He has pretty strong sexual desires, and says he can perform in either character.'[58] However, the eyewitness account of Peter Handyside, who saw

---

[54]   Ibid., p. 279. On the maternal imagination, see for example Herman W. Roodenburg, 'The Maternal Imagination: The Fears of Pregnant Women in Seventeenth-Century Holland', *Journal of Social History*, 21 (1988); Marie-Hélène Huet, *Monstrous Imagination* (Cambridge, MA, 1993); Valeria Finucci, 'Maternal Imagination and Monstrous Birth: Tasso's *Gerusalemme liberata*', in Valeria Finucci and Kevin Brownlee (eds), *Generation and Degeneration: Tropes of Reproduction in Literature and History from Antiquity to Early Modern Europe* (Durham, NC and London, 2001).

[55]   A. Pope, 'To a Lady in the Name of her Brother', p. 279. Gilbert, *Early Modern Hermaphrodites*, does not take up the issue of the individual's desire when discussing Pope's example.

[56]   Geertje Mak, 'Hermaphrodites on Show. The Case of Katharina/Karl Hohmann and its Use in Nineteenth-Century Medical Science', *Social History of Medicine*, 25 (2011), p. 15 citing Paul F. Mundé, 'A Case of Presumptive True Lateral Hermaphrodism', *American Journal of Obstetrics and Diseases of Women and Children*, 8 (1876), pp. 615–31; p. 617, n. 1. The interpretation of this primary source is my own, but Mak too argues that a hermaphrodite could be tailoring her response to the person asking the question ('Hermaphrodites on Show', p. 17). Mak has also looked at late nineteenth-century cases where the physician chose not to tell the patient the 'true sex', or colluded with the patient in retaining the 'sex at birth' despite clinical findings indicating that this was not the 'true sex'; Geertje Mak, 'Doubting Sex from Within: A Praxiographic Approach to a Late Nineteenth-Century Case of Hermaphroditism', *Gender & History*, 18 (2006), p. 336.

[57]   *Certificates of a very rare specimen of hermaphroditism, Dublin 5 July 1835*, British Library Cup.366.e.20.

[58]   Ibid.

Göttlich in Edinburgh, presents a different picture, stating that 'he has not much passion for women, and ... his amative desires are still directed towards his own sex' (that is, men).[59]

The individuals discussed so far in this chapter were seen as significant because they were not easy to classify in terms of the different models that existed. Was menstruation necessary to be a woman? Was a penis always definitive proof of being a man, or was evidence of ejaculation – or, indeed, of generation – needed? Laqueur's model does not help us to analyse the attempts that have been made to classify people whose sex was considered uncertain; their mixture of external genitalia, internal organs, secondary sex characteristics and personal preferences go far beyond a 'one-sex'/'two-sex' model of the body. In many cases, the accounts of their bodies concern an initial impression which is then challenged, in its turn challenging the sexual dichotomy that is assumed to be normal. While much of the medical and legal literature concerns attempts to force individuals into categories, those individuals could also actively resist categorisation.

Reading the *Epidemics*

How well does Phaethousa fit into these collections of individual stories? She featured as the first of Taruffi's examples because she is the oldest written medical case that could be interpreted as sex change or hermaphroditism, but also because she emerges under the aegis of the Father of Medicine himself; she appears in the Hippocratic *Epidemics*, at the very end of the sixth book of this seven-volume collection, and probably dates to the late fifth or early fourth century BC. Her sole appearance is in this case history and, whatever we may think of the details of her symptoms today, like the individuals we have already discussed, she originally appears as a real woman. But what is an ancient 'case history', and how far should we automatically assume her reality? To what extent is she a medical construct?[60] Examining this story will take us further into both the theories and the practices of the ancient world, helping us to understand how the body was understood in Greek and Roman medicine and again demonstrating that Laqueur's claims for a dominant 'one-sex' body do not do justice to the complexity of the evidence.

---

[59]   Peter D. Handyside, 'Account of a Case of Hermaphroditism', *Edinburgh Medical and Surgical Journal*, 43 (1835), p. 318.

[60]   Ivan Crozier, 'Pillow Talk: Credibility, Trust and the Sexological Case History', *History of Science*, 46 (2008): pp. 375–404 discusses the relationship between the 'case' and the 'individual' from whom it is 'written up'; p. 377 explores the extra level of editing that takes place in sexologists' case histories, so that the voice of the patient is further removed. In a valuable survey article, Flurin Condrau, 'The Patient's View Meets the Clinical Gaze', *Social History of Medicine*, 20 (2007): 525–40 analysed the move in the social history of medicine to 'the patient's point of view' and examined the argument that case histories show us the doctor's construction rather than that of the patient.

I suspect that calling the story of Phaethousa a 'case history' immediately lulls us into a false sense of security. Reading of people from the past who, like ourselves, experience pain, run fevers, have indigestion, and – if they are female – menstruate and give birth, we feel that we should easily be able to make sense of what they say and do. The body is where we meet the problems of history most acutely; doing the history of medicine involves walking a tightrope between recognition and over-familiarity, between knowing 'the same' and failing to understand 'the other'. Either we make the past in our own image, or we are struck dumb by its difference, unable to say anything about it whatsoever. As with modern viewers' reactions to Vesalius' Figure 27, we should beware of any feeling of familiarity, and instead contextualise the source and perform a close reading of it. Rather than 'case history', I would prefer here to use the term 'case story', for reasons that will become clear.

Unlike a case history, an ancient case story is not a document prepared within a modern context of hospital records, noting test results and dosages, facilitating communication between other health care workers who will encounter the same patient, or avoiding possible litigation by relatives. Instead, as Iain Lonie showed, it is a piece of writing from the earliest stage of the development of ancient Greek prose, where compiling lists led to the grouping together of similar items, thus opening up the possibility of thinking about why they are similar; for example, the third section of *Aphorisms* begins with a comment on the changing of the seasons being the main cause of disease, and then brings together various reflections on seasonal patterns, such as 'Autumn is bad for those with *phthisis*.'[61] The most recent editor of *Epidemics* 6, Wesley Smith, characterised the *Epidemics* collections in particular as 'technical prose from the time when prose was coming into being and authors were realizing its potential; unique jottings by medical people in the process of creating the science of medicine'.[62] He noted that one particular section, which lists things that should be investigated, was read by Galen as comprising topics needing further work when the notes were rewritten for publication, but is assumed by modern readers – academics used to lecturing – to be 'a list of lecture topics'.[63] In each case, our preconceptions about what kind of text this is influence how we interpret it.

The physicians who wrote the descriptions of disease in *Epidemics* travelled from community to community across the Greek world; while there was a chance that they would pass through the same town twice, this was not inevitable, and what we have here may be 'notes to self' which record significant points in order

[61]   Iain M. Lonie, 'Literacy and the Development of Hippocratic Medicine', in François Lasserre and Philippe Mudry (eds) *Formes de pensée dans la collection hippocratique: Actes du Colloque hippocratique de Lausanne 1981* (Geneva, 1983); *Aphorisms* 3, Loeb IV, p. 122 ff. *Phthisis*, 'wasting away', is often identified with tuberculosis.

[62]   Wesley D. Smith, 'Introduction' to Loeb Classical Library, *Hippocrates* VII (Cambridge, MA and London, 1994), p. 2.

[63]   Ibid., p. 9 on *Epid.* 6.8.7 ff.

to jog the writer's memory later on so that he can recall further details. Sometimes these take the form of questions for further consideration; for example, 'Noses and ears always cold. Is the blood thin because of that?'[64] Significantly, observation is not necessarily given priority; what is seen may then be recorded in such a way that it does not challenge the prior theory.[65] These physicians formed a literate, and self-consciously literate, group, writing about writing, including remarks such as 'As I have written ...'.[66] Ann Hanson has discussed the different levels of literacy within medicine, pointing out that from the third century BC onwards physicians were signing for illiterates or witnessing documents, and arguing that, at least in the Roman period, they would write down new recipes they heard about.[67] In a striking image, the writer of the Hippocratic treatise *Regimen* discussed *hê grammatikê* – which can mean grammar, scholarship, or the alphabet – as enabling us to 'recall past events, to set forth what must be done'.[68] The writer draws an analogy between the vowels, and the different senses through which the physician reads the patient's body: diagnosis is 'reading'. Both those who know their letters, and those who do not, gain their knowledge of the body by hearing, seeing, smelling, tasting, speaking, touching and 'passages outwards and inwards for hot or cold breath'.[69] The 'grammar' with which this writer was concerned brings together the *schêmata* – a word which can mean 'structures', but also something like 'organs'[70] – and the signs of the human voice; this could suggest that the physician uses what the patient says as a way of uncovering what is happening in the unseen parts of his or her body.

Earlier in *Epidemics* 6, a list of significant signs opens with 'Things from the small tablet (*ek tou smikrou pinakidiou*), to be observed'.[71] As Smith notes, 'already by Galen's time' this reference had 'generated much discussion as to what it might tell us about the mode of composition of *Epidemics* 6, and of *Epidemics* 2 and 4 as

---

[64] *Epid.* 6.2.20 (Loeb VII, p. 232).

[65] Langholf, *Medical Theories in Hippocrates*, pp. 186–90 and 209.

[66] *Epid.* 6.7.1 (Loeb VII, p. 272).

[67] Ann Hanson, 'Doctors' Literacy and Papyri of Medical Content', *Studies in Ancient Medicine*, 35 (2010), pp. 187–204.

[68] *Regimen* 1.23 (Loeb IV, p. 258).

[69] *Regimen* 1.23 (Loeb IV, p. 260).

[70] See *On Ancient Medicine* (22): some structures (*schêmata*) are hollow, 'some solid and round, some flat and suspended, some are stretched out, some large, some thick, some are porous and sponge-like'. Those that are wide at one end and narrow at the other – such as the bladder, the skull and the womb – are best able 'to attract and absorb moisture from the rest of the body', 'and are always filled with fluid'.

[71] *Epid.* 6.8.7, Loeb VII, p. 278. In the case of Callimachus, the *pinakes* appear to have been catalogue entries; see Francis J. Witty, 'The *Pinakes* of Callimachus', *Library Quarterly*, 28 (1958), pp. 132–7; Alexia Petsalis-Diomidis, *Truly Beyond Wonders: Aelius Aristides and the Cult of Asklepios* (Oxford and New York, 2010), pp. 219–20.

well'.[72] Does it imply a prior stage of note-taking? For remedy collections, we now have a better sense of how these were compiled. Laurence Totelin has recently argued that the treatises on treatments for disease which survive were created by merging small personal collections of written remedies.[73] In the Hippocratic treatise *Affections*, drug handbooks or *Pharmakitides* are mentioned in passing; following Elizabeth Craik, Totelin argues that each physician would have had his own personal handbook of this kind, arranged either by disease or by action, such as 'warming drugs', 'cooling drugs' and so on.[74] While no example of such a handbook now survives, the character of these lost books can be detected not just from passing references in Hippocratic treatises, but also from meticulous analyses of groups of recipes within the treatises, and from comparisons with papyri which give remedies. With case stories, in contrast, it is very difficult to know how the collections were put together. However, some case stories occur in more than one book of the *Epidemics*, suggesting that the treatises we have were built up from earlier collections, perhaps in the same way as those concerning treatment.

Naming Phaethousa

One of the features most striking to a modern reader of the *Epidemics* is the naming of patients, which increases our sense of them as real people, accessible to us across the centuries. Phaethousa is very unusual in having three identifying tags: her name, her husband's name and her place of residence making her 'Phaethousa of Abdera, wife of Pytheas'. Nanno, too, has three tags. Unlike men, women are rarely named in these collections; they are usually 'wife of' or 'sister of', or left entirely anonymous, but with some feature of their case or their place of residence included as an identifier, such as 'the girl who fell from the cliff' or 'the woman who lived over the gate'.[75] Similarly, as minors, children too could be referred to by the name of their father: Callimedon's son; Parmeniscus' child.[76] While some men, too, are nameless – such as 'the man at the house of the niece of Timenes in Perinthos' or 'another man, in the upper town' – the more consistent reluctance to name women suggests that these texts conform to a cultural convention by which only women who are dead, or of

---

[72]   Smith, Loeb VII, p. 279 note b.

[73]   Laurence Totelin, *Hippocratic Recipes. Oral and Written Transmission of Pharmacological Knowledge in Fifth- and Fourth-Century Greece* (Leiden, 2009).

[74]   Ibid., p. 98; Elizabeth Craik, *Two Hippocratic Treatises: On Sight and On Anatomy* (Leiden, 2006), p. 17.

[75]   'The girl who fell from the cliff', *Epid.* 7.77 (Loeb VII, p. 374); 'the woman who lived over the gate', *Epid.* 7.8 (Loeb VII, p. 310).

[76]   Callimedon's son, *Epid.* 5.68; Parmeniscus' child, *Epid.* 5.66 (Loeb VII, p. 198).

ill-repute, can be named.[77] Phaethousa and her companion in this case story, Nanno, both die, thus falling within this convention; however, in addition, their level of masculinisation may also move them out of the category of 'respectable woman'.

While commentators have assumed that there was a real woman behind this story, some initial caveats are in order here. Phaethousa shares her name – 'Shining One' – with a daughter of the sun-god, Helios; in Renaissance dictionaries, this was the Phaethousa one would most easily encounter. Like our Phaethousa, she experienced a bodily transformation – into a poplar tree.[78] So we may wonder whether this name is a little too appropriate for a woman who seems to be suffering from the effects of excess heat; similar questions arise with Agnodice's name, which means 'Chaste before justice', but we should remember that Greek and Roman names, like our own, had meanings, and we should probably not be too suspicious here.[79] Furthermore, although Phaethousa's town, Abdera in Thrace, was the birthplace of three philosophers – Protagoras, Democritus and Anaxarchus – it was proverbial for the stupidity of its inhabitants; 'no more sense than the people of Abdera' recalled their foolishness in thinking that Democritus' symptoms showed he was mad, when in fact he was merely laughing at the folly of human existence.[80] Is this story about failure to understand? However, other case stories too are associated with the people of Abdera, and so it is more likely simply to have been somewhere that the anonymous author of this case story regularly visited.

If we ignore the convenient name and location, is there anything to indicate that the person who wrote this case story actually met Phaethousa? In general, the level of detail given in many case stories makes us assume that the writers of these texts saw the patients, and noted down day-by-day accounts of the changing symptoms. But other case stories, such as this one, are far sketchier. Rather than a day-by-day account, we find a time frame that is difficult to quantify. The vague timing already discussed – 'in the preceding time', 'beforehand', 'for a long time' – may suggest that the story we are given comes from something other than *autopsia*. The vocabulary used elsewhere in the *Epidemics* often suggests that eyewitness evidence plays an important part; for example, an earlier section of *Epidemics* 6

---

[77] 'The man at the house of the niece of Timenes in Perinthos', *Epid.* 6.2.19 (Loeb VII, p. 232). He is also identified as 'the one with dark skin'. 'Another man, in the upper town' features in *Epid.* 7.15 (Loeb VII, p. 322). On the convention with regard to women, see David M. Schaps, 'The Woman Least Mentioned: Etiquette and Women's Names', *Classical Quarterly*, 27 (1977).

[78] Apollonius Rhodius, *Argonautica* 4. 965 ff.

[79] See below, p. 131.

[80] Charlton T. Lewis and Charles Short, *A Latin Dictionary* (Oxford, 1879), s.v. Abdera; Martial 10.25; Thomas Burton, *The Anatomy of Melancholy* 1.114; on the Hippocratic pseudepigrapha in which the story is told, Thomas Rütten, *Demokrit – lachender Philosoph und sanguinischer Melancholiker. Eine pseudohippokratische Geschichte* (Leiden, 1992).

includes the comment 'I did not see (*ouk eidon*) kidney disorders get better beyond [the age of] fifty years.'[81] Sometimes the wording of a case story includes direct contact with a patient through his or her words, reporting something the physician had not seen, or would never be able to see; for example, 'He said that ...', in *Epidemics* 7.117, where the child (or slave; the Greek word *pais* can mean either) of Deinias said that bilious matter came out of his fistula, or *Epidemics* 7.11, where a female patient, the wife of Hermoptolemos, sick with a fever in the winter, 'said that her heart had been damaged'.[82] On other occasions the information given concerns earlier experiences, and must derive from the patient or her family; for example, Agasis' wife who 'had breathing difficulties as a child'.[83] However, it is far from clear that all the cases in these collections originate from personal observation or from patient accounts given to the writer. In some cases the writer may be repeating the observations made by an assistant, but other stories may have been heard from other practitioners, or even constructed to illustrate a theory.[84]

In ancient medical writing, personal observation and stories from other people could easily interweave without any clue to the reader that this was happening. In early modern medicine, while stories from books read by the author were interwoven with first-hand observation, it is easier to see that this is happening, as sources are usually named; Brian Vance has traced the emergence of the *Observationes* genre in the sixteenth century as a progression from editions of the ancient texts most concerned with case stories (such as the Hippocratic *Epidemics*), to commentaries on these, and finally to the *Observationes* that start from the author's own cases rather than from the classical ones.[85]

The complexity of the relationship between *historia* and *autopsia* in ancient medicine is illustrated very effectively by Armelle Debru's discussion of the relationship between Galen's description of a woman who was affected by retained 'female seed', told in his *On Affected Places* 6.5, and a section, closely based on Galen, in the sixth-century AD writer Aetius' book on diseases of women.[86] In the

----

[81]   *Epid.* 6.8.4 (Loeb VII, p. 279); I have modified Smith's translation of *ta nephritika* as 'kidney *infections*' because it is too modernising.

[82]   *Epid.* 7.117 (Loeb VII, p. 408); *Epid.* 7.11 (Loeb VII, p. 314).

[83]   *Epid.* 6.4.4 (Loeb VII, p. 246).

[84]   Lesley Dean-Jones, '*Autopsia, Historia* and What Women Know: The Authority of Women in Hippocratic Gynaecology', in Don Bates (ed.), *Knowledge and the Scholarly Medical Traditions* (Cambridge, 1995), pp. 43–4: 'sometimes a physician will report what he learned through historia as if he had learned it through autopsia', suggesting that this could be because he knew it from an assistant or apprentice left with the patient.

[85]   Brian Nance, 'Wondrous Experience as Text: Valleriola and the *Observationes medicinales*', in Elizabeth Jane Furdell (ed.), *Textual Healing: Essays on Medieval and Early Modern Medicine* (Leiden: Brill, 2005), p. 115.

[86]   K 8.413 ff; Aetius of Amida, *Aetii Amideni medici ... Libri sexdecim nunc primum Latinitate* (Venice, 1534), 16.68; James V. Ricci, *Aetios of Amida: The Gynaecology and Obstetrics of the VIth Century A.D.* (Philadelphia, PA, 1950), p. 71; Skevos Zervos, *Aetii*

Galenic version, contrary to what some commentators have assumed, there is no suggestion that Galen ever saw the patient. The story is introduced by a statement that this story 'came into Galen's mind' while he was thinking about the topics he discusses in this chapter.[87] This, then, is simply a story that helps Galen to think about the broader topic of this section, namely the idea that seed needs to be eliminated for there to be health, and that in the female body retained seed is more dangerous than retained menses. But Aetius moved Galen's story of the widow into his own personal experience, introducing it with 'I myself saw a woman ...' (Lat. *Ego quidem mulierem vidi*).[88] Debru used this example to illustrate that even the appearance of the first person in a medical account does not necessarily mean that the writer really 'saw' what is described; as stories moved from one writer to another, they could pick up an 'I myself saw' that was not in the original. Galen sometimes used the ambiguous 'I know' (Gk *oida*) rather than 'I saw'; for him, a 'case' may be representative, exceptional, or taken from his own first-hand experience.[89]

How does Phaethousa's case story fit into this? There is nothing in the text to indicate the first-hand experience of the writer as an individual; no verbs of seeing, or reporting of the patient's words. Instead, there is one first-person plural reference: 'we did everything to bring forth menses'. The 'we' in turn picks up an unusual reference to 'all the other physicians I met/talked to';[90] it seemed to them that the only hope of restoring a woman's identity as a *gynê*, a wife/woman (the Greek word means both), is to restore normal menstruation. While this could suggest a number of physicians at the bedside, it is also possible that the story was an exceptional one that was widely discussed; perhaps Phaethousa and Nanno had been seen by different physicians, with the writer himself having seen neither woman. The inclusion of both women shows that, although exceptional, this situation could arise again and any physician should be prepared for it.

---

sermo sextidecimus et ultimus (Leipzig, 1901), p. 190: 98 line 1. Ricci's translation is based on the Latin of Cornarius' 1542 translation; a better edition of the final volumes of Aetius is in preparation in the *Corpus Medicorum Graecorum* series.

[87]   Gk *En tautais mou pote tais ennoias ontos ephanê toionde symban* ..., characterised by Armelle Debru, 'La Suffocation hystérique chez Galien et Aetius: réécriture et emprunt de "je"', in Antonio Garzya (ed.), *Tradizione e ecdotica dei testi medici tardoantichi e bizantini* (Naples, 1992), 79–89, p. 87 as indicating that Galen only knows this story indirectly.

[88]   Aetius, *Aetii Amideni medici*, p. 131, here given as 16.70; Debru, 'La Suffocation hystérique', pp. 85–9.

[89]   Debru, 'La Suffocation hystérique', p. 86; see further Helen King, 'Galen and the Widow. Towards a History of Therapeutic Masturbation in Ancient Gynaecology', *EuGeStA: Journal on Gender Studies in Antiquity*, 1 (2011), p. 222. On a similar case which Galen takes from Rufus of Ephesus, but presents as his own, see Peter Pormann, 'New Fragments from Rufus of Ephesus' *On Melancholy*', *Classical Quarterly*, 64 (2014).

[90]   The verb used is 'to meet' or 'to talk with' (here, the aorist singular, *enetychon*). There is a further plural reference to 'doing everything' in an attempt to cure Nanno.

Reading Phaethousa

One of the earliest medical writers to focus on Phaethousa's death was du Laurens, already discussed in Chapter 2, as part of his discussion of the reliability or otherwise of the beliefs of 'the ancients'; in 1593 he called it an 'elegant tale', *elegans historia*, phrasing later repeated by Helkiah Crooke. It is interesting to speculate on what makes it 'elegant', a term which later was applied even to medicines; in the late eighteenth century the educationalist and writer of conduct guides, Vicesimus Knox, compared the work of moralists to that of physicians, and wrote that they should sugar their message to make it taste better, as 'The physicians call a medicine which contains efficient ingredients in a small volume, and of a pleasant or tolerable taste, an elegant medicine.'[91] The description of Phaethousa as an 'elegant tale' seems to have a similar sense; the story is concise, but vividly memorable. But du Laurens insisted that the story should not be misread: this was not a one-sex story, as the insides did not move outside. In particular, he recognised the importance of Phaethousa's previous fruitfulness, meaning that she must have had all the female reproductive parts.[92]

To interpret this 'elegant' case story in its original context, we could draw on theories and remedies found in other treatises on women; the *Epidemics* collections do not stand alone, but reflect complex relationships with other treatises of the Hippocratic corpus. On women's diseases, Ann Hanson has shown considerable overlap between remarks in *Epidemics* and comments in the Hippocratic treatises on the diseases of women, so that we can use treatises such as *Diseases of Women* 1 and 2 to explain the thinking behind case stories.[93] But other connections exist. For example, *Epidemics* and *On Superfetation* share a belief that swelling in the face, calves, feet and thighs, with a lack of appetite, show that a second foetus has remained in the womb after a birth.[94] Not only are some parts of the *Epidemics* treatises set out in the form of aphorisms – the section immediately before the case of Phaethousa states 'Melancholics tend to become epileptic generally and epileptics melancholic'[95] – but there are also links between *Epidemics* and the treatise *Aphorisms* itself. The statement about kidney disorders and the

---

[91]   Vicesimus Knox, *Winter Evenings: or lucubrations on life and letters: In three volumes* (London, 1788), vol. 1, p. 67.

[92]   *Opera anatomica* (Lyon, 1593), pp. 262–3 and p. 275 (*nihil profecimus, sed interijt*). Laqueur, 'Sex in the Flesh', p. 305 comments that du Laurens regards stories of 'organs popping out of girls to make them boys, [as] a minor sideline of the question of difference'. I find his discussion of this text too simplistic.

[93]   Ann Hanson, 'Diseases of Women in the *Epidemics*', in Gerhaad Baader and Rolf Winau (eds), *Die Hippokratischen Epidemien: Theorie–Praxis–Tradition, Sudhoffs Archiv*, Beiheft 27 (Stuttgart, 1989).

[94]   *Superfetation* 1 (Littré 8. 476; Loeb IX, p. 318); compare *Epid.* 5.11 (Loeb VII, p. 160). This link is pointed out by Paul Potter in Loeb IX, p. 319 n. 1.

[95]   *Epid.* 6.8.31 (Loeb VII, p. 288).

impossibility of recovery in patients aged over fifty mentioned in the previous section echoes one in *Aphorisms*, where we read 'Kidney disorders, and those of the bladder, are cured with difficulty in older patients (*toisi presbuteroisi*)'.[96] The precise direction of the relationship between treatises remains unclear. Here, was the writer of the *Epidemics* statement aware of the aphorism, noting here that it seemed to be borne out in practice? Or was he refining its claims from 'older' to 'over fifty': from 'with difficulty' to 'not that I saw'? Or did *Aphorisms* draw on the particular cases in the *Epidemics* collections? However, it seems legitimate to use other Hippocratic treatises to reconstruct the thinking behind Phaethousa's diagnosis.

Within a case story, what is written down, from the mass of experiences and observations, and how can that help us to understand what is happening in the writer's mind? In the case of Phaethousa, her previous childbearing, the departure of her husband, and the cessation of menstruation appear as the most significant of the features thought important enough to note. No details of the actions taken by the physicians – 'we did everything' – are given; this is standard in the *Epidemics*, which assume that the reader knows what treatments to administer, but the intention here is explicitly to bring on menstruation. This is the only hope for Phaethousa; the word for 'hope' here is *elpis*, the same hope that was the only thing left in Pandora's womb-jar after the evils contained in it – including disease – went out into the world.[97] In this cultural context, however, hope is not something optimistic; it carries the sense of waiting for an uncertain future.[98] For the ancient Greeks, waiting for a woman to give birth was a matter of uncertainty; instead of a child, she may produce the shapeless mass of flesh known as a uterine mole.[99] It is difficult to know whether this selection of events – and the implied link between the missing husband, and Phaethousa's inability to hold a properly female form – results from the physician's questions, or the patient's offering of information. But a connection does appear to be made here between cause (absence of husband/absence of menstruation) and effect (becoming masculine). The husband's departure is expressed as a causal genitive – *because* her husband fled/was exiled – giving a clear sense of where the problem began.

---

[96]   *Aphorisms* 6.6 (Loeb IV, p. 180).

[97]   On Pandora's womb-jar in Greek culture and in later art, see King, *Hippocrates' Woman*, p. 26.

[98]   Jean-Pierre Vernant, 'À la table des hommes: Mythe de fondation du sacrifice chez Hésiode', in Marcel Detienne and Jean-Pierre Vernant, *La Cuisine du sacrifice en pays grec* (Paris, 1979), pp. 125–32; Pietro Pucci, *Hesiod and the Language of Poetry* (Baltimore, MD, 1977), p. 105.

[99]   On the mole and its classical origins see Helen King and Cathy McClive, 'When is a Foetus not a Foetus? Diagnosing False Conceptions in Early Modern France', in Véronique Dasen (ed.), *L'Embryon humain à travers l'histoire: Images, savoirs et rites*, Actes du colloque international de Fribourg, 27–29 octobre 2004 (Gollion, 2008), pp. 223–38.

Where does Phaethousa fit into Laqueur's claims for the dominance of a 'one-sex' body in the pre-modern world? In this case story, the body is about fluids rather than organs; a woman's sexual identity is presented as being easily disrupted if she ceases to menstruate. The female body seems to depend on the presence of the male body to keep it properly female. The reddening of the joints may suggest increased heat, and it is in them that the Greek suggests she experiences pain. The term used here is not *odynê* (as in our 'an-odyne', without pain), but *ponos*, a word meaning not only 'pain' but also 'work' or 'labour'. I argued some years ago that *ponos* was used to indicate not only long-lasting, dull pain, but also pain that would not be treated because it was seen as a necessary part of the process; so, for instance, in childbirth the pains can be *ponoi*.[100] Nicole Loraux suggested that, in classical Greece, *ponos* was a glorious sensation linked to war and to childbirth, the ways in which men and women respectively served the *polis* or city-state, while in other contexts, picking up on the features the poet Hesiod associated with the present 'Age of Iron', it was more like 'hard work', linked to the fatigue of bodily labour.[101] So why are Phaethousa's pains *ponoi*? Is this her own word, a reference to the pains of childbirth, which of course she knows from her own experience from having previously had many children? This seems unlikely, as the pain is apparently in her joints.

If this Hippocratic case story concerned a 'one-sex' body, it should be easy for the organs to shift position to the outside, but this does not appear to be the case for Phaethousa, or for Nanno. The *ponos* Phaethousa suffers could be mentioned as an implied criticism of those physicians who took a 'one-sex' approach to her case and assumed that the beard was part of a process, with the pain being necessary to the work of becoming male; instead, this reference suggests that any movement from female to male is not something that her body can easily bear, as what is inside cannot readily come outside. The 'two-sex' reading of the story is the one that is consistent with the assertion in the Hippocratic *Diseases of Women*, already discussed in Chapter 1, that 'the diseases of women and those of men differ very much in their treatment', and that the key difference of menstruation arises from the fact that women have flesh that is wet and spongy, while men have flesh that is dry and firm. The story as we have it, with the deaths of Phaethousa and Nanno showing that women who stop menstruating and grow a beard will die, may represent an example of a two-sex model in debate with a one-sex model, thus suggesting that both models already existed in the fourth century BC.

---

[100]   Specifically *gynaikeioi ponoi*, in Aeschylus fr.99.7–8 Nauck; King, *Hippocrates' Woman*, pp. 123–6.

[101]   Nicole Loraux, '*Ponos*. Sur quelques difficultés de la peine comme nom du travail', *Annali dell'Instituto Orientale di Napoli* 4 (1982): 171–92.

Chapter 4

Phaethousa and Sex Change in Early Modern Europe

The previous chapter argued that, in her original appearance in the Hippocratic corpus, Phaethousa challenged any 'one-sex' model, since her increased heat did not in fact lead to a change of sex, but instead to her death. The way in which the case story was told may include a hint at a 'one-sex' model, if that is how we understand the suggestion that her pain is *ponos* and thus part of a process, but the focus throughout is on restoring menstruation: the *gynaeikeia* that define the *gynê*, and the one hope of her salvation. The difference between men and women lies in the fluids of the body and the direction they take out of it. Early modern writers who included Phaethousa in their lists of sex changes read this case story in very different ways. In 1614, in a chapter on hermaphrodites in one of his two collections of amazing stories, Heinrich Kornmann noted that, 'Hippocrates writes that Phaethousa the wife of Pytheas was turned into a man, and had a beard, a hairy body and a harsh voice.'[1] No explanation was given, other than a brief reference to 'Hippocrates and Galen' holding the opinion that women have testicles and genitalia just like those of men. By this date, this statement looks somewhat old-fashioned. It was more common in the sixteenth century for readers to leave out her death, and instead to imply that she completed the transition to male shape, and remained alive in her revised bodily form.[2] But 'two-sex body' readers, increasingly familiar after the 1520s with the Hippocratic corpus and with the model of complete difference between men and women, retained her death as an essential part of the story, demonstrating that the line between male and female cannot be crossed; they also noted that it was her previous childbearing that proved she was definitively female. This history of having given birth also acted as an obstacle for anyone wanting to propose that her 'true sex' was late-revealed male; men do not give birth, so acknowledgement of her functioning womb either puts her firmly into the category of 'woman' or makes her that rare beast, the 'perfect

---

[1]   Heinrich Kornmann, *De miraculis vivorum* (Frankfurt, 1614), p. 42: *Hippocrates scribit Phaetusam Pythaei uxorem in marem fuisse conversam, barbam, hirsutum corpus et vocam asperam habuisse.*

[2]   A point missed by Beecher, 'Concerning Sex Changes'; Beecher does not seem to have read the original story. For example, Jean Riolan, *Discours sur les Hermaphrodits* (Paris, 1614), p. 38 and see further below, pp. 115–16 on readers who leave out her death and have her complete the change.

hermaphrodite'. Again, the womb, always a challenge to a 'one-sex' body, led to a greater emphasis on the gap that separates women from men.[3]

In this chapter, I shall further explore the meaning of Phaethousa in her original classical context, before going on to consider the contrasting ways of reading Phaethousa found in early modern writers. In the process, I shall also introduce some readings which cannot easily be classified as either 'one-sex' or 'two-sex'. These provide evidence for models of the body which went beyond Laqueur's simple dichotomy. They could be created by users trying to make sense of Phaethousa by linking her story to further ancient accounts, whether these were other Hippocratic texts or accounts of sex change in classical writers. In some cases, the links made may seem to us quite tenuous, but for those creating these variants, they allowed a connection to be made to the authority either of the classical tradition, or of contemporary medical writers, or both.

For example, in 1599 *Wits Theatre of the Little World* was published, perhaps compiled by Robert Allott.[4] The book described itself as 'a collection of the flowers of antiquities and histories', and included in the section on 'Marriage' the statement: 'Phaethusa, the wife of Pytheus, thought so earnestly vpon her husbands absence, that at his returne, she had a beard growne vpon her chinne. *Hier. Merc.*' (p. 110).[5] Other than the identity of its central figure, this version seems a long way from the Hippocratic corpus. Its location, a relatively unstudied collection of moral sayings and anecdotes from history – a printed commonplace book – could act as a handbook to enable anyone to sound learned. What should we make of the reference to Hieronymus Mercurialis? As Adam Smyth has pointed out, many references in *Wits Theatre* are 'altered, unascribed, or wrongly attributed'.[6] So is this medical humanist really the origin of this variant and, if not, why is he mentioned?

The previous collections of stories available to Allott, and to which *Wits Theatre* acted as a continuation volume, did not include Phaethousa. *Politeuphuia, Wit's Commonwealth* (London, 1597), compiled by Nicholas Ling, combined sayings, such as 'When the Mermaides daunce and sing, they meane certaine death to the Marriner'; precepts, such as 'Give place to thy betters and elders'; and historical

---

[3]   Christian Billing, *Masculinity, Corporality and the English Stage 1580–1635* (Aldershot, 2008), p. 32: 'By 1600, the womb is almost ubiquitously considered as an entity in itself, belonging only to women and having its own proper function in the act of gestation.'

[4]   *Wits Theatre of the Little World* (London, 1599). The reference in the title is to the human world, the microcosm; this is a common image in medicine at the period. Compare Sadler, *The Sick Woman's Private Looking-Glass*, p. 2.

[5]   The 'flowers' reference is to the ancient and medieval genre of the florilegium on which, in relation to humanism, see Ann Blair, 'The Rise of Note-Taking in Early Modern Europe', *Intellectual History Review*, 20 (2010), p. 309.

[6]   Adam Smyth, *'Profit and Delight': Printed Miscellanies in England, 1640–1682* (Detroit, 2004), p. 20.

facts, such as 'Tarpeia a Romaine Lady, to avoyde lust, pulled out her own eyes.'[7] It rarely gave the sources for these statements; however, classical authorities were mentioned for some, such as Dionysius of Halicarnassus, Cicero, and Plato.[8] It included a section on 'women', but not one on 'marriage'. A year after the publication of *Wit's Commonwealth* there appeared Francis Meres, *Palladis Tamia, Wits Treasury, being the second part of Wits Commonwealth* (London, 1598). Here, the list of authors cited included Hippocrates, but Phaethousa still did not feature. Like the first volume, its overall structure moved from God to Hell, but drawing on very different material; it included sections on both 'women' and 'marriage', as well as others on 'a wife' and 'matrimonial society'. Allen's study of this text characterizes Meres as 'a hack who had a contracted obligation to fulfil'[9] and notes that all the historical examples came from Ravisius Textor, *Officina*, where the section on 'Wonders of Nature' included the cases of sex change compiled by Pliny, who was very familiar to sixteenth-century writers. Pliny's *Natural History* included stories taken from another first-century AD writer, whose work is now lost, Licinius Mucianus. The list Pliny produces, and which early modern writers took over wholesale, has a case of a virgin transforming to a boy, dated to the consulship of Licinius Crassus and Cassius Longinus; the married woman Arescusa, who grew a beard and a penis and became Arescon; and a case that Pliny says 'I myself saw' in Africa, a woman who became a man on the day of her marriage.[10] *Wits Theatre* was thus the third in a series, although there is no sense in which each successive volume followed on from the previous one. Instead, all went over similar ground, but differed in the sources on which they drew. *Wits Theatre*, like *Wits Treasury*, included a list of its sources, but these do not include the one authority mentioned for Phaethousa: the sixteenth-century humanist physician, Hieronymus Mercurialis.

Like its predecessors, the structure of *Wits Theatre* began with 'God' but, unlike them, the material given consisted almost entirely of *exempla* rather than proverbs or precepts. *Wits Theatre*'s short version of Phaethousa aimed at general readers raises three points. First, here the story is reduced to a statement on the power of the imagination, already mentioned in Chapter 3 as featuring in Pope's later account of the hermaphrodite, where the physician suggested that the presence

---

[7]   Pp. 194r, 91r and 251v.

[8]   P. 194r (Cicero); p. 174r (Plato).

[9]   Don Cameron Allen (ed.), *Palladis Tamia (1598)* (New York, 1938), p. vii.

[10]   Pliny, *NH* 7.36; on Arescusa/Arescon, *nupsisse etiam, mox barbam et virilitatem provenisse uxoremque duxisse*; 'even though she had been married, she grew a beard and became a man'. On his own experience, *ipse in Africa vidi* ...see Mary Beagon, *The Elder Pliny on the Human Animal. Natural History Book 7. Translation with Introduction and Historical Commentary* (Oxford, 2005), pp. 66–7 with commentary, pp. 173–7; Beagon cites the various (very rare) conditions which can cause apparent change from the female to the male, noting that the difference in these ancient stories is the suddenness with which it is supposed to occur. She does not challenge Laqueur's model of the ancient world.

of a penis was due not to the individual's own imagination, but to that of their mother.[11] The power of the imagination of an individual to cause a full sex change also features in a story told by Simon Goulart in the year after *Wits Theatre* was published; first published in French in 1600, Goulart's collection of 'admirable and memorable' tales was translated into English in 1607. Goulart says he is inspired to tell this particular story because he has just read the story of Phaethousa (here, 'Phetula') in Hippocrates; he does not say any more about the details of her case. In fact, as the reference he gives at the end of the paragraph makes clear, he was reading not Hippocrates, but another collection of marvellous tales, the *Jardin de floras curiosas* of Antonio de Torquemada, published in 1570 and translated into English in 1600 and French in 1625.[12] Torquemada told the stories from Pliny, the modern one of Marie – who became Manuel – Pacheco, and then 'Phetula muger de Piteo'; Hippocrates was cited as the source of this final story, in which Phaethousa/Phetula 'miraculously changed sex'. Torquemada then went on to give a story of the woman whose imagination and desire to be a man enabled her to grow a penis.[13] It was this that Goulart copied, including Torquemada's words that the story was passed on to him by his 'friend ... of good authority, and worthy of belief'. This incident involved a woman in Spain who once argued with her husband, and the argument 'grew so hot' that she found a man's clothes, dressed in them, and went to live as a man. Indeed, she actually became a man, and married a wife, her transformation being due either to the 'powerful working of Nature in her, or the burning and excessive imagination'. She is, for Goulart, 'this woman made man'.[14] Goulart and Torquemada in turn took the story from Amatus Lusitanus, whose version of Phaethousa will be discussed later in this chapter.

---

[11]   A. Pope, 'To a Lady in the Name of her Brother', p. 279; above, pp. 85–6.

[12]   I am using here the 1575 edition: Antonio de Torquemada, *Jardin de floras curiosas* (En Enveres, 1575; full text at <http://www.biblioteca-antologica.org/wp-content/uploads/2009/09/TORQUEMADA-Jard%C3%ADn-de-flores-curiosas.pdf> accessed 18 November 2012). The English is *The Spanish Mandeuile of miracles. Or The garden of curious flowers* (London, 1600), p. 34v which tells the story as follows: 'There was, sayth he, in his 6. booke *De morbis popularibus,* a woman called Phaetula in the Citty of Abderis, wife to Piteus, which beeing of young and tender yeares, when her husband was banished from thence, remained many months without hauing her flowers, which caused her to feele an exceeding payne in her members, whereupon her body shortly after miraculously changed sexe, her voyce became manly & sharpe, and her chinne was couered with a beard. The selfe fame hapned in like sort in Tafus to Anamisia, wife to Gorgippus.' The French is *Histoires en forme de Dialogue sérieux* (Rouen, 1625), p. 125.

[13]   Torquemada, *Jardin de floras curiosas*, pp. 115–7. 'Phetula' 'se le hizo el cuerpo de varón, todo velloso, y le nació la barba, y la voz se le hizo áspera'. See Sherry Velasco, '*Marimachos, hombrunas, barbudas:* The Masculine Woman in Cervantes', *Cervantes*, 29 (2000), p. 73.

[14]   Simon Goulart, *Thresor d'histoires admirables et memorables de nostre temps* (Paris, 1600); I am here citing 1610, pp. 237–8, with the translation of Edward Grimeston, *Admirable and memorable histories containing the wonders of our time* (London, 1607), p.

So, around the time that *Wits Theatre* was compiled, some still believed that the imagination could cause more than a beard to grow; complete sex change could occur, and this is associated with increased heat.

The other two points raised by *Wits Theatre*'s version are, firstly, that it does not even nod in the direction of Hippocrates; instead the sole authority given is Hieronymus Mercurialis. This is unusual; as we saw in Chapter 3, it was the connection with the Father of Medicine that made Phaethousa so important. Indeed, Torquemada's version cited precisely this authority; in the English translation, the character Ludovico, on hearing the story, exclaims 'Truly these things which you have rehearsed are mervailous, and the onely authoritie of Hippocrates sufficeth to give them credit.'[15] Secondly, unlike in the Hippocratic original, in *Wits Theatre* Phaethousa's husband returns. This appears to be a unique twist to the story; we shall meet other twists later in this chapter. This one may remind the reader of the 1560 case of the return of Martin Guerre but, unlike his wife Bertrande, Phaethousa does not take another 'husband' while Pytheas is away.[16] In the rest of this chapter I shall investigate Mercurialis' discussions of her, claimed as the origin for *Wits Theatre*'s version. As with the reference to *Wits Theatre*, I shall also expand the evidence base further, beyond the canonical medical writers on whom Laqueur's story relied, concentrating here on sixteenth- and seventeenth-century English texts and on the texts by which Phaethousa's story came to the attention of writers on sex change.[17]

Being *oikouros*

Wits Theatre is not the only early modern reading of the story to present Phaethousa as a 'good' wife, who misses her husband so much that she starts to look like him. Jacques Ferrand proposed that the cause of the transformation was 'passionate love': she 'loved her husband dearly, but was not able to enjoy him due to his long

---

275. On Grimeston see G.N. Clark, 'Edward Grimeston, the Translator', *English Historical Review*, 43 (1928): 585–98.

[15]   *The Spanish Mandeuile*, p. 34v.

[16]   Natalie Zemon Davis, *The Return of Martin Guerre* (Cambridge, MA, 1984). In Davis' reading, subsequently criticised as too modernising, Bertrande is not an innocent woman taken in by the deceitfulness of the man who claims to be her husband, but instead someone who sees the social and economic advantages of having a man, even if this means accepting an imposter into her bed.

[17]   Beecher, 'Concerning Sex Changes', p. 994 notes that previously scholars have simply looked at 'the most accessible authors' on sex changes. As Park, 'The Rediscovery of the Clitoris', p. 173 noted, 'gender was produced and maintained in many different sites in early modern Europe', not only in medical texts.

absence'.[18] But he insists, despite Galen and modern editors of the text 'tak[ing] [Hippocrates] quite literally' that 'this metamorphosis was one of behavior and complexion only and not of sex'. Ferrand notes the inside/outside model and the possibility it offers – according to Galen – of being 'overheated by the fury of love' so that the female genitals are 'pushed outside the body, because those parts are the same as the male parts reversed', but he adds that Galen is 'contradicted in this by our modern anatomists' such as du Laurens.

While so much about *Wits Theatre*'s condensed version appears anomalous, the emphasis on Phaethousa as 'good wife' is also found in the original. In Chapter 1, we met the wife of Diognetos, who in Artemidorus' second-century AD guide to the interpretation of dreams had a dream of growing a beard on only one side of her face, and was subsequently left to keep the house – *oikourein* – when her husband was travelling abroad. In the *Epidemics*, Phaethousa is introduced as 'the wife of Pytheas, *oikouros*'. Before looking further at early modern readings, in this section I shall explore the meaning of *oikouros*, and then that of another label for Phaethousa: *epitokos*. Based on analysing these two terms, I shall be suggesting that, in Hippocratic terms, Phaethousa's failure to replace Pytheas in her bed may be the origin of her problems.

What does it mean for a woman to be *oikouros*? Wesley Smith translates it as 'who kept at home': Brooke Holmes prefers 'who kept to the house'.[19] In the sense of keeping watch over the house, the *oikos*, it could also be 'the housekeeper'.[20] In some manuscripts, it was replaced by *hê kouros*, meaning 'the maid-servant', but there is no reason to prefer this reading; it may simply reflect the copyist not understanding *oikouros*. The modern translation of 'keeping at home' could suggest to a reader that Phaethousa was housebound either by illness or by choice; we may read it and wonder if perhaps she simply did not want to be seen in public with her beard. But a different possibility emerges if Phaethousa's case story is read alongside an ancient story of sex change, found in Diodorus Siculus.

As we have noted already, in this case story Phaethousa and Nanno do not in fact become men: they die. Nevertheless, in early modern collections of amazing tales, such as those of Torquemada and Goulart, they were often found alongside accounts of sex change, taken from Pliny and other ancient writers on natural history, and from the *Book of Marvels* of Phlegon of Tralles, an older contemporary of Galen.[21] Some stories of hermaphrodites and sex change that appeared in these accounts were clearly flagged as myth; for example, the seer Teiresias who was changed into a woman after wounding a snake he saw having sex on a mountain in

---

[18]   Ferrand, *De la maladie d'amour* (Beecher and Ciavolella, *Jacques Ferrand*), p. 230.

[19]   ... *hê Pytheou gynê oikouros*; Loeb VII, p. 289; Holmes, *Gender*, p. 14.

[20]   Manetti and Roselli, *Ippocrate*, pp. 194–5 has her as 'la massaia (housekeeper) di Pitea'.

[21]   Warren T. Treadgold, *The Nature of the Bibliotheca of Photius* (Washington, DC, 1980), pp. 100–101.

Arcadia, and returned to his male form after the god Apollo advised him to wound the other one, and Kainis who, after having sex with the god Poseidon, asked to be transformed into a man, Kaineus, and to become invulnerable.[22] As William Hansen observes, often in these stories 'a change of gender prompts a change of name'; this is true both for stories told as myth, and those told as reality.[23] In the *Book of Marvels*, after telling the mythical sex change stories, Phlegon identified his next sections as reality, by giving precise dating based on the names of the magistrates of the year: the Athenian archon or the Roman consuls.

One of Phlegon's true stories, set in 45 AD, concerns an attractive *parthenos*: a young unmarried girl, the Greek *parthenos* probably being the original word behind Hyginus' description of Agnodice as *puella virgo*. The girl, who came from a wealthy family, was aged thirteen; this is a significant year in terms of ancient medicine, as it is ideally in the 'fourteenth year' – that is, at age thirteen – that girls were expected to marry. As she was about to leave the house for her wedding, this girl experienced severe pain which was assumed to be colic.[24] The term used for 'pain' here, as in the case story of Phaethousa, is *ponos*, and here it is a necessary part of a process; in this context, it certainly cannot refer to her own memories of labour pain, as she has never given birth. The girl remained in pain for three days, and doctors were unable to find out what was causing this. On the fourth day her *ponoi* became stronger and suddenly 'male parts' burst out 'and the girl became a man'.[25] Phlegon's fourth historical story is from 116 AD and concerns a woman called Aitete who experiences 'a change in form (*tên morphên*) and name' 'even while she was living with her husband', becoming the male Aitetos; the 'even while' suggests that Phaethousa's situation, with change occurring once her husband is away, is the more usual scenario. Here, Phlegon – like Pliny, describing sex change in his *Natural History* – adds 'I myself have seen this person', a phrase repeated in many sixteenth-century writers listing ancient cases of sex change.[26] These stories were in turn copied by Galen's contemporary, Aulus Gellius, who agreed with Pliny that 'the change of women into men is not a fiction'.[27] With regard to these claims of *autopsia*, already challenged in the

---

[22]   Phlegon, 4.4–5.

[23]   William Hansen, *Phlegon of Tralles' Book of Marvels* (Exeter, 1996), p. 117.

[24]   Phlegon, 4.6 (ed. Antonio Stramaglia, Phlegon Trallianus, Opuscula de rebus mirabilibus et de longaevis. Bibliotheca scriptorum Graecorum et Romanorum Teubneriana (Berlin and New York: Walter de Gruyter, 2011), pp. 31–2).

[25]   ... *arsenika moria proepesen ... kai hê korê anêr egeneto.*

[26]   Pliny, *NH* 7.4.34: *touton kai autos etheasamên.*

[27]   *Attic Nights* 9.4.15; *Ex feminis, inquit, mutari in mares, non est fabulosum*; Hansen, *Phlegon of Tralles*, p. 122. Aulus Gellius takes the following stories from Pliny: the events of 171 BC in the consulship of Q. Licinius Crassus, where a girl at Casinum became a boy at the house of her parents; Arescusa who became Arescon; a boy in Smyrna; and L. Cossutius whom 'I saw' changed into a man on her wedding day, and who is 'alive today'. These words, *vivebatque cum proderem haec*, given by Aulus Gellius, appear to fill the

previous chapter of this book, Donald Beecher has noted that at least one of Pliny's stories – Lucius Cossitius who became a boy on the day of his marriage – is 'so close to an Ovidian tale that we may wonder whether it is not displaced from an underlying mythological tradition'.[28]

However, in terms of their connections to Phaethousa – and indeed to Agnodice, to whom I shall return in the next chapter – the most interesting ancient sex change stories are two linked to the first-century BC historian, Diodorus Siculus: the cases of Heraïs and Callo.[29] These were not known to sixteenth-century writers, as the volume of Diodorus' *Universal History* in which they featured had by then been lost; it still is. However, sections – including these particular stories – survived in the *Bibliotheca* of Photius, ninth-century patriarch of Constantinople. Probably composed in 845 AD, the *Bibliotheca* summarises the 279 books Photius had read, 55 per cent of which no longer survive in the condition in which he read them. It is 'an untidy compilation of various elements composed in different ways'; in some cases Photius had the texts in front of him, but in others he relied on his memory.[30] This means that the stories may not be as Diodorus originally told them, but may instead survive as re-imagined by Photius in the light of his other reading. Photius was first published in 1601 and translated into Latin in 1606.

While Diodorus originally seems to have told the sex change stories to prove that sexual ambiguity was not evidence of divine wrath, they survive until today because of Photius' love of accounts of marvels, provided that he thought they were

---

lacuna in Pliny's text at 7.4.36; see Holford-Strevens, *Aulus Gellius*, p. 78, who notes that 'Even when Gellius does identify his source, he may not quote exactly.'

[28]   Beecher, 'Concerning Sex Changes', p. 996.

[29]   Peter Green (tr.), *Diodorus Siculus: Books 11–12.37.1. Greek History, 480–431 BC, the Alternative Version* (Austin, TX, 2006) notes, p. 4, that these stories have been 'studiously avoided by most modern scholars'.

[30]   Treadgold, *The Nature of the Bibliotheca of Photius*, p. vii and pp. 4, 5, 36; Paula Botteri, *Les fragments de l'histoire des Gracques dans la Bibliothèque de Diodore de Sicile* (Geneva, 1992, pp. 28–32); Ann Blair, *Too Much to Know: Managing Scholarly Information before the Modern Age* (New Haven, CT, 2010), p. 22–3. The stories of sex change feature in codex 244, which Warren Treadgold argues were 'probably copied by Photius' secretary from reading notes taken before the *Bibliotheca* was compiled', Cod. 244: 377a line 29–379a line 33; Treadgold, *Bibliotheca of Photius*, p. 184. See also Gerhard Wirth, *Diodorus. Griechische Weltgeschichte Fragmente Buch XXI–XL*, vol. 1 (Stuttgart, 2008), pp. 9–10. A complete copy of the 40 books of Diodorus Siculus existed in 1453, when it was seen by Constantine Lascaris in the imperial library in Constantinople; its fate is not known but it was probably lost in the sack of Constantinople (Nigel G. Wilson, *From Byzantium to Italy: Greek Studies in the Italian Renaissance* (London, 1992), p. 162, n. 4; Botteri, *Les Fragments de l'histoire des Gracques*, pp. 13–16). As well as Latin translations, editions of Diodorus existed in different European languages in the late sixteenth century; in the 1480s John Skelton translated Diodorus Siculus into English from the Latin translation of Poggio Bracciolini. But that version only includes Books 1–5. Seven books of Diodorus were published in 1554 in French translation.

true; he had also read Phlegon and in addition had what Treadgold characterises as a 'substantial, and practically professional' knowledge of medicine, with his reading including the medical works of, among others, Dioscorides, Galen, Alexander of Tralles, Paul of Aegina and Oribasius.[31] Photius regarded stories of 'men born with the physical characteristics of women' as 'trustworthy'; his wording suggests that he saw this not as real change, but rather the emergence of the male 'true sex' later in life.[32] For him, such stories did not conform to a 'one-sex' model, because the true sex was male, even though the outward appearance was initially female.

The two sex-change stories which Photius preserves from Diodorus Siculus suggest to me that one of these men knew the story of Phaethousa, and perhaps also that of Agnodice. In one of these stories Callo, from Epidauros, was born without an 'opening' in 'the orifice with which women are naturally provided', so when she married she could only have 'unnatural' – presumably, anal – intercourse.[33] She then developed a tumour on her genitals, which none of the physicians called in could treat, but when 'a certain apothecary' cut into it he revealed testicles and an imperforate penis inside. She 'laid aside her loom-shuttles and all other instruments of women's work' and dressed as a man, now known as Callon. But because she had previously been a priestess, her sex change led to a charge of impiety, 'because she had witnessed things not to be seen by men'. The 'out of the frying pan, into the fire' nature of this story recalls Agnodice's display of innocence on one charge leading to prosecution on another, although as we shall see in the following chapters Agnodice avoids punishment on the charge of seducing women by revealing her *absence* of a penis to the assembled court.

The story preceding that of Callo/Callon in Diodorus Siculus is that of Heraïs; the text flags up this story as a 'marvel', opening with the distancing device of 'they say that …' (*phasin*), and being labelled as *paradoxos* (contrary to expectations; incredible) and *pantelôs apistoumenêi* (completely beyond belief). As in the case of Callo, a tumour appeared, this time at the base of her abdomen, and the area continued to swell, with high fevers occurring.[34] This is an interesting feature, as it suggests that her body was 'hotter' than normal for a woman, thus assimilating her to the male; it thus recalls Phaethousa's reddened joints. Heraïs' physicians

---

[31]   On Diodorus' motives, P. Green, *Diodorus Siculus*, p. 4; on his knowledge of medicine, Treadgold, *Bibliotheca of Photius*, p. 103.

[32]   Robert Garland, *The Eye of the Beholder: Deformity and Disability in the Graeco-Roman World* (London, 1995), p. 130.

[33]   Diodorus Siculus, 32.11. In some versions of her story she was supposed to have served as a priestess of Demeter. See here John J. Winkler, 'Laying Down the Law: The Oversight of Men's Sexual Behavior in Classical Athens', in David M. Halperin, John J. Winkler and Froma I. Zeitlin (eds), *Before Sexuality: The Construction of Erotic Experience in the Ancient Greek World* (Princeton, NJ, 1990), p. 175 on 'unnatural' in an ancient Greek context not functioning in the same way as it would in the Enlightenment; that is, not as an equivalent of 'abnormal' or 'monstrous'.

[34]   Diodorus Siculus, 32.10.3.

thought that this condition could be an ulcer at the mouth of the womb, and applied remedies to reduce the inflammation. However, 'on the seventh day, the surface of the tumour burst, and projecting from her groin there appeared a male genital organ with testicles attached'.[35] This description, almost a 'birth' of the male organs, although it predates Galen, sounds like a very 'one-sex' and Galenic story – the innate heat drives out the previously internal organ. Yet if it is 'one-sex', then this is a 'one-sex' body as something doubted, challenged, and hedged around with distancing devices, another one of which features when the maleness bursts out of Heraïs' body, as this event happens when only 'her mother and two maidservants' are present, not the physicians who are treating her.

Like Agnodice, Heraïs appears before a court. In an element that has strong resonances instead with the story of Phaethousa, Diodorus tells us that Heraïs had been married to 'a man named Samiades. He, after living in wedlock with his wife for the space of a year, went off on a long journey.' For both women, it was after their husbands left that their bodies became masculine, suggesting that this triggered the transformation. But, unlike Phaethousa's husband, Samiades returns, and he takes the case to court after her refusal to sleep with him is supported by her father (who knows her secret). When the court agrees with Samiades, Heraïs then reveals to them all the 'truth' beneath her clothing; loosening her clothing, she showed her 'masculinity'.[36] This visual demonstration of the truth to an audience contrasts with her earlier shame (*aischynê*) at coming into her husband's presence; literally, 'into his view'.[37]

Before her husband's return, when she was still trying to pretend nothing had happened, Diodorus tells us that those in the know assumed that Heraïs must be a hermaphrodite. She continued to dress as a woman, and to act like a normal woman; in fact, perhaps, to over-act. And it is the wording here that provides another echo of the Phaethousa story and connects to *Wits Theatre*'s version of her as a good wife who misses her husband; Diodorus states that Heraïs 'continued to conduct herself as *oikouros* and as one subject to a husband'. In the 1814 translation by George Booth, s/he 'managed the affairs of the house as usual' while for the 1933 Loeb, Francis R. Walton translates as 'conduct herself as a

---

[35]   Diodorus Siculus, 32.10.3; out of her *gynaikeia* came a penis (*aidoion andreion*) with testicles (*echon didymous*). George Booth, *The Historical Library of Diodorus the Sicilian, in Fifteen Books*, vol. II (London, 1814), p. 539: a 'man's yard with the testicles complete'.

[36]   Diodorus Siculus, 32.10.6: *to tês physeôs arren*, 'male/masculine in nature'. The 1933 edition changed the order of words here; in an earlier edition these words came immediately after 'revealed the truth', so that the penis becomes 'the truth' here.

[37]   Diodorus Siculus, 32.10.5: *eis opsin. Aischynê* appears again at 32.10.7. I shall address further the issues of shame and the gaze when discussing Agnodice in Chapter 7. Bernadette Brooten, *Love between Women: Early Christian Responses to Female Homoeroticism* (Chicago, IL, 1996), p. 278 argues that it is speaking in public, rather than showing, that marks the point at which she becomes 'a man'.

homebody'.[38] Phaethousa's label of *oikouros* contributes as much to her identity as do her name, her husband's name and the town where she lives. Heraïs seems to be adopting the *oikouros* model only *after* the event, to make her behaviour seem more 'womanly', and to deny the terrible secret her clothes conceal.

But there is an important difference between Phaethousa and Heraïs: while Heraïs develops a penis, Phaethousa remains a woman. While Heraïs seems to be posing as 'a good stay-at-home wife', Phaethousa is the real thing, and the terminology used in the case story for her menstruation may not be accidental here; not the most common terms of 'monthlies', *ta katamênia* or *ta epimênia*, which would put the focus on regularity, but *ta gynaikeia* – 'women's things' – and later *ta kata physin*, the 'natural things'.[39] As we have seen in Chapter 1, menstruation is essential to being a woman, and these labels serve to contrast her previously established and stable femininity with her later transformation. The fact that they are still used even while she is bearded suggests that her 'true sex' remains female. This femininity contrasts with her body becoming 'masculine' (Gk *êndrôthê*), which I would interpret in this context as meaning firm-textured rather than soft; as well as growing a beard, she becomes hairy all over, with a rough voice.

Being *epitokos*

Both Heraïs and Phaethousa develop male characteristics while their husbands are away. A brief comparison between Phaethousa and another woman with an absent husband – Bertrande, the wife of Martin Guerre – helps us to understand the significance of another word that, like *oikouros*, is central to her identity. That word is *epitokos*; Phaethousa was 'formerly *epitokos*',[40] which is today normally taken to mean simply that she had previously given birth. In this section I shall be suggesting that it was Phaethousa's high fertility that made her particularly susceptible to this condition once her husband was no longer with her, in contrast to Bertrande, who did not even have any children until eight years after her marriage to Martin Guerre. This statement of Phaethousa's child-bearing history was not always included in early modern versions; for example, it does not feature in Amatus Lusitanus who, as we shall see later in this chapter, brought Phaethousa

---

[38] Booth, *Diodorus the Sicilian*, p. 539. 'One subject to a husband' is *hypandros*, which can also simply mean 'married'.

[39] Smith's choice of translations in Loeb VII, pp. 289–91, is interesting here; for *ta kata physin* he gives 'normal menstruation' while for *ta gynaikeia* he simply gives 'menses'. While the logic of his choice is clear – what the unspecified treatments aim to produce is indeed 'normal menstruation' – there is perhaps more significance in *ta gynaikeia* than he acknowledges.

[40] Gk *epitokos eousa tou emphrosthen chronou*.

into the standard list of 'sex change' cases.[41] In the most commonly available English version of Phaethousa's case story, that of Wesley Smith, this description of Phaethousa is translated as 'having borne children in the preceding time'. This echoes the mid-nineteenth century French translation of Emile Littré, 'avait eu des enfants auparavant'.[42] But I would argue that the Greek *epitokos* is stronger than simply 'having children'. This in turn means that the case story is not about what happens to 'women' in general; in contrast to Laqueur's model of the movement of genitalia in a 'one-sex' model, Phaethousa suggests that different female bodies will behave differently.

To demonstrate this, we need to look at the earliest example of the reception of Phaethousa: Galen's interpretation of this case story. Galen considered *Epidemics* 1, 2, 3 and 6 to be genuine works of Hippocrates, and therefore wrote commentaries on them in which he explained what the texts meant; however, in the extant Greek, his commentary on *Epidemics* 6 only goes up to section 6.6.5. But the text of the rest of *Epidemics* 6 survives in Arabic commentaries, so far unpublished, by the eleventh-century Ibn Ridwan and the thirteenth-century Ibn al-Nafis, and even more importantly in the translation of Galen's own *Commentaries* by Ḥunayn ibn Isḥāq (died *c.*873).[43] Using the modern German translation of Ḥunayn, Rebecca Flemming has noted that, in his commentary on Phaethousa's case, Galen 'generalizes from a case in which a husband's exile following prolific child production has lethal consequences'.[44]

Galen read this not as a story of a woman who had previously had children, but rather as a woman whose health was, or had become, entirely dependent on regularly giving birth. Without her husband to make her pregnant, her route to health is blocked. We may speculate that, if she had been a widow, she would have been able to remarry; but this route is not open to her, as her husband is not dead, only absent. Here is Ḥunayn's version, in Peter Pormann's translation: the format is that Ḥunayn gives the text of Hippocrates, followed by that of Galen.

---

[41]   See below, p. 114–16; Beecher, 'Concerning Sex Changes', p. 998 does not realise that there is any omission in Amatus' version, simply saying that in Amatus the 'fertility rate' of Arescusa, Maria Pacheco and Phaethousa 'went unrecorded'.

[42]   Loeb VII, p. 289; Littré 5. 357.

[43]   Peter Pormann, 'Case Notes and Clinicians: Galen's Commentary on the Hippocratic *Epidemics* in the Arabic Tradition', *Arabic Sciences and Technology*, 18 (2008): 247–84. The Epidemics Project at Warwick is working on these Arabic commentaries; see <http://www2.warwick.ac.uk/fac/arts/classics/research/dept_projects/epidemics/> accessed 16 May 2012.

[44]   Flemming, *Medicine and the Making of Roman Women*, p. 334 on Galen, *Hipp. Epid.* 6.8 (*CMG* V 10.2.2, p. 506.21–38); Pfaff translates as 'oft schwanger gewesen'.

Hippocrates said: 'The woman of 'xwx'rs[45] in a previous age was bearing-many-children [*walūd*]. Then her husband went away from her, and her menstruation was retained for a long period of time. After this had occurred to her, her body [194b] turned into the state of the body of a man ['*ilā ḥāli badani r-raǧuli*], her hair grew strong in her whole body,[46] and she grew a beard [*wa-nabatat lahā liḥyatun*]. Her voice became hard [*ṣulb*] and rough/coarse [*ḥašin*].[47] Then we tried every method that one uses to stimulate menstruation, yet it was not freed [?]. But she [only] lived for a while. Then she died not a long while afterwards.'

Galen said: 'Hippocrates means by 'bearing-many-children [*walūd*]' the woman who is pregnant and gives birth continually [*mutawātiran*]. [Such a woman] is called 'having-many-children [*an-nātiq*]' and 'having-many-children [*al-muntiq*]'.[48] After this woman had lost her husband, her menstruation was retained. Then it first happened to her that her state changed into the state of a man ['*ilā ḥāli r-raǧuli*]. Then it only took a short while until she died. This case story is beneficial in that you learn that when women lose their husbands, this causes them to suffer great damage, especially when they used to get pregnant before. We ourselves also saw a large number of women who suffered damage for this reason, and some of them died.'

Galen adds in evidence presented as deriving from his own observations – 'We ourselves saw' – thus giving his own support to the Hippocratic case story although of course such accounts of *autopsia* may not reflect real observations. In several ways, this version diverges from the Greek text of *Epidemics* as we have it today, most notably by omitting Phaethousa's identity as *oikouros*, leaving out the clause about 'afterwards, pain and reddening in the joints', and not mentioning Nanno.[49] But we can clearly see that Galen chose to focus on Phaethousa's previous childbearing; it is 'especially [women who] used to get pregnant before' who suffer when their husbands are no longer there. Flemming links this view

---

[45]   Peter Pormann notes, 'The name is not dotted; x stands for an undotted 'hook' that could be b/t/ṯ/n/y.' In Pfaff's German translation, *CMG* V 10, 2, 2 p. 506, line 21, the Arabic is rendered 'Die Frau des Pytheas'. As Pormann notes, 'Difficult Greek names may simply have been omitted or corrupted by later scribes' (pers. comm. July 2011).

[46]   [*Q*]*awiya š-ša'ru fī badanihā kullihī* lit. 'the hair was/became strong in her whole body' for the Greek *edasynthê panta*.

[47]   This suggests that Galen's manuscript was one of those in which *kai sklêron* was added here; Manetti and Roselli, *Ippocrate*, p. 195.

[48]   Pormann, pers. comm., notes 'Not translated in Pfaff; it might be a gloss. Basically, Ḥunayn is giving two Arabic synonyms for *walūd*.'

[49]   Gk *meta de, es arthra ponoi kai erythmata*. Pormann notes that *es arthra* can easily be amended into *es andra*, 'into a man', so perhaps this clause was left out because it was wrongly assumed to be repeating the previous clause on 'turning into the body of a man'. The omission of the *oikouros* reference could be because it was not understood.

to Galen's comments in *On Affected Parts* where he singles out women who have previously menstruated and had babies 'well' (Greek *kalôs*), and who have been used to having sex with men, as most likely to suffer from suffocation of the womb.[50] The very womanly woman appears more at risk of disease if she is prevented from fulfilling her functions.

In contrast to Smith's more general 'having borne children', Ḥunayn's text thus suggests that Galen read the Greek *epitokos* as more than a statement of having given birth; instead, it is 'the woman who is pregnant and gives birth continually'. Earlier translators of the *Epidemics* seem to have recognised this sense of *epitokos*; for example, in an early nineteenth-century French translation Phaethousa 'had had many children during her youth'.[51] This was in turn based on a sixteenth-century Latin translation, that of Anuce Foës in 1596, which gave 'before this, during her youth, she had been fruitful'.[52] Cornarius had translated slightly differently, losing the reference to her 'youth' but retaining her previous fecundity.[53]

Galen's interpretation of Phaethousa is thus that this is a woman whose body was used to being pregnant virtually all the time, and it is because of this that she suffers so much when her husband is not there. The sense of the prefix *epi-* can be one of accumulation, so that *epitokia* and *epitokos* can also mean 'compound interest'. The only other use of *epitokos* in the Hippocratic corpus is in the treatise *On Superfetation*, which opens by discussing how a woman can become pregnant again while already carrying one child; this theory was used to account for the birth of twins where one was clearly larger than the other, or for a non-viable foetus being born alongside a living child.[54] After an initial chapter on this possibility, the treatise then discusses other topics concerned with childbirth. In Chapter 17, the writer discusses a woman who is *epitokos*, and whose body swells up, presenting this as likely to lead to a stillbirth, a non-viable birth, or a premature birth. Potter translates *epitokos* here as 'approaching childbirth', perhaps following Littré who gives 'près d'accoucher', near to giving birth. However, it is possible that here too *epitokos* should be translated as 'who is always pregnant'.[55] A similar concern about these highly fertile women occurs later in *Superfetation*: 'Let any woman who was once prolific (*arikumôn*) but has ceased becoming pregnant, be

---

[50]   Flemming, *Medicine and the Making of Roman Women*, p. 334; Galen, *Loc. Aff.* 6.5 (K 8. 417).

[51]   *Traduction des Oeuvres Médicales d'Hippocrate* vol. 4 (Toulouse, 1801), p. 495: 'avoit fait plusieurs enfans dans sa jeunesse'; *antea per iuuentam foecunda erat*, based on the text of Foës.

[52]   Anuce Foës, *Hippocrates: Opera omnia, quae extant* (Frankfurt, 1596), p. 184.

[53]   Janus Cornarius, *Opera quae nos extant omnia* (Basle, 1558), p. 543, *priore quidem tempore foecunda erat*.

[54]   *Superfetation* 1 (Littré 8.476; Loeb IX, p. 318). Littré discusses animal and human cases of this occurring; vol. 8, pp. 472–5.

[55]   *Superfetation* 17 (Littré 8.485; Loeb IX, pp. 328–9).

phlebotomized twice a year from the arms and legs.'[56] Perhaps if Phaethousa had taken another man to her bed, or undergone this treatment, she would not have grown a beard.

In the Hippocratic original, then, as correctly interpreted by Galen, Phaethousa was not Everywoman. What happened to her was specific to the very fertile woman whose health has come to depend on regularly giving birth. This discussion demonstrates again that, just because the genre in which we meet Phaethousa appears easy to identify as a 'case history' or, as I have proposed, a 'case story', we should not stop interrogating the text. As I have indicated both here and in the preceding chapter, despite a long history of being seen as materials on which later readers can perform retrospective diagnosis, Hippocratic case histories are not straightforward documents and, like any other ancient sources, they respond to close reading. It is not clear how much of what we read in *Epidemics* comes from Phaethousa, or from her family, and how much is the physician's interpretation of her body; while some of the principles of selection used can be understood, we do not know how much editing has taken place on the story to make it into the form in which we have it now. There are similar themes found in this Hippocratic passage and later sex change narratives; both can include either statements of 'I myself saw', or distancing devices. But Phaethousa was not originally a story of sex change; her body remains female. In terms of where Phaethousa's sexual identity resides, while her visible body sends out messages of maleness, it is in the hidden, fertile womb of this *epitokos* that her femaleness resides, even when circumstances prevent it from functioning at its normal level. *Wits Theatre*'s condensed version of Phaethousa, in which her bodily change is simply a beard and the causative agent is her imagination, picks up the *oikouros* theme of the original text, but not the *epitokos* theme; as we have already seen, the story is highly adaptable to the needs of its users.

Mercurialis: Four Shades of Phaethousa

In the previous sections I have hinted that early modern translations of this case story into Latin can be nearer to the sense of the original than those made more recently. There was a considerable amount of interest in Hippocratic gynaecology in the sixteenth century in particular. As I have already mentioned, the first Latin translation of the gynaecological treatises appeared in 1525, made by Marco Fabio Calvo; another, by Janus Cornarius, came out in 1546. In both cases these were complete translations of the Hippocratic corpus. Both the gynaecological texts and the *Epidemics* (or, as they were often called in Latin, *De morbis popularibus* or *De morbis vulgaribus*), also circulated outside such complete editions of the Hippocratic corpus, versions of the latter often excluding Book 6 because most interest in this period lay in Books 1 and 3, seen as 'genuine' works of the historical

---

[56]   *Superfetation* 23 (tr. Paul Potter, Loeb IX, p. 331).

Hippocrates. However, as we have seen, the story of Phaethousa quickly became independent of the editions of the *Epidemics* and circulated alongside an existing standard list of Greco-Roman 'sex change' stories.

In this section I shall return to the alleged source for *Wits Theatre*: Hieronymus Mercurialis (Geronimo Mercuriale, 1530–1606). Was it really Mercurialis who was the source of this version's particular variations, namely the power of the imagination and the return from exile of Phaethousa's husband, Pytheas? This attribution shows something of the complexity of the relationship between vernacular and Latin medical sources on the female body in the second half of the sixteenth century, a time that, as I have argued elsewhere, was particularly critical for the history of women's diseases and their treatment, in the aftermath of the Latin translations of the gynaecological treatises becoming available. Mercurialis' work was included in the later editions of a large compilation of gynaecological texts first published in 1566 and later reissued with additions in 1586–88 and 1597: the *Gynaeciorum libri*.[57]

Mercurialis, who held chairs of medicine at Padua, Bologna and then Pisa, was a medical humanist; rather than seeking the truths of the body in anatomy, he believed that a better study of Greek and Roman medicine, locating superior manuscripts and making more accurate translations, was the route to improving practical medicine. It is to this approach – contrasting very clearly with that of Vesalius, discussed in Chapter 2 – that Christine Nutton attributes the relative neglect of Mercurialis in the history of medicine.[58] Nancy Siraisi has suggested that, even among medical humanists, Mercurialis was exceptional in the breadth of his interests.[59] He told the story of Phaethousa on four different occasions that I have been able to identify, but never in the way that *Wits Theatre* says he does. His four discussions of Phaethousa appeared as follows: first, when he examined variant readings and explained difficult passages in some ancient medical texts, in *Variarum lectionum in medicinae scriptoribus et aliis libri*, the first version of which appeared in Venice in 1570;[60] second, in his treatise on the diseases of women, the work that was printed in 1586 as part of the *Gynaikeia* collection of medical treatises;[61] again in his edition of the complete works of Hippocrates,

---

[57]   King, *Midwifery, Obstetrics and the Rise of Gynaecology*; on Mercurialis, see Siraisi, *History, Medicine, and the Traditions of Renaissance Learning*, pp. 42–55.

[58]   Christine Nutton, 'Introduction' to *Hieronymus Mercurialis, De arte gymnastica* (Stuttgart, 1978), p. 3; p. 5 underlines the point that the purpose of better editions was to improve actual treatment.

[59]   Nancy Siraisi, 'History, Antiquarianism, and Medicine: The Case of Girolamo Mercuriale', *History of Ideas* 64 (2003), p. 232.

[60]   Ibid., p. 233; Italo Paoletti, *Gerolamo Mercuriale e il suo tempo* (Lanciano, 1963), p. 7 has this as 1571.

[61]   On the gynaecological treatise, see Alessandro Simili, *Gerolamo Mercuriale lettore e medico a Bologna* (Bologna, 1966), pp. 22–3. Paoletti, *Gerolamo Mercuriale e il suo tempo*, p. 7 dates the Basle first edition of *De Morbis Muliebribus* to 1583; whereas Simili

printed in 1588; and finally in the *De hominis generatione* which appears in the Pisa lectures (*Pisanae Praelectiones*) of 1597.

The 1570 *Variae lectiones* was an important work for Mercurialis; with *De arte gymnastica*, Siraisi argues that it was the *Variae lectiones* that enabled him to get the Bologna chair in 1587.[62] But it was not in this first edition, which only ran to four books, that Mercurialis mentioned Phaethousa. In the 1576 edition, a fifth book was added,[63] and then in the 1585 edition Book 6 appeared, Chapter 20 of which combines stories of people turning into wolves with those of women becoming men.[64] This dating still makes this the earliest of Mercurialis' discussions of Phaethousa.

This suggests that Mercurialis became interested in the case story in 1585, probably because he was working on his 1586 gynaecology book at that time. The combination of lycanthropy and sex change – suggesting that these were equally worrying transformations – is also found in Johannes Wier's famous treatise on demons, and here Mercurialis may be using either Wier, or Wier's own source, Amatus Lusitanus. Wier's book featured Phaethousa from the 1564 Latin first edition, and the French translation of 1567 also included this section.[65] The elements

---

p. 23 dates it to 1582. Monica H. Green, *Making Women's Medicine Masculine: The Rise of Male Authority in Pre-Modern Gynaecology* (Oxford, 2008), p. 355 has the first edition outside the *Gynaeciorum libri* as the 'authorized' Venice edition of 1587.

[62] Siraisi, 'History, Antiquarianism, and Medicine', p. 251; Simili, *Gerolamo Mercuriale*.

[63] *Variarum lectionum libri* (Basle, 1576; only five volumes, the fifth being new); *Variarum lectionum libri* (Venice, 1588); here the story is on p. 129r and a further seven new chapters follow it.

[64] In the edition printed at Paris by Nicolaus Nivellius, Mercurialis wrote, *Verum Hippocratem huiuscemodi sexus mutationem (quod aliqui male conscii putarunt) voluisse significare, cum in fine lib vi epid Phaetusae Pythei uxoris, nec non Namysiae Gorgyppi coniungis corpora virilia effecta esse, pilosque ac barbam emisisse scribit, tantum a vero abest quantum verissimum est huiuscemodi conversionem solis virginibus contingere, atque tum dumtaxat, cum menses profluere, et libidinis aestus incendere (cuiusmodi commemoratae ab Hippocrate iam vetustiores et diu nuptae haud quaquam erant) incipiunt. Voce enim WNDRWTHE non solum 6 Epid. verum etiam in lib. de articulis, atque alibi usus invenitur Hippocrates, non cum mutationem sexus, sed corporis ad robur et virilitatis profectum indicare intendit.*

[65] *De praestigiis daemonum, et incantationibus ac veneficiis libri sex* (Basle, 1564), Book 3, Chapter 18, p. 359 *De naturali sexus humani mutatione.* In the 1566 edition it is Book 4, Chapter 22, pp. 455–6 and in 1568 it is Book 4, Chapter 24: *Hippocrates autem scribit, Phaetusae cuipiam Pythei uxori corpus virile, et in universum hirsutum et pilosum fuisse redditum, barbamque; eam emisisse, vocem item asperam fuisse effectam. Quod ipsum etiam Namysiae Gorgyppi uxori in Thaso evenisse, subiungit.* In the French edition of 1567, this is Book 3, Chapter 22, p. 281r. The French translation of Wier in 1567 also included the story, at Book 3, Chapter 22, p. 281r; this version (presumably because it is later than the Latin so more has happened) has an extra story inserted between the Hippocratic stories and those attributed to Amatus Lusitanus, concerning events that

mentioned by Wier were her hairiness and beard, and harsh voice; there was no reference to her previous childbearing, her husband's exile, her absent menses, or her death. There is nothing 'one-sex' about Wier's version of the story, which instead featured in a list of stories which were all taken to show that an enlarged clitoris becomes the penis,[66] but which moved Phaethousa outside the world of medical writers working in Latin, and into collections of amazing phenomena published in various vernacular languages, such as those of Torquemada and of Goulart.

Discussions of witchcraft, as much as any other early modern scientific writing, formed an aspect of the quest for the explanation of mysterious phenomena such as metamorphosis, and 'the mutation of the sexes' was one of many curiosities that had been – and continued to be – attributed to demons.[67] Wier, rejecting this explanation, in turn drew on earlier collections listing sex change stories but, immediately after Pliny's 'I myself saw' case, he added in Phaethousa. He also gave the case of Maria/Manuel Pacheca who, at the time of life in which women first emit the menses 'in place of menses' (*vice mensium*) pushed out a penis which was 'at that time lurking inside' (*ad id tempus intus latitantem extra eiecit*). In this story, what comes out is not a reversed womb, but a completely different organ.

Wier, like Torquemada in 1570, took all these stories wholesale from a book published in 1552: the *Centuria secunda* of the physician Amatus Lusitanus (João Rodrigues de Castelo Branco).[68] In the history of medicine, Amatus is associated with an increased interest in observation, but this does not mean that he was no longer interested in telling the traditional stories. He used them, however, not as the prime evidence, but as part of his discussion of the contemporary account of Maria/Manuel Pacheca, of whom he wrote that, 'out of a woman a male was made'.[69] Like Photius on Callo and Heraïs, Amatus was clear that this was not

---

happened 'in our time' in the reign of Ferdinand I of Naples (1423–94): Louis Garne of Naples had five daughters, two of whom grew a penis at age 15, and during the reign of the same king, a girl of Ebulo grew one on her wedding night.

[66]   Beecher, 'Concerning Sex Changes', p. 1001.

[67]   The quotation is from Gaspar Schott, *Physica curiosa* (Würzberg, 1667) cited in S. Clark, *Thinking with Demons*, p. 276.

[68]   Wier, *De praestigiis daemonum*, 1568, p. 423. The centuriae were published between 1551 and 1566. For the various editions, see Maximiano Lemos, *Amato Lusitano. A sua vida e a sua obra* (Porto, 1907), pp. 200–203.

[69]   *Et sic ex femina factus est masculus*, Amatus Lusitanus, *Centuria secunda (Venice, 1552)*, Cur. 39, p. 423. Gianna Pomata, 'Observation Rising: Birth of an Epistemic Genre, 1500–1600)', in Lorraine Daston and Elizabeth Lunbeck (eds), *Histories of Scientific Observation* (Chicago, IL, 2011), 45–80 contrasts Amatus' foundation in first-hand observation of cases with Schenck von Grafenberg's method of compiling excerpts from other people's works, both published treatises and letters from his 71 correspondents who shared what they had found in their own reading, but also notes of cases they had seen. She characterises Schenck as having 'scoured the texts of the medical tradition to retrieve, so to speak, the fragments of observation scattered in a great sea of doctrine' (p. 61).

a true transformation, but the emergence of a previously hidden male organ; unlike Photius, however, he suggested on the following page that apparent 'sex change' may be due to what is really a very large clitoris.[70] The renewed interest in the clitoris in the mid-sixteenth century was clearly shifting the terms of the debate; Laqueur's lack of interest in anatomy as driving change is odd here, as regarding a large clitoris as resembling a penis is very different from seeing a penis and testicles as a womb and its neck moving to the outside.[71] But Amatus also expresses the possibility of real change, here sounding more 'one-sex'; normally, he stresses, it only occurs from the female to the male, because Nature 'always adds, and never takes away: she always drives out, and never sends back: she is always moved towards the more worthy form, never the unworthy'.[72] So, 'one-sex', but only one-way.

When Amatus told the story of Phaethousa, he omitted her death: and so, copying him, did Wier. This omission seems consistent with a belief in previously hidden penises, of the 'true sex' emerging late, *without* any danger to life, and this version where she survives went on to have a long history. It dominated the second half of the sixteenth century, precisely because it was on Amatus' version that so many later writers relied; not just Wier in 1564, and Torquemada in 1570, but also for example du Laurens in 1593, Goulart in 1600 and Duval in 1612. In all these, Amatus' Maria Pacheca features alongside Phaethousa, and there is no mention of Phaethousa's death.[73]

Giulia Pomata has shown how broadly influential Amatus' work was, his 700 cases not only showing the *varietas* of human experience, which appealed to Renaissance tastes, but also providing a model for how those cases were presented, in that he separated the case from the commentary, or *scholia*.[74] In the *scholia* that

---

[70]   Amatus Lusitanus, *Centuria secunda*, p. 424. On the view of the clitoris as part of the urinary system in this period, see Park, 'The Rediscovery of the Clitoris', pp. 176–7.

[71]   Laqueur insists that 'one might have thought [the discovery of the clitoris] would have shaken the foundations of the old view as much as the other Columbus's voyages unsettled European views more generally. But this did not happen' ('Sex in the Flesh', p. 300). On the debates between Laqueur and Park over the impact of the discovery of the clitoris on the 'one-sex' model, see Traub, 'The Psychomorphology of the Clitoris', pp. 157–8.

[72]   Amatus Lusitanus, *Centuria secunda*, p. 424: ... *semper addit, nunquam demit: semper expellit, nunquam reprimit: semper movetur versus dignius, nunquam indignius.*

[73]   Du Laurens, *Opera anatomica*, pp. 262–3. After giving Maria Pacheca, Goulart claims to be taking Phaethousa not from Amatus, but direct from the text, with 'Ce que i'ay leu en Hippocrate au 6. livre des maladies populaires' (*Thresor d'histoires admirables*, 1610, pp. 237–8), translated by Edward Grimeston (1607, p. 275), 'That which I have read in Hypocrates ...'; Duval, *Des Hermaphrodits*, pp. 368–9.

[74]   See Pomata, 'Observation Rising', p. 58 and Nance, 'Wondrous Experience as Text', p. 109 on Amatus providing a model for others in his method of presentation of cases, in that he separated the case from the commentary, or scholia, and of the format of *observationes* with *scholia* more generally.

follow this particular section, Amatus gives his explanation of the stories he has summarised from Pliny:

> From these stories not much is missing that Hippocrates had already mentioned in the sixth book of *Epidemics*, in this matter, that in Abdera Phaethusa the wife of Pytheas had formerly been fertile; however when her husband went into exile, her menses were suppressed for a long time: afterwards pain and reddening arose in her joints: while these things happened her body was made manly, and became completely hairy and brought out a beard: and her voice was made harsh, and this same thing also to Namysia the wife of Gorgippos in Thasos.[75]

It is worth looking a little more carefully at Amatus's version of Phaethousa. What did *he* use as a source? What he gives is simply the 1546 Latin translation of Hippocrates by Cornarius up to *vox aspera facta est*, 'her voice became harsh'.[76] He then omitted altogether the sentence in the original about how attempts were made to bring down the menses, but she died; instead, he moved straight on to Namysia (Nanno). Whereas Cornarius correctly included the ending of the story, Amatus thus appears to have deliberately softened it into something closer to a sex change story. Although it is not complete, Amatus' version still represents a much fuller version than that of Wier. It includes the previous fecundity of Phaethousa, evidence that she *is* a true woman, not a true man whose sex appears late in life.

Returning to Mercurialis, he could have taken the story of Phaethousa from Wier, or from the much fuller version of Amatus that included her previous fertility (but still omitted her death). But in 1585 the humanist Mercurialis did rather more than his sources had done with the story of Phaethousa. After mentioning Pliny's eyewitness account of seeing a person in Africa who had turned into a man, he told the story of Phaethousa and Nanno and used it to discuss virgins in whom the flame of lust begins to burn at the point when menstruation first begins. He then noted that these two women were instead older, and had been married for a long time. He examined the Greek phrase *to te soma êndrôthê* 'her body was masculinised', and linked the verb here to another use in the Hippocratic treatise *On Joints*.[77] His conclusion was that this is *not* a reference to actual sex change, but to a stronger,

---

[75]   Amatus Lusitanus, *Centuria secunda*, p. 222: *A cuius historiis non multum absunt quae Hippo. praedixerat libro sexto de morbis popularibus, ad hunc modum, in abderis Phaethusa Pytheae uxor priore quidem tempore foecunda erat: quum autem maritus ipsius in exilium abiisset, menses multo tempore suppressi sunt: postea dolores, et rubores ad articulos oborti sunt: Haec autem ubi contigissent: et corpus virile factum est, et hirsuta penitus evasit, et barbam produxit: et vox aspera facta est, et subdit, idem hoc contigit, etiam Namysiae Gorgippi uxori in Thaso.* 'Namysia' is the vulgate's version of 'Nanno'.

[76]   Janus Cornarius, *Hippocratis Coi medicorum omnium longe principis, opera quae apud nos extant* (Paris, 1546), p. 355.

[77]   In *On Joints* 58 and 60, the verb *androô* is used to mean 'to become adult'. In *On Virgins*, *êndrômenai gynaikes* has the sense of 'to have had sex with a man'. Within

more mature body.[78] Already, then, Mercurialis was doing something very different to the other writers who based their discussion exclusively on Amatus Lusitanus, and coming to a different conclusion.

In 1586, in a treatise on the diseases of women appearing in the second edition of the *Gynaeciorum libri* collection, Mercurialis' focus was more medical than philological.[79] He used the story of Phaethousa in a section on defective menstruation to show how, if the menses are suppressed, the humours are spread around the body, causing changes to the hair, beard and voice.[80] This was followed by a discussion of the illnesses suffered as a result of retention; for example, he referred to the Hippocratic *Diseases of Women* Book 1, saying that if the menses are suppressed for six months this becomes incurable. Here Mercurialis was showing his familiarity not with the usual stories from Pliny, but with the details of the Hippocratic corpus; this pattern was repeated at the end of the section, where he referred to Hippocrates on the wife of Gorgias in *Epidemics* 5.4.[81] She suffered from menstrual suppression for four years, but was cured. She 'became pregnant, and became pregnant again', a reference which appears to concern not the fertility of the *epitokos*, but superfetation, the situation in which a woman becomes pregnant while already carrying a child, as the children were then born 40 days apart, the first healthy but the second 'simply flesh'.[82]

This method of understanding Phaethousa, not by comparing her with other sex change stories, but by bringing her into conjunction with other Hippocratic passages, is also found in Jean Liébault, who published his first book in 1582, before Mercurialis' first engagement with Phaethousa. But for him this does not

the Hippocratic corpus, only in this passage of *Epidemics* does it have the sense 'become masculine'. However the Liddell-Scott-Jones lexicon also points to Lycophron 176, 943.

[78]   P. 378 ... *non cum mutationem sexus, sed corporis ad robur et virilitatis profectum indicare intendit.*

[79]   Phaethousa also features in two of the other works included in Israel Spach, *Gynaeciorum sive de Mulierum tum communibus, tum gravidarum, parientium et puerperarum affectibus et morbis libri Graecorum, Arabum, Latinorum veterum et recentium quotquot extant, partim nunc primum editi, partim vero denuo recogniti, emendati* (Strasbourg, 1597), p. 751 (Akakia) and p. 833 (Mercatus).

[80]   On the gynaecological treatise, see Simili, pp. 22–3. The dating he gives is wrong; as M.H. Green, *Making Women's Medicine Masculine*, p. 355 notes, the *Gynaeciorum* version is 1586, followed by the Venice edition of 1587 as the 'authorized' version. Mercurialis, *Muliebrium libros IV* (the first edition, by Bauhin, in 1586–88 *Gynaeciorum libri*), p. 110 (in Spach, p. 262): from retention of the menses, *Mulieres habitum virilem contrahere et deformari, ita ut pili varii et barba oriatur, quod testum habemus non modo ab Avicenna, sed etiam ab Hippoc. 6 Epid. circa finem, ubi exemplum affert Phaelusae et Namesiae, quae ob retentos Menses barbam acquisierunt.* On the importance of humoral theory in Mercurialis, see C. Nutton, 'Introduction', p. 4.

[81]   In current editions, this is *Epidemics* 5.11.

[82]   The most recent editor, Wesley D. Smith, inserts a reference to superfetation into the text (Loeb VII, p. 161).

seem to have been a conscious decision to use one story to understand another. The Phaethousa of the *Epidemics* appears in the section on monstrous conceptions, in a discussion of sex change as being due to an excess of seed accompanied by heat. She comes after a young boy with one leg larger than the whole of the rest of his body, and before references to Amatus on Maria Pacheca and to the Pliny stories.[83] But within the section on menstrual suppression – where one may expect to find her – we encounter instead 'the maidservant of Phaethousa' who had no menstrual period for seven years but recovered and resumed menstruation.[84] In the Hippocratic original, *Epidemics* 4.38, this is simply 'the newly purchased maidservant'; there is no reference to Phaethousa, and Liébault seems to be eliding the two cases. This indicates something of the power of Phaethousa's name in the late sixteenth century, but also acts as a warning: we should read these texts with care and try to understand what is going on in them, and why she appears where she does. John Sadler's version of Phaethousa, appearing in 1636 in *The Sick Woman's Private Looking-Glass*, has already been discussed in Chapter 3 as having Phaethousa, not her husband, as the one being exiled. Sadler's version in other respects followed Mercurialis' insistence on the immediate cause of the condition as being menstrual suppression.[85] Later in this section, Sadler looked to the Hippocratic *Aphorisms* 5.57; Hippocrates, he said, speaks of the serious dangers of menstrual suppression.[86] In such a grave condition, Sadler insisted, one should reverse the normal order of medical interventions, in which surgery is the last resort, and instead begin with blood-letting, only then moving on to drugs and dietary recommendations. Yet, despite his dire warnings concerning this condition, he did not mention Phaethousa's *death* here. For him, Phaethousa, as a virago, 'consumes' her blood; it was not suppressed, and that is why the medical interventions mentioned in her case story in *Epidemics* were unsuccessful.

---

[83]   This is Book 3, Chapter 12; Chapter 13 is on hermaphrodites. See Jean Liébault, *Trois Livres appartenant aux infirmitez et maladies des femmes, pris du Latin de M. Jean Liebaut* (Paris, 1582), pp. 632–3: 'Pareillement de l'abondance de semence accompaignee de chaleur abondante peut advenir que les femmes degenerent en hommes, ainse que recite Hipp au 6. des epid. partic. 8 aph. 45. du corps de Phaetusa femme de Pithee qui devint velue part tout, mesme que la barbe luy creust au menton, et parloit d'une voix virile: ce qu'il dict estre aussi advenu en Thase en Namisie femme de Gorgippe.' The book is based in some sections on Giovanni Marinello, *Le Medicine partenenti alle infirmità delle donne* (Venice, 1563), but not to the extent of being a copy or translation; see King, *Disease of Virgins*, p. 152, n. 2. Liébault also cites Wier.

[84]   Liébault, *Trois Livres*, p. 343, 'ainsi qu'il advint à la servante de Phaëtusa (comme il est recité au 4. des epid.) laquelle fut sept ans avoir ses mois, parce que tout son sang menstrual s'estoit diverti au ventre et vers les parties droites de son corps'. A further reference to her appears on p. 349.

[85]   Sadler, *The Sick Woman's Private Looking-Glass*, p. 17.

[86]   Ibid., p. 21. This aphorism is equally a warning about the dangers of too heavy a flow.

In 1588, Mercurialis had a different focus again; in his edition of the complete works of Hippocrates, we find the Greek text and Latin translation of the text and then, two pages later, a discussion of the passage in *Epidemics* 6.[87] Again he insisted that it is menstrual suppression that leads to the bodily fluids moving all over the body, causing excess hair and a beard to grow; his discussion concluded with an even more emphatic rejection of the tradition of listing Phaethousa with 'sex change' stories, as he stated that 'nobody of sound mind would have said that these women truly become men'.[88] While his Latin translation included the full text of the story – including her death, *sed mortua est* – in his discussion he did not address this aspect directly.

When he returned to Phaethousa for a final time with *De hominis generatione* in the 1597 *Praelectiones Pisanae*, he was arguing against a different interpretation put forward by Matthiolus in 1558, against Amatus.[89] He referred to Phaethousa – although he did not give her name, maybe not surprisingly as this is the fourth time he has discussed her in print – in Chapter X, 'On the causes of similarity and dissimilarity according to sex'.[90] Here he discussed what had been claimed about sex change by other writers.[91] He noted that 'Hippocrates said that a certain woman, whose husband was away for a long time, grew a beard, and was made into a man', and that some said this is not contrary to reason, since men and women are formed from a mixture of male and female 'seed'.[92] But this, Mercurialis insisted, was nonsense; his language here recalls the contemporary objections to the idea that the homology between the womb and the penis was 'ridiculous' or 'absurd'.[93] In a typically humanist move, Mercurialis continues to insist on a return to the original Hippocratic text. Matthiolus, he writes, thought that the woman became a man, but that is not in fact what Hippocrates said: *non dicit Hippocrates mulierem illam factam esse virum.* Instead, Hippocrates said that she produced a beard,

---

[87] *Opervm Hippocratis Coi qvae Graece et Latine extant* (Venice, 1588), p. 180 and p. 182.

[88] Ibid., p. 180; discussion, p. 182; ... *non tamen vere eas fieri viros quisquam mentis compos dixerit.*

[89] I have not been able to identify this passage in Matthiolus; this is not *Apologia adversus Amathum Lusitanum, cum censura in eiusdem enarrationes* (Venice, 1558), which is taken up with the violent disagreements between the two men concerning Dioscorides, on whom Amatus published in 1553. The *Praelectiones Pisanae* (Venice: apud Iuntas, 1597) also include *In Epidemicas Hippocratis Historias* where Mercurialis takes 42 specific case histories and analyses them; Phaethousa is not included here.

[90] *Praelectiones Pisanae*, p. 29: *De causis similitudinis, et dissimilitudinis secundum sexum.*

[91] ... *scio a nonnullis relatum fuisse hoc quandoque visum esse: Scio etiam relatum esse foeminam quandam fuisse, quae evasit vir circa decimumquartum annum.*

[92] ... *imo Hipp. narrat quandam mulierem, cuius vir diu abfuerat, emisisse barbam, et virum factam esse* ...

[93] *Sed nugae sunt* ... On the womb and the penis, see above, p. 67.

on account of the retained menses, and that she had the 'form' of a man (Lat. *effigies*). Mercurialis distinguished Phaethousa from cases where a woman does indeed appear to have become a man; but such cases are not real 'changes'. A man has his genitalia outside, a woman inside, but what should be outside can be briefly retained inside, and later be 'thrust out'.[94] Despite the inside/outside statement, even this is not sex change, but a revelation of the 'true sex'. In none of these versions does Mercurialis focus on Phaethousa's death, even though he was clearly aware of it.

What then of the variant version in *Wits Theatre*? It was published after all four of Mercurialis' discussions of Phaethousa, and within a period in which Phaethousa's story is very commonly found, in medical treatises and also in collections of tales of wonder. The nearest match for its version is Mercurialis' 1597 summary, 'Hippocrates said that a certain woman, whose husband was away for a long time, grew a beard, and was made into a man'; but this does not name Phaethousa, says nothing about the power of the imagination, and does not have her husband return, unless we stretch the point and argue that 'was away' would imply that her husband did indeed come back. More probably, the *Wits Theatre* version does not come from Mercurialis; but did the compiler know that he had told the story on four different occasions, or is it an entirely random attribution? *Wits Theatre* has in common with Mercurialis a removal of Phaethousa from the list of sex change stories into which she had been placed by Amatus Lusitanus and his imitators; all Mercurialis' versions hinge on the cause, suppressed menses, but this is not mentioned by *Wits Theatre*. Bearing in mind what I have said about Diodorus Siculus' story of Heraïs as echoing Phaethousa, but with the husband's return, *Wits Theatre*'s motif of the return of Phaethousa's husband may suggest that the compiler is merging these two stories; but the relevant parts of Diodorus Siculus were not available at this time, so if he was thinking of another story of return it is more likely to be that of Martin Guerre.[95] The origin of this variant thus remains something of a mystery. Most probably, like Liébault's elision of the maidservant with no menstruation for seven years and the case of Phaethousa, *Wits Theatre* is simply merging a range of stories, heard or read. In any case, it shows that her story had escaped from medical literature and had moved into other types of writing, in the vernacular.

Other Phaethousas

The Latin medical texts of the sixteenth century included those that set Phaethousa in a sex change context, but also work like that of Mercurialis who sought to

---

[94] ... *cum proprium viri fit habere genitalia extra: foeminae vero intra ... illa membra genitalia, quae extra debebant esse sint paulisper intro retenta.*

[95] The collection does use Diodorus elsewhere, but only the earlier books, which existed in English translation.

understand her as a medical case. While *Wits Theatre* is interesting in terms of showing the presence of Phaethousa in English vernacular literature, it is not the earliest reference to this case that I have found here. In his recent book *Beard Fetish in Early Modern England*, Mark Johnston mentioned Phaethousa by name – as cited in a lecture given to barber-surgeons by Alexander Read in the 1630s – but did not realise that another of the passages he quotes is also about her.[96] This passage predates both *Wits Theatre*, and Mercurialis; it comes from 1578, in *The Historie of Man, Sucked from the Sappe of the most Approved Anathomistes*, where the surgeon/physician John Banister mentioned her – but *not* by name – in a section on monstrous deviation.[97] While the standard position on Banister is that his work was 'compiled from the standard authorities', Johnathan Pope has recently argued that he is more than simply a compiler, and 'represents the emergence of a particularly English post-Vesalian narrative of the body that combines religion and anatomy'.[98] Banister described human variation between geographic regions – he made considerable use of the Hippocratic treatise *Airs Waters Places* – and also across time; so, for example, in Galen's time eunuchs *did* suffer from gout, whereas 'in the tyme of Hipocrates it was not so'.[99] Clearly thinking of Phaethousa, Banister wrote:

> It is straunge to us that women have beardes, albeit not so every where: for in Caria it is a thyng familiar: whereas some of them beyng a while frutefull, but after widowes, and for that suppressed of natural course, put on virilitie, being then bearded, hoarie,[100] and changed in voyce. Shall it be counted a fable that toucheth the transformation of one kinde into an other, as the Male into the Female and so contrariwise? surely Plinie saith. No: since him selfe to haue sene a woman chaunged into man, in the day of mariage, he playnly auoucheth. And agayne, a child of a yeare old, from a mayden to a boy.[101]

While keeping the unnamed Phaethousa in the company of the Pliny sex change cases and their claim to autopsy, Banister is mixing quite a full version of her story (previous fertility, absence of husband – here refigured as 'widows'[102] – menstrual suppression, beard, hairy all over, voice change) with a brief reference

---

[96] Mark Johnston, *Beard Fetish in Early Modern England* (Aldershot, 2011), p. 174.

[97] John Banister, *The Historie of Man, Sucked from the Sappe of the most Approved Anathomistes* (London, 1578).

[98] New DNB, s.v. Banister; Johnathan H. Pope, 'Religion and Anatomy in John Banister's *The Historie of Man* (1578)', *LATCH*, 3 (2010), 1–33.

[99] Proeme B3v; also noted by J.H. Pope, 'Religion and Anatomy', p. 14.

[100] This has the sense of 'hairy', as in body hair, rather than referring to age.

[101] Proeme B2v. On the following page he has as a separate category 'those that are both Male & Female'.

[102] Here it seems to be Pytheas rather than Phaethousa who dies. This is another unique variant.

to another woman with a beard that appeared in the classical Greek historian Herodotus. In fact, Herodotus was not talking about 'a thyng familiar', but something that only happens to one person or role, and only a limited number of times: 'whenever any disaster was about to happen to the people of Pedasa or their *perioikoi*, the priestess of Athene grew a large beard. This only happened three times' (Herodotus 1.175.104).[103] So, *contra* Johnston, the reference to women who have been 'frutefull' and are then widowed, explicitly taken from Hippocrates (the marginal note, apparently not noticed by Johnston, clearly points the reader to Book 6 of the *Epidemics*), is not about Caria. Phaethousa's town of Abdera is in northern Greece (Thrace): Caria is now a part of south-western Turkey. Banister thus merges Phaethousa with another ancient story, but unlike the strategies used by Liébault, Mercurialis and later Sadler, this is not one from the Hippocratic corpus.

Many other variations on the story existed in the early modern period. For some writers, Phaethousa was not suffering from a sex change, and the causative factor was not her lust or her sorrow, or diverted menses, but a physical and mechanical condition. Despite there being no reference in the original case story to anything being visible on the exterior of the body apart from Phaethousa's facial and body hair, some writers included her in their sections on the prolapse of the womb. There is a hint of the Laqueur 'one-sex' model here, but it is mixed up with other ways of seeing the body, and when prolapse occurred the first reaction was not to see the emerging womb as a penis.

Sixteenth-century writers such as Jean Liébault based their general comments on prolapse on the sixth-century AD physician Aetius and on Avicenna. In 1582, Liébault distinguished between different levels of prolapse. In the second level of severity, the entire body of the womb comes outside; he cited Aetius as saying that this looked like a goose or ostrich egg, but went on to note that it was more like 'the pouch of the testicles, which in Latin is the scrotum'.[104] Here, then, there was no suggestion that this was more than a visual resemblance, and nor was it the first that came to his mind; a similar use of the image occurs in the Hippocratic treatise *On the Nature of Woman*, where the author described a 'full prolapse' of the uterus: 'If the uterus descends completely out of the genitals, it hangs like (Gk *hôsper*) a scrotum.'[105] In the next level of severity on an ascending scale, a prolapse could involve what was formerly inside the cavity of the womb being outside it; Liébault commented that he had seen this when a midwife pulled on the afterbirth and pulled out the womb and, despite the involvement of surgeons to replace the womb, the woman died two days later.[106] Clearly, in a woman who

---

[103]   *The famous hystory of Herodotus* (London, 1584), p. 55 has this as 'Minerva's Priest' rather than specifying the gender. *Perioikoi*, 'those who live around', is a Greek political term for freeborn non-citizens in an area.

[104]   Liébault, *Trois Livres*, p. 445.

[105]   *On the Nature of Woman* 5 (Littré 7.216–8; tr. Potter, Loeb X, p. 199).

[106]   Liébault, *Trois Livres*, p. 446.

had given birth, there was no sense that this could be a penis emerging. For this third level of severity, no analogies with the male body were offered; instead the appearance was described as being like turning a bag inside out, so the outside is inside, the base is down, and the neck at the top.[107]

Jacques Ferrand, who used Liébault, quoted Mercado and Castro, who at one point had attributed the condition of Phaethousa and Nanno to 'the protrusion or descent of the matrix that bore a certain resemblance to the male member', but elsewhere had followed Wier in regarding what they could see as an enlarged clitoris instead.[108] In addition to mentioning Phaethousa in his chapter on 'erotic melancholy' as a possible example of prolapse, Ferrand also included her under 'melancholy in married persons'.[109] Here the context was the need to check that a woman's body has not closed up, a condition that can happen not only in young girls but also 'in widows or in married women whose husbands are away for long periods'. He asserts that Hippocrates 'claimed ... that Namysia and Phaëtusa were changed into men', but adds that his own view concerning their condition is that they were 'unperforated', an ailment 'often responsible for the breakdown in marital relations'.[110] Again, this moves the case story into the realm of the surgeon, rather than the physician who would try to restore the menstrual flow.

Phaethousa also featured as an example of prolapse in the surgeon Jacques Guillemeau's *Child-Birth*, published in 1609 in French and 1612 in English; here the chapter on prolapse appeared in the section on what can happen after childbirth, so that her status as *epitokos* took on a very different meaning, her many confinements having put her at risk of this condition. One of the 'internal causes' of prolapse in general which Guillemeau listed was the desire of a woman to have sex; another was long-standing menstrual suppression; the third was having intercourse too soon after childbirth, while the lochia still flow. All of these could have been imagined to apply to Phaethousa, but in fact it was the second which Guillemeau linked to her.[111] He thus merged the medical and the surgical explanations for her condition.

The frequent avoidance of any mention of Phaethousa's death, taken with her appearance alongside sex change cases, suggests that, in the mid-sixteenth century,

---

[107]   Ibid.

[108]   Beecher and Ciavolella, *Jacques Ferrand, A Treatise on Lovesickness*, pp. 230–31 and, on uses of Liébault, p. 585, n. 34; Luis Mercado, *De mulierum affectionibus* Book 2 (Venice, 1587); in the 1594 Madrid edition, p. 236. Castro in turn used Mercado; see *De universa mulierum medicina* (Hamburg, 1603) Book 2, ch. 9 *De uteri prurito*.

[109]   Beecher and Ciavolella, *Jacques Ferrand, A Treatise on Lovesickness*, p. 340.

[110]   Ibid.

[111]   Jacques Guillemeau, *De l'heureux accouchement des femmes* (Paris, 1609), pp. 423–4; *Child-Birth or, the Happy Deliverie of Women* (London, 1612), p. 238: '... the long suppression of the naturall courses, which sometimes makes a woman grow Viril, or mankind [*sic*], as Hippocrates witnesses of Phaëtusa, wife of Pitheus, who became like a man, with a beard, and a man's voice'.

she could function within a 'one-sex' model rather than the 'two-sex' model which, I have argued, was originally associated with her: the Hippocratic case story is dominated by a 'two-sex' perspective in which one is either fully male or fully female, and where intermediate categories cannot be sustained. Over the second half of the sixteenth century, however, she was being taken out of the then-standard list of sex change stories, and instead read alongside other Hippocratic material, and other classical texts; the medical humanist engagement with the text, represented by Mercurialis, also worked towards a closer understanding of the original text. As I noted in Chapter 3, in 1596 Schenck von Grafenberg included her death and explicitly warned of the danger to a woman's life if she grew a beard.[112] All this supports the argument that any debate between one- and two-sex models was happening not at the start of the eighteenth century, but in the sixteenth. It is clear that genre matters: in the translations of the Hippocratic corpus published from 1525, she still died, showing that sex change could not happen, and the example of Mercurialis shows that one person could function with both one- and two-sex readings. The wide range of contexts in which she could feature in medical works, the various types of writing in which she appeared, and the very different explanations for her condition, all suggest that she was a surprisingly blank canvas on which early modern discussions of sex change and of gender identity could be played out. While in the original version her status as the very feminine *oikouros* and the highly productive *epitokos* account for her extreme reaction to the absence of her husband, for early modern readers she was of interest far more widely. There was no simple correlation between the public display of people displaying the characteristics of both sexes in a single body, and readings of Phaethousa that ignored her death and focused on her living with a beard.

Other sixteenth- and early seventeenth-century uses of Phaethousa's story, however, go far beyond Laqueur's basic dichotomy. Variants such as those of Sadler, in which she was exiled, or *Wits Theatre*, in which her husband returned, were able to sit alongside theories of causation linked to the power of the imagination, passionate love, or mechanical changes in the body. None of these variants are 'mistakes'; instead, they show us the vitality of the Hippocratic texts as used by sixteenth- and seventeenth-century writers, and the need for writers with conflicting views about the possibility of sex change and bodily transformation to anchor their work in that of the Father of Medicine.

In Laqueur's 'one-sex' period, among the range of explanations for apparent sex change, there were thus some observations that a prolapsed womb looked like the scrotum, but I have found no interest in suggesting that it resembled a penis. However, in the nineteenth century – in Laqueur's 'two-sex' period – I have found a case where prolapse was presented, by a sufferer, as an inside-out reversal of the body. In 1833, Everard Home discussed the various reasons for apparent hermaphrodites, in very much the same terms as sixteenth-century writers had used. It could be due to a large clitoris, or prolapse, where 'The womb, thus

---

[112]   Schenck von Grafenburg, *Observationes Medicae*; see above, p. 74.

displaced, has put on an appearance resembling a penis.' He described how he himself had seen a French woman, aged 25, with a long-standing prolapse; 'This woman was shown as a curiosity in London; and in the course of a few weeks, made four hundred pounds.' However, 'To render herself still more an object of curiosity, she pretended to have the powers of a male. As soon as the deception was found out, she was obliged to leave England.'[113] In this period, people were still prepared to pay to see evidence of a 'one-sex' model, but the question remained of whether the organs they were shown were capable of reproductive function.

In the next chapter we shall return to the story of Agnodice. Told and retold at much the same time as that of Phaethousa, it featured in an even wider range of genres of material; it thus gives us further evidence from which to challenge Laqueur's picture of the early modern period. As with Phaethousa, I propose to examine the text in some detail in order to understand what it says to our understanding of ideas about the body in the classical world, as well as considering how it was told in later history. In the next chapter, I shall consider the genre of the classical text in which Agnodice features. I shall then discuss the role of Herophilus, firm supporter of the 'one-sex' body, as her teacher. How has their relationship been seen by later users of the story? The following chapter will focus on her gesture of revelation of her own sex to her patients and her accusers, and will re-examine the issue of what is wrong with her first patient, to whom she first performs this gesture. I shall examine how she demonstrates her 'true sex' in different versions of her story told in the period from the 1590s onwards, and discuss how key sections of the original Latin text have been reinterpreted by Agnodice's supporters and enemies – both male and female – over the early modern period, and beyond.

---

[113] Everard Home, *Lectures on Comparative Anatomy*, vol. 3 (London, 1823), p. 318.

PART III
Agnodice

Chapter 5
Agnodice: Gender and Genre

Agnodice's story was first printed in the 1535 edition of Hyginus' *Fabulae*, only a decade after Phaethousa's story became available in the first Latin translation of the full Hippocratic corpus. While Phaethousa is a patient, Agnodice practises medicine; her story invites us to move beyond theories of how the body works and to reflect on women's actual medical roles in the ancient world and beyond, as it was used to think about the female body and about women's involvement in the history of midwifery, gynaecology and medicine. As we shall see in this and the following chapters, it was retold many times, often in the context of debates about whether men or women should assist in childbirth and, by the nineteenth century, about whether women could train as physicians. If there is only one sex with the same organs in different locations, or if there are two radically different sexes with entirely different organs, what are the implications for how medical care is gendered? In a possible echo of Agnodice's story, but one which also repeats the concern of the fourth-century BC Hippocratic *Diseases of Women* with those female patients who are ashamed to speak to a man, the fifth-century AD Caelius Aurelianus claimed that 'it was finally decided by the ancients to institute female physicians (Lat. *medicae*), so that the diseases of a woman's private parts (Lat. *pudenda*), when they needed to be examined, would not have to be exposed to male eyes'.[1] So do the female genitalia, normally discreetly hidden but displayed by Agnodice, always provide a rationale for segregated medical care, or can knowledge of the 'outside' male organs be applied, by analogy, to the 'inside' female organs?

As I have already argued, if we are going to understand the ways in which the body was understood and sexual difference produced in the classical and early modern worlds, we need to go beyond Laqueur's analysis in two key ways: by performing close readings of our texts, and by reading a wider range of texts. Although he made reference to the broader context in which the mostly medical/scientific sources he used existed, for example mentioning in passing 'the world of Hippocrates', Laqueur did not consider how that world was constructed and

---

[1] Caelius Aurelianus, *Gynaecia* in Miriam F. Drabkin and Israel E. Drabkin, *Caelius Aurelianus, Gynaecia: Fragments of a Latin Version of Soranus' Gynaecia from a Thirteenth Century Manuscript* (Baltimore, MD, 1951), p. 1: *hinc denique consultum est ut medicas instituere antiquitas providisset, ne femine pudendorum vitia virilibus offerrentur oculis perscrutanda.* See M.H. Green, *Making Women's Medicine Masculine*, p. 33. This passage does not feature in the other Latin works based on Soranus: Muscio and Theodorus Priscianus. See also above, Chapter 1.

experienced outside his limited range of evidence; in his chapter on the classical world, in the midst of discussion of the 'big names' such as Galen, Hippocrates, Aristotle, Lucretius and Augustine, there is just one brief mention of Greek 'art and drama' and another to unreferenced 'poetry and prose'.[2] As Jack Winkler pointed out in another context, it is normally the case that 'Behind sentences that begin "The Greeks believed ..." there lies a fairly small set of elite canonized texts';[3] with his limited range of source material and his apparent assumption that those sources he does address are straightforward to use, Laqueur is no exception to this. The story of Agnodice and the case history of Phaethousa each exist in only one ancient source, but the genres in which they appear are very different and – as we saw in the previous chapter – in the case of Phaethousa changed as the stories went on being told. Even Laqueur's medical/scientific texts are not an undifferentiated category, but work with their own rules; the case (hi)story genre, in which we find Phaethousa, is still so familiar that we risk bringing to it inappropriate assumptions about how it was composed and used. While ancient case (hi)stories are certainly not transparent sources, in comparison with Phaethousa it is clear that Agnodice is far more difficult to place in terms of genre. But it is important to consider the various options because the decision affects how different readers have interpreted her story; is it fiction, or is there anything 'historical' in it?

The trial of Agnodice on the charge of learning medicine despite being a woman has much to say to the case against Laqueur that I am constructing here. In contrast with Phaethousa's passivity as her body produces a beard and moves towards death, Agnodice has agency; she chooses to play with the boundaries of sexual identity by disguising herself as a man in order to learn medicine, and then revealing herself as a woman when this is necessary. The ease with which she passes as a man challenges Galen's comments about how simple it is to recognise whether someone is a man or a woman, even if fully clothed.[4] This recalls a comment made by Donald Beecher, 'if sex is grounded in the essences of nature, as the medical record from the late sixteenth century supports, then gender play becomes a safe and harmless form of self-expression to social ends. A disguise is merely a disguise.'[5] But how 'safe' is Agnodice's decision to disguise herself, when at the end of the story she is put on trial? Its safety must depend on the certainty that her eventual revelation of her genitals will be decisive.

In the story, she is taught by Herophilus; interestingly, as we saw in Chapter 1, a known supporter of a 'one-sex' body. In the reception of Agnodice, his presence in the story has often been discounted. Scholars argue that the phrasing 'a certain

---

[2]   Laqueur, *Making Sex*, p. 25; Aristophanes features in a sentence on 'Greek art and drama' on p. 31 but without any sense of Aristophanes as a comic playwright, and on p. 34 there is a passing mention of the 'great abundance of poetry and prose praising or making fun of the male or female organs', but with no references given.

[3]   Winkler, 'Laying Down the Law', p. 203.

[4]   Above, pp. 37–8.

[5]   Above, p.21; Beecher, 'Concerning Sex Changes', p. 1012.

Herophilus' (Lat. *Herophilo cuidam*) suggests that Hyginus did not in fact know who he was. It is possible that he was added to the story to give it a date, rather than because of his specific views; as his work has been lost, and survives only in fragments quoted in writers including Galen, his role as a promoter of a 'one-sex' body may not have been appreciated. In Chapter 6, I shall discuss the representation of Herophilus in terms of the different interpretations of Agnodice's gesture of revelation in the period from 1535 onwards. In 'one-sex' terms, she is showing that her organs of generation are firmly inside her body; she is not a man and so cannot have seduced women patients. In Chapter 7, the focus will be on Agnodice's identity – midwife, or physician? – and I shall investigate there how different ideas about sexual difference have influenced notions about who is the proper person to give care to women, and how Agnodice's story has been rewritten to fit different historical contexts. How has she been read by those supporting women as physicians – and men as midwives? First, however, it is important to think about what sort of story that of Agnodice is.

Reading Agnodice

Agnodice's story is notoriously difficult to fit into any one genre. In this chapter I shall consider its relationship to lists of inventors, novels, saints' lives, and historical writing, arguing that it is precisely the lack of a definite genre that has made the story so flexible for its subsequent users. It is known from only one ancient source, the elusive Latin writer Hyginus, who cannot be tied to any firm dates within the period of the early Roman Empire; while he used to be conveniently identified with Caius Julius Hyginus, freedman of the emperor Augustus, this is no longer thought likely.[6] His *Fabulae* or 'Stories', in which Agnodice features, must have been written before 207 AD, when an anonymous writer copied a Greek version of parts of the text. The Latin version we have is clearly based on a Greek one, sometimes transliterating a Greek word where the writer could not readily find a Latin alternative.[7] The Greek name of the heroine, presumably from *hagnos* and *dikê*, so 'Chaste-before-justice',[8] seems rather convenient bearing in mind the

---

[6]   As early as 1766, Jean Astruc doubted the link to Augustus' freedman, and argued that the 'solecisms and barbarisms' (Fr. p. xlii: Eng. p. xxv) in the Latin would put it into the seventh or eighth century: Jean Astruc, *L'Art d'accoucher réduit a ses principes* (Paris, 1766), pp. xl–xliii; English, *Elements of Midwifery. Containing the most Modern and Successful Method of Practice* (London, 1767), pp. xxiv–xxv.

[7]   An example features in the story of Agnodice; see further below, p. 133, n. 16.

[8]   Tilde A. Sankovitch, *French Women Writers and the Book: Myths of Access and Desire* (Syracuse, NY, 1988), p. 64, writing about Catherine des Roches' 1578 version, suggests a different reading, using the Greek *agnôs*, 'unknown', to make Agnodice's name mean 'The Unknown'. Des Roches' version will be discussed further below. Naoko Yamagata (pers. comm. 22 April 2012) has suggested that the name could come from

story of Agnodice's appearance in court on a charge of seduction. A modern editor of Hyginus, H.J. Rose, argued that the text was not taken direct from its Greek sources, but instead from summaries of them given in compendia, thus introducing another level of distance from the originals.[9]

The work preserves some ancient myths that are otherwise unknown, alongside unique variants of well-known stories. All that survived from antiquity was a crude copy, or perhaps summary, of the Latin version of Hyginus' work, probably made around the fourth or fifth century AD, before being copied again; from its simple style, some scholars have assumed this to be the work of a schoolboy.[10] Within this sole example of the *Fabulae*, Agnodice featured in a list of 'who invented what'.

Unusually for a work from Greco-Roman antiquity, the text that we have today is based on only a single manuscript, written in around 900 AD, now lost, and labelled by modern scholars as φ. The 1535 first printed edition of Jacob Molsheim (usually known by his Latinised name, Micyllus), identified by scholars as F, was in turn based on this one manuscript. It was through F that the simple story of Agnodice re-entered the Western tradition and it was quickly popularised through the work of André Tiraqueau (often known by the Latin form of his name, Tiraquellus) in the 1550s and Charles Estienne (Stephanus) in the 1590s.[11] As I have already noted, this is a significant period in terms of changing ideas about the female body; the time during which Agnodice became familiar coincided with the years in which a Hippocratic 'two-sex' model of the body, with women as fundamentally different from men, became better known. At some point after Micyllus used it, φ was dismantled, so the other printed editions of Hyginus that followed were restricted to copying Micyllus.[12] In modern times, in a further twist to this story, fragments

---

the verb 'to ignore' (*agnoein*), making Agnodice the one who 'ignores/defies the law' by becoming a physician.

[9]   H.J. Rose, 'An Unrecognized Fragment of Hyginus, *Fabvlae*', *Classical Quarterly*, 23 (1929), p. 99.

[10]   Ibid, p. 98, describes the style as 'poor and jejune', commenting on the Latin writer's 'gross carelessness and his atrocious mistakes in translating the simplest Greek' (p. 99). Rose noted that the version of the *Fabulae* which we now have is a fourth- or fifth-century abbreviation of the original Latin work.

[11]   André Tiraqueau, *De nobilitate, et de iure primigeniorum* was first published in 1549. It includes a section on *Foeminae medicae*, 'Women doctors', starting from the goddess Diana/Artemis. He repeats Hyginus' account, correctly situating it as concerning 'the art of medicine' rather than simply midwifery; his purpose is to show that no loss of nobility ensues from practising this noble art; *De nobilitate* (Basel, 1561), p. 410. Charles Estienne's *Dictionarium historicum ac poeticum* was first published in 1553, and went into 20 editions: Agnodice does not enter this encyclopaedia until the 1590 edition printed by Jacobus Stoer.

[12]   The Latin of Micyllus was reprinted in Hieronymus Commelinus, *Mythologici Latini* ([Heidelberg], 1599), pp. 143–4. There seem to have been more manuscripts of Hyginus available in the Middle Ages, but these had apparently disappeared by the sixteenth century. For example, Arnulf of Orleans, a twelfth-century writer, gives some extracts from

of a manuscript of Hyginus have been found and recognised as belonging to the lost φ.[13] Judging from these, the textual problems in the Latin we now have derive from the fact that 'frequently Micyllus simply could not read what was in front of him'.[14] The text, then, has a particularly complicated history, copied many times by intermediaries who did not understand what they had in front of them, and abridged. But it is important to remember that there was a Greek original; and, in the absence of any full manuscripts to consult, if we find that the words we have make little sense, the answer may be to speculate as to what the Greek original would have said.

Lists of Inventors

Within Hyginus' *Fabulae*, the story of Agnodice appears in a list of *Quis quid invenit*, 'who invented/discovered what'.[15] This raises the question of why we would want an 'inventor' or 'discoverer' for midwifery. Within this section of the *Fabulae*, the story follows a short passage summarising the contributions to medicine made by Chiron the centaur, the god Apollo, and his part-mortal son, Asclepius, who was also one of Chiron's pupils. Chiron, we are told, was the first to establish the surgical side of medicine, 'as a result of herbs'; Apollo first developed medicine for the eyes; and Asclepius 'discovered the art of clinical medicine'.[16]

---

parts of Hyginus that are more comprehensible than the equivalent passages in Micyllus; this may mean that he was more able to understand the hand in which manuscript φ was written (Beneventan, a particularly difficult type of handwriting used from the eighth century AD onwards), but perhaps hinting that he had access to another manuscript, one superior to φ; see H.J. Rose, 'Second thoughts on Hyginus', *Mnemosyne*, 11 (1958), p. 45, discussing a 1943 article.

[13]   They have turned up in book bindings, used to stiffen the spines of other books; the first at Regensburg in 1864 and subsequently at Munich in 1942. These have led to revised editions of small parts of the text; edition by Moritz Schmidt, *Hygini Fabulae* (Jena, 1872); edition by H.J. Rose, *Hygini Fabulae* (Lugduni Batavorum, 1936). On the manuscript transmission and first publication, see M.D. Reeve, 'Hyginus', in Leighton D. Reynolds (ed.), *Texts and Transmission: A Survey of the Latin Classics* (Oxford, 1983), pp. 189–90.

[14]   As noted in Peter Marshall's highly critical review of Jean-Yves Boriaud (ed.), *Hygine*, Fables (Collection Budé; Paris, 1997), 'The Budé Hyginus', *Classical Review*, 49 (1999), p. 411. The other fragment is Vatican Pal. lat. 24 (known as N).

[15]   Hyginus, *Fabula* 274.

[16]   Chiron *artem medicinam chirurgicam ex herbis primus instituit*; Apollo *artem ocularium medicinam primus fecit*; Asclepius *clinicen repperit* (the phrase *artem medicinam* is understood here, from the two previous clauses); Hyginus' use of the Greek ending *–en* in *clinicen* shows that he took this summary from a Greek original. In the ancient world Apollo is a god widely associated with healing in general, but Hyginus' specific association of Apollo with eye disease is found in the early modern period, perhaps based on this passage of Hyginus itself; for example, in Robert Barret's *A Companion for Midwives,*

After Agnodice, the list moves on to Perdix, son of the sister of Daedalus, who invented the compass. Other than the logical connection between listing the founders of medicine and describing the first midwife, the catalogue of topics given seems to be random; the discovery of the mixing of wine, metal production, music, the trumpet, dye, and chariot racing. Modern editors of Hyginus assume that there was once more text at the beginning of the section.

Stories of 'who invented what' were a popular genre in the ancient world. Different cities and areas contested each other's primacy, but many activities or institutions had a named *prôtos heuretês* or 'first finder'; from Prometheus who discovered fire, to Cecrops who instituted monogamous marriage.[17] An influential list, probably known to Hyginus, was that of the Roman encyclopaedist Pliny, whose work was based on over 2000 sources, more than two-thirds of which were Greek, and who described more than 200 inventions: he did not name an inventor of midwifery.[18] Pliny was the basis for the versions of 'who invented what' in circulation at the time when Micyllus published his edition of Hyginus; most notably, Polydore Vergil's 1499 *De rerum inventoribus*, 'On the Inventors of Things'.[19] As it predated Micyllus' publication of Hyginus, this of course did not include Agnodice; indeed, it did not feature midwifery at all, although it

---

Child-bearing Women, and Nurses Directing them how to Perform their Respective Offices (London, 1699), preface, we read that 'Appolo [*sic*] was an Oculist'.

[17]   Adolf Kleingünther, *Prôtos Heuretês: Untersuchungen zur Geschichte einer Fragestellung*, *Philologus* Supplement 26.1 (Leipzig, 1933). Kleingünther emphasises the competing claims of different geographical areas to 'own' these discoverers and discoveries. On the later tradition, including Polydore Vergil, see John K. Ferguson, *Bibliographical Notes on Histories of Inventions and Books of Secrets*, 2 vols (Glasgow, 1895; reprinted London, 1959). In the final chapter of the *Fabulae*, 277, a further eclectic list of inventions features; the letters of the Greek alphabet, wrestling, taming animals, domesticating crops, some sacrificial customs, and sails.

[18]   Pliny, *NH* 7. 191–215, which 'draws on a variety of Greek sources'; see Beagon, *The Elder Pliny on the Human Animal*, p. 419 and Brian P. Copenhaver, 'The Historiography of Discovery in the Renaissance: The Sources and Composition of Polydore Vergil's *De inventoribus rerum*, I–III', *Journal of the Warburg and Courtauld Institutes*, 41 (1978), p. 197. Roger French, *Ancient Natural History* (London, 1994), p. 210 notes that, for medicine, only one-eighth of Pliny's sources were in Latin. On how our interest in his sources, and the notion of Pliny as 'compiler', obscures our understanding of Pliny the 'author', and on the cultural context of the Roman empire as a locus for collecting, cataloguing and displaying facts and objects, see for example Sorcha Carey, *Pliny's Catalogue of Nature: Art and Empire in the Natural History* (Oxford, 2003) and Trevor Murphy, *Pliny the Elder's Natural History: The Empire in the Encyclopaedia* (Oxford, 2004).

[19]   *De rerum inventoribus* (Venice, 1499); a translation is available, Brian P. Copenhaver, *Polydore Vergil On Discovery* (Cambridge, MA, 2002); see also Copenhaver, 'The Historiography of Discovery'; Catherine Atkinson, *Inventing Inventors in Renaissance Europe: Polydore Vergil's De inventoribus rerum*, Spätmittelalter und Reformation Neue Reihe 33 (Tübingen, 2007).

covered the invention of 'physic, and the parts therof' (Book 1, ch. XVI), and of herbal remedies (ch. XVII).[20] For the section on medicine, Vergil relied to a large extent on Giovanni Tortelli, the first librarian of the Vatican Library, whose 1449 *Orthographia*, first printed in 1471, included a short history of medicine within the entry for 'Hippocrates'; he too had used Pliny.[21] Hyginus' list of inventors thus provided an alternative, and supplement, to the popular lists taken from Pliny.

For Hyginus, the inventors or discoverers are mostly gods, or the children of gods. Agnodice, whose story is by far the fullest of any told here, is anomalous, being a mortal woman rather than a figure from mythology; other than the goddess Demeter/Ceres, who discovered grain, she is also the only female discoverer listed. Reading the story carefully, the reader will note that the verb 'to invent/discover' (Lat. *invenio*) features only once in it, and what Agnodice 'invents/discovers' is not in fact midwifery – she learns that from studying with Herophilus – but rather 'health'. When the Athenian women address the court they say 'You are not husbands but enemies, for you are condemning the woman who *discovered* health for us.'[22] Monica Green suggests that the 'discovery' here takes place in the sense of 'making the knowledge of men available to female patients in a form they could accept'; while this makes sense to a modern reader, it does not work so well within the list of 'discoverers' itself.[23]

Historically, midwives and medical men have taken a range of positions on whether midwifery needs to be 'discovered', as this story suggests, or whether it is entirely natural, simply a matter of women assisting each other and in most cases waiting for Nature to take her course. For early modern writers, such as the French surgeon Pierre Dionis, who wrote his treatise on midwifery in 1718, Adam was the first midwife; as the only other person in the world, he must have helped Eve, if she had any difficulties. Adam then taught 'the Women the Art of it, so far as he understood it'.[24] For Hyginus, too, midwifery or medicine needs to be learned, and from a man. The boundary between men's knowledge and women's

---

[20]   See William A. Hammond (ed.), *Polydori Virgilii de rerum inventoribus; translated into English by John Langley* (New York, 1868), pp. 43 ff. Vergil based his structure on the seven liberal arts, one of these being medicine. Copenhaver, *Polydore Vergil*, p. 165; Hammond, *Polydori Virgilii*, p. 46; using Pliny *NH* 25.30 and *NH* 7.196, *herbariam et medicamentariam [medicinam]*. On Vergil's use of Pliny as his favoured source in Books 1–3, see Atkinson, *Inventing Inventors*, p. 105.

[21]   Tortelli, *De orthographia dictionum e Graecis tractarum*, Book 1, ch. 20 ff.; see Copenhaver, 'The Historiography of Discovery in the Renaissance', p. 208. On Tortelli in general, see Gemma Donati, *L'Orthographia di Giovanni Tortelli. Percorsi dei classici, 11* (Messina: Centro Interdipartimentale di Studi Umanistici, 2006).

[22]   Lat. *vos coniuges non estis sed hostes, quia quae salutem nobis invenit eam damnatis.*

[23]   M.H. Green, *Making Women's Medicine Masculine*, p. 32.

[24]   Pierre Dionis, *Traité general des accouchemens* (Paris, 1718), p. 438; *A General Treatise of Midwifery* (London, 1719), p. 353.

health needs to be crossed, and in his story the one who negotiates this boundary does so by disguising herself so convincingly as a man that her potential patients need to have evidence of her real femininity, while her male enemies assume she must be gaining patients by seducing them; an interesting conclusion to draw, as it raises other issues of crossing the boundaries of the body, and suggests that this is a scenario with which these men are familiar from their own experience. This seamier side of male interest in women's healthcare was taken up by Elizabeth Nihell, a midwife who wrote in 1760 against men-midwives. In the 1771 French edition, Nihell told the story of Agnodice in full, then returned to it at a later point in her book, saying that some accoucheurs – the French term for what in English were called 'men-midwives' – seduce women under the pretext of saving them. She questioned whether the accoucheurs of her own day were people of known integrity, of watertight virtue and above gossip.[25]

Novels

But why is the story of Agnodice so different in content and length from the other items in Hyginus' list of 'who invented what'? One possibility is that the compiler was using a source not from the established literature on inventions and discoveries, but from a very different genre: the ancient novel. The novel was a literary form that originated in the Hellenistic Greek world and was later developed by Roman writers. The earliest of the five novels in Greek that survives in full, Chariton's *Chaireas and Callirhoe*, is dated somewhere between 1 AD and 100 AD, and the genre peaked in the second century AD, so Hyginus would have been writing at a time when the novel was well established.[26] Most scholars today regard these novels as having been written for the elite, although Helen Elsom noted that the novels which survive in full seem to be 'at the more literary end of the spectrum', with those for which we only have papyrus fragments apparently being considerably more sleazy.[27] She has drawn attention to a passage in the work of Theodorus Priscianus, a physician writing in around 400 AD, where he advised novels as part

---

[25]   Elizabeth Nihell, *La Cause de l'humanité, référée au tribunal du bon sens et de la raison: ou traité sur les accouchemens par les femmes: ouvrage tres-utile aux sages-femmes, & tres-interessant pour les familles* (London and Paris, 1771), p. 197: 'Dira-t-on, pour se disculper, que les Accoucheurs d'aujourd'hui sont gens d'une probité connue, d'une vertu à toute épreuve et au-dessus de la médisance?' This section is not in the English version of 1760.

[26]   Helen Elsom, 'Callirhoe: Displaying the Phallic Woman', in Amy Richlin (ed.), *Pornography and Representation in Greece and Rome* (New York and Oxford, 1992), p. 221.

[27]   Ibid., p. 215. For the translated texts of complete and fragmentary novels, see Bryan P. Reardon, *Collected Ancient Greek Novels,* 2nd edition (London and Berkeley, CA, 2008), and for discussion of the genre, Tomas Hägg, *The Novel in Antiquity* (Berkeley and Los Angeles, CA, 1983); Stelios Panayotakis, Maaike Zimmerman and Wytse Hette Keulen,

of the medical treatment for impotence; in the later history of European medicine, a strong link was made between novels and immorality, with nineteenth-century medical writers forbidding entrance to public libraries for the under-twenties, because imagining scenes from novels would lead to the premature development of the sexual organs.[28]

All five of the ancient Greek novels that we have in full take as their central theme a romantic boy–girl relationship, although we know of lost novels with other themes. The story of Agnodice, at least in the summary of the plot that Hyginus seems to be supplying, is not a romance. In other ways, however, it has much in common with the surviving Greek novels; like them, it features a feisty young heroine and themes of long journeys, legal battles, disguise, chastity and the display of the female body.[29] If we are to see the story behind Hyginus' version as concerned with placing midwifery in the nature/culture divide – presenting midwifery not as something that comes naturally, but as something that needs to be learned from male culture – then it could connect with another ancient Greek novel from the early Roman Empire, Longus' *Daphnis and Chloe*. As Froma Zeitlin has shown, that novel challenges the idea that knowledge about sex 'comes naturally', portraying its hero and heroine as being unsure what to do when they are alone together.[30] Perhaps Hyginus' source is giving us a situation in which women simply did not know what to do to help other women giving birth – taking 'the ancients had no midwives' as a statement imagined to apply to all previous human experience – until Agnodice found out on their behalf. Perhaps, for its ancient readers, this was as preposterous a scenario as suggesting that people need to be taught how to have sex. But, one could object, Herophilus *does* know how to practise midwifery; the issue lies with how that knowledge can be transmitted to women, as these are the

---

The Ancient Novel and Beyond, Mnemosyne supplement 241 (2003); Tim Whitmarsh (ed.), *The Cambridge Companion to the Greek and Roman Novel* (Cambridge, 2008).

[28]   Elsom, 'Callirhoe: Displaying the Phallic Woman', p. 215 (citing Theodorus Priscianus, *Euporiston* 2.11 in Valentin Rose, *Theodori Prisciani, Euporiston libri III* (Leipzig: Teubner, 1894), p. 133). Sex manuals also existed in the ancient world; see Helen King, 'Sowing the Field: Greek and Roman Sexology', in Roy Porter and Mikuláš Teich (eds), *Sexual Knowledge, Sexual Science. The History of Attitudes to Sexuality* (Cambridge, 1994). On novels in the later history of medicine, see King, *The Disease of Virgins*, p. 41.

[29]   The possible 'journey' theme exists in the mention of Herophilus as teacher, as he was based in Alexandria but Agnodice in Athens; see further below, Chapter 6. Katharine Haynes, *Fashioning the Feminine in the Greek Novel* (London, 2003), pp. 4–10 critically examines recent claims for a female readership for the Greek novel. See also Elsom, 'Callirhoe: Displaying the Phallic Woman', p. 221 on the pornographic display of Callirhoe's body to the reader. Elsom usefully discusses how the 'act of looking at a woman … confirms the manhood of the looker', p. 228.

[30]   Froma Zeitlin, 'The Poetics of *Eros*: Nature, Art, and Imitation in Longus' *Daphnis and Chloe*', in David M. Halperin, John J. Winkler and Froma I. Zeitlin (eds), *Before Sexuality: The Construction of Erotic Experience in the Ancient Greek World* (Princeton, NJ, 1990), pp. 417–64; King, 'Sowing the Field', p. 35.

only helpers women in childbirth are prepared to accept. As we have already noted, the problem here is that Agnodice learns from him not midwifery, but 'medicine'; however, as we shall see in the next chapter, the name of Herophilus was linked very closely to midwifery.

Hagiography

In addition to its connections with the genres of the 'first finders' and the ancient novel, commentators on the story of Agnodice have also proposed a connection with another genre: hagiography. In 1920, Campbell Bonner argued for a connection between Agnodice and the story of St Eugenia, who avoids marriage by entering a monastery in male disguise, on the grounds that both shared a plot in which 'A young woman who has been led by some stress of circumstances to adopt male attire is accused of immoral conduct and obliged, in order to establish her innocence, to disclose her sex to her judges.'[31] In contrast to Agnodice, Eugenia does this by showing her breasts; in the courtroom context, this was also the gesture used by Phryne – a pagan courtesan rather than a Christian saint – who displayed her breasts when tried for impiety in the fourth century BC.[32] There are some similarities too with the Biblical story of Susanna and the Elders, which was added on to the book of Daniel when it was translated into Greek, probably in the first century BC; here too the female body is displayed, false accusations of improper sexual conduct are made, and a death sentence pronounced on the heroine but avoided after the truth is revealed.[33] Eugenia died in the mid-third century BC, and the first surviving account of her life, written in Armenian, has been provisionally dated to 275 or 280 AD; perhaps those writing her story were familiar with that of Agnodice, rather than Agnodice being the precursor of St Eugenia, but the basic plot of exposure is so widespread that it is impossible to demonstrate a direct link.[34] Like the story of Agnodice, that of Eugenia was first written in Greek; a joke about the 'black and gloomy' name of the character Melanthia, whose name derives from the Greek *melanos*, 'black', would otherwise not work.

A closer similarity between Agnodice and Eugenia – not one drawn out by Bonner, but noted recently by E. Gordon Whatley – is that both of these stories

---

[31]   Campbell Bonner, 'The Trial of St Eugenia', *American Journal of Philology*, 41 (1920), p. 256.

[32]   On the many stories about Phryne, see especially Athenaeus 13.590f–591a and Quintilian, *Institutes* 2.15.9 and Laura McClure, *Courtesans at Table: Gender and Greek Literary Culture in Athenaeus* (London, 2003), pp. 132–6.

[33]   Susanna features in *Daniel* 13:1–64. On the reception of the story and the range of degrees of exposure of her body, see Dan W. Canton, *The Good, the Bold, and the Beautiful: The Story of Susanna and its Renaissance Interpretations* (New York and London, 2006)

[34]   Bonner, 'The Trial of St Eugenia', p. 255.

involve medicine as well as law.[35] Eugenia is accused by a frustrated patient; as 'Eugenius', she heals a woman, who falls in love with 'him' and then accuses 'him' of assault when her passions are not reciprocated. If 'Eugenius' had revealed to patients that 'he' was really a woman, as Agnodice did, this charge could not have been made. In Agnodice's case, of course, although the patients are in on her secret, the rival physicians are not, so it is they who bring her to court. Both stories suggest that the practice of medicine is not only an area of sexual unease but also a key site for the negotiation of gender uncertainty, a central theme of this book.

Phaethousa too has her parallel saints. St Wilgefortis, later known as 'St Uncumber', was killed by her father after her wish to preserve her virginity and avoid marrying her intended husband was granted, and she grew a beard on the morning of her wedding. Popular all over Europe in the fifteenth and sixteenth centuries, she was supposed to have lived in the second century AD. Another saint, too, took this route to purity: St Paula of Avila.[36] As a symbol of militant feminism today, Wilgefortis remains potent; the French feminist group, La Barbe, members of which appear at major events wearing fake beards, has posted a video in which 'bearded' members go on pilgrimage to a statue of the bearded Wilgefortis. Founded in 2006, La Barbe uses the image of the bearded woman as a challenge to male dominance in a range of fields: business, the arts, politics, religion, the public arena, media, sports and sciences.[37] This playful, but also serious, engagement with the image of the body suggests that beards, display, disguise and boundary crossing continue to concern us. Unlike Wilgefortis, however, Phaethousa is not trying to avoid marriage, but is adversely affected by the absence of her husband. The theme of growing a beard thus has a very different meaning in her story.

Art, Myth and Ritual

Modern scholars, including Bonner, have sometimes tried to see the story of Agnodice as a misguided attempt to explain otherwise puzzling physical objects;

[35]   E. Gordon Whatley, 'More than a Female Joseph: The Sources of the Late-Fifth-Century *Passio Sanctae Eugeniae*', in Stuart McWilliams (ed.), *Saints and Scholars. New Perspectives on Anglo-Saxon Literature and Culture in Honour of Hugh Magennis* (Suffolk, 2012), pp. 104–5; he considers that the parallels are 'too numerous to be coincidental'.

[36]   Harry S. Lipscomb and Hebbel E. Hoff, 'Saint Uncumber or La Vierge Barbue', *Bulletin of the History of Medicine*, 37 (1963), pp. 523–7; Brett D. Hirsch, '"What are these Faces?" Interpreting Bearded Women in *Macbeth*', in Andrew Lynch and Anne M. Scott (eds), *Renaissance Poetry and Drama in Context, Essays for Christopher Wortham* (Newcastle-upon-Tyne, 2008), pp. 95–6.

[37]   <http://www.labarbelabarbe.org/La_Barbe/Religion.html> accessed 13 May 2012; <http://www.youtube.com/watch?v=3RWld9elUBE> accessed 6 May 2011. 'La barbe [à la fin]' also means 'enough' in French slang. See <http://www.guardian.co.uk/commentisfree/2011/jun/29/la-barbe-feminism-france> accessed 10 July 2011.

for example, the 'Priene terracottas', found in Turkey in 1898, which date to the early second century BC and merge a female lower torso and a face.[38] Others have looked not to art but to myth, and have tried to tie Agnodice's gesture to that made by the old woman Baubo, when she exposed her lower body to cheer up the mourning goddess Demeter, after the abduction of Demeter's daughter Persephone by the god of the underworld.[39] A further possibility would be to link Agnodice to other stories from the ancient Mediterranean that feature the display of the female body: in addition to those already mentioned, these could include the Egyptian women worshipping the god Apis by lifting their skirts, assumed by scholars to be a fertility ritual; another Egyptian custom described by the historian Herodotus, where women travelling by barge to a festival at Bubastis lift their skirts and shout abuse at the women of the towns through which the river passes (Figure 5.1); and a group of stories in which women lift up their clothes to their fleeing husbands in order to shame them into returning to the battlefield.[40] All of these have some

---

[38]   Overall, Bonner, 'The Trial of St Eugenia', favoured an object as the explanation, arguing that the plot may 'have been suggested by a statue or figure of some sort representing a woman in the act of uncovering her sexual parts' (pp. 258–9). For a summary of the context of the Priene terracottas see Lucia Nixon, 'The Cults of Demeter and Kore', in Richard Hawley and Barbara Levick (eds), *Women in Antiquity: New Assessments* (London, 1995), pp. 84–5. On the terracottas see Maurice Olender, 'Aspects de Baubo: textes et contextes antiques', *Revue de l'Histoire des Religions*, 202 (1985): 3–55; an abbreviated English translation, 'Aspects of Baubo: Ancient Texts and Contexts' appears in David Halperin, John J. Winkler and Froma Zeitlin (eds), *Before Sexuality: The Construction of Erotic Experience in the Ancient Greek World* (Princeton, NJ, 2001), pp. 83–113.

[39]   In the *Homeric Hymn to Demeter*, lines 203–4, the old woman Iambe makes the goddess laugh after Persephone's abduction, although the details of how Iambe does this are not specified here; these come from Clement, *Protr.* 20.1–21.1 and Arnobius, *Adv. Nat.* 5.25–6, where the old woman is called Baubo. On the images linked by modern scholars to Baubo, see Georges Devereux, *Baubo. La Vulve mythique* (Paris, 1983); Olender, 'Aspects de Baubo'. See also Th. Karaghiorga-Stathacopoulou, 'Baubo', *Lexicon Iconographicum Mythologiae Classicae* (*LIMC*) (Zürich and München, 1986) III.1, pp. 87–90. Bonner, 'The Trial of St Eugenia', pp. 260–61 rejected Baubo as a likely source, because images of her were 'monstrous grotesques'. On the myth, see Monique Broc-Lapeyre, 'Pourquoi Baubo a-t-elle fait rire Demeter?', in *Pratiques de langage dans l'Antiquité* (Paris, 1985), pp. 59–76. A recent discussion of the meaning of Baubo's gesture can be found in Laurie O'Higgins, 'Women's Cultic Joking and Mockery', in André P.M. Lardinois and Laura McClure (eds), *Making Silence Speak: Women's Voices in Greek Literature and Society* (Princeton, NJ, 2001), pp. 139–42; developed in Laurie O'Higgins, *Women and Humor in Classical Greece* (Cambridge, 2003), pp. 51–4.

[40]   The Egyptian women are described in Diodorus Siculus 1.85.3; the Bubastis festival is in Herodotus, *Histories*, 2.60; on the 'war stories', best known in Plutarch, *Moralia* 241b (Spartan women) and 246a (Persian women), see Helen King, 'Agnodike and the Profession of Medicine', *Proceedings of the Cambridge Philological Society*, 32 (1986), pp. 63–7. In the war stories the central characters are mature women, unlike the young virgin (Lat. *virgo*, so originally Gk *parthenos*) Agnodice, but the speech they make to their men – in essence,

elements in common with Agnodice: none of them, however, provides an exact parallel.

The gesture shown in images such as the Hellenistic terracotta admits of many possible interpretations, and I shall return to it in Chapter 8; in the context of the history of medical illustration, it also recalls medical texts that illustrated female external anatomy by showing a woman unveiling herself, alongside a discarded Grecian urn, in a classicising pose that seems to recall Agnodice (Figure 5.2).[41]

History

Other aspects of the story make it sound as if it should fall into the category of historical writing; these have contributed to a long tradition of reading it as an accurate account of the past. In 1869 – the year in which, after a long struggle, she was finally admitted to Edinburgh University to study medicine – Sophia Jex-Blake published an essay, 'Medicine as a Profession for Women' in a volume edited by Josephine Butler.[42] Here she argued that women should be physicians to other women, and men to men, using as one piece of her evidence Hyginus' '*history* of Agnodice, the Athenian maiden whose skill and success in medicine was the cause of the legal opening of the medical profession to all the freeborn women of the State' (my italics).[43] Kate Hurd-Mead, who received her MD from the Woman's Medical College of Pennsylvania in Philadelphia in 1888, wrote a history of medicine after she retired in 1925.[44] This book was very much the product of

---

'Where are you running to, worthless men? Are you trying to sneak back inside the place you came out from?' – places the focus on the womb, as well as their straight talking making them not unlike the leading women of Athens in the Agnodice story.

[41]   The urn could also suggest the womb, seen as a jar in ancient Greek medicine; see King, *Hippocrates' Woman*, pp. 26, 34–5.

[42]   Sophia Jex-Blake, 'Medicine as a Profession for Women', in Josephine Butler (ed.), *Woman's Work and Woman's Culture. A Series of Essays* (London, 1869), 78–120. Jex-Blake and her fellow women medical students had to attend separate lectures in Edinburgh; on the cohort see Margaret A. Crowther and Marguerite Dupree, *Medical Lives in the Age of Surgical Revolution* (Cambridge, 2007), pp. 38–44.

[43]   Jex-Blake, 'Medicine as a Profession for Women', pp. 81 and 84–5. While 'history' can simply mean 'account', in this context it implies rather more. When she gives the full story of Agnodice (p. 85, n. 1) she uses Elizabeth Cellier's 1688 version, 'now to be found in the British Museum', rather than any of the published versions in male-authored books; Cellier will be discussed in detail in Chapter 6.

[44]   Originally published in parts in the journal *Annals of Medical History*, it was issued as a book in 1938; further volumes were to follow, but were not completed at the time of her death. On Hurd-Mead see Montserrat Cabré, 'Kate Campbell Hurd-Mead (1867–1941) and the Medical Women's Struggle for History', *Collections. The Newsletter of the Archives and Special Collections on Women in Medicine. The Medical College of Pennsylvania* 26 (1993), pp. 1–4, 8.

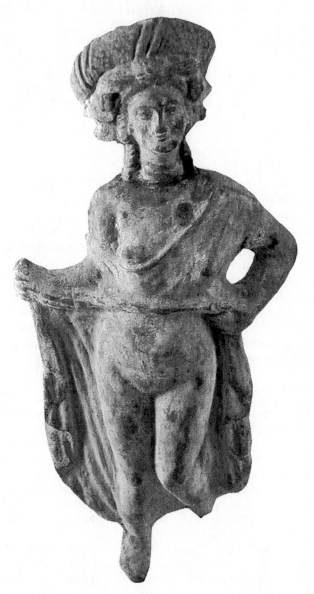

Figure 5.1   Hellenistic terracotta, from Memphis, Egypt, third century BC; the figure has been identified on the basis of the headdress as the goddess Aphrodite, but the gesture may relate to the Bubastis festival in Herodotus (Amsterdam, Allard Pierson Museum. Credits: Barbara McManus, 2003, <http://www.vroma.org/images/mcmanus_images/tcwoman_uncoveringself.jpg>)

the first women physicians looking to history to support their very existence, 'presenting the conquest of the new space as a re-entry ... to give women the strength offered by tradition'.[45] Alongside other women of the classical world, mythical and real, they would include Agnodice. Hurd-Mead argued that Hyginus had taken the story of Agnodice from 'an old book dealing with the history of medicine', possibly Menon, a suggestion she said came from the eighteenth-century writer, Johann Zacharias Platner.[46] Platner had himself added further weight to the historicity of Agnodice by quoting from Samuel Petit's comprehensive and authoritative *Leges Atticae*, 'The Laws of Athens', of 1635.[47] Petit had used the story as evidence of a firmly established ancient Athenian law, 'That no servant, or woman, should learn medicine'. After repeating the story from Hyginus, he added that this was the earlier law, which was then abolished to be replaced with another, that freeborn women could learn medicine.[48] Once the story had settled into place in books on ancient law, Agnodice seemed even more to be a real historical figure.

While any attempt to treat the story as history needs to cope with the lack of a firm date, its geographical context and the proper names have been used in attempts to narrow this down; 'the Athenians' and the Areopagus as the court that tries the heroine suggest a classical Greek context in the fifth century BC. Later commentators on the story noted the role of this court; for example, in an encyclopaedia published in French in 1697, and translated into English in 1702, and which was in print for over 200 years, Pierre Bayle told the story of Agnodice

---

[45]   Cabré, 'Kate Campbell Hurd-Mead', p. 2.

[46]   Kate Hurd-Mead, 'An Introduction to the History of Women in Medicine 1. Medical Women before Christianity (continued)', *Annals of Medical History*, 5 (1933), p. 190 and n. 2, citing Polycarpus F. Schacher and Joannes H. Schmidius, *Dissertatio historico-critica de feminis ex arte medica claris* (Leipzig, 1737), p. 10, who in turn cited Johann Zacharias Platner, *Commentatio de arte obstetrica veterum, in Facultatis medicae in academia lipsiense* (Leipzig, 1735), pp. 9–10; reprinted in Platner, *Opusculorum: Tomus 1: Dissertationes* (Leipzig, 1749), pp. 62–3. However, Menon is not mentioned here, and there are no grounds for Hurd-Mead's suggestion. In Platner, the setting is that the law means the Athenians have no midwives, or more specifically only 'the most unskilled' of midwives (*nullae, vel imperitissimae habuerunt obstetrices*), because they relied solely on experience rather than on anatomical demonstrations. He praises Agnodice for having been taught by a man; in the context of eighteenth-century midwifery, this was a situation that did exist in this period. On men-midwives and their female patients, see further below, pp. 145–6, 161, 197–8.

[47]   Samuel Petit, *Leges Atticae* was first published in 1635. I am using here the 1742 Leiden edition, p. 387, *Veteri olim Atheniensium Lege cautum fuerat, Ne quis servus, neve qua femina, artem Medicam disceret*; Platner cited this passage in *Commentatio de arte obstetrica veterum*, p. 10.

[48]   Petit, *Leges Atticae*, p. 387: *Est igitur prior Lex, quod ad feminas ingenuas spectat, abrogata, et haec altera ei suffecta* (Therefore the earlier law, which dealt with freeborn women, was repealed, and this other was appointed).

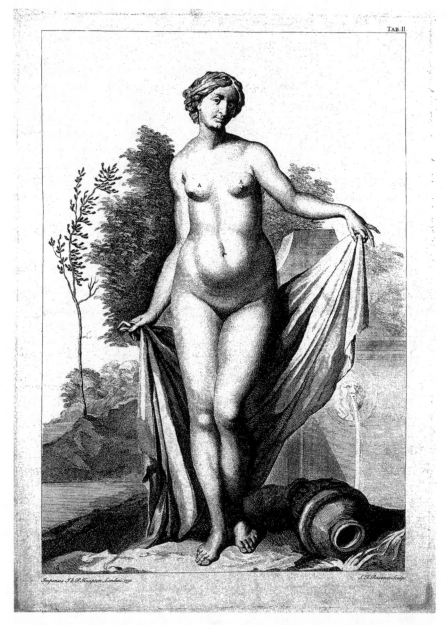

Figure 5.2   Superficial anatomy of the woman: anterior view. Engraving by
S.F. Ravenet after G. Bidloo (London: J. and P. Knapton, 1750)

Note: On Govard Bidloo, see Tim Huisman, *The Finger of God: Anatomical Practice in Seventeenth-Century Leiden* (Leiden, 2009), pp. 108–15; Bidloo intended his anatomical atlas to be a successor to the *Fabrica*.

as being 'too curious a piece of history not to be related in a remark'. He described the Areopagus as 'the most grave and most venerable tribunal that was then in the world'; even the use of the word 'then' suggests the historicity of the story.[49] Anyone with a classical education – that is to say, anyone with an education – would have been very familiar with Aeschylus' play *The Eumenides*, produced in 458 BC. Here the Areopagus tries Orestes for the murder of his mother; the votes being equal, the goddess Athena gives her casting vote in favour of Orestes. The anger of the defeated Erinyes, or Furies, is placated by them being given a cult at Athens, at the north-eastern end of the Areopagus hill, and being renamed the Kindly Ones; their new remit includes the fertility of land and people. The connection with fertility in the original version of the story could perhaps be seen as making this an appropriate place for a midwife to be tried.[50]

In persuading generations of readers that the women-free context with which the story opens represented historical fact, highly influential was the second volume of the very widely read history of ancient Greece compiled by John Potter, who was to become the Regius Professor of Divinity and eventually the Archbishop of Canterbury. Published in 1698–99, translated into Latin and into German, and reprinted many times until 1840, this contains a full retelling of Agnodice's story that opens by reversing the focus of the Latin opening, 'The ancients had no midwives', to make it 'It is observable that the ancient Athenians used none but Men-Midwives'; a negative statement becomes a positive affirmation of men-midwives.[51] In the first half of the nineteenth century, Potter remained the standard work in English on ancient Greece, the obvious place to turn as much

---

[49] Pierre Bayle, *Dictionaire Historique et Critique* (Rotterdam, 1697); the entry for 'Hierophile' is in vol. 2, H–O, p. 83. It was translated into English as *A General Dictionary, Historical and Critical*, 1710, vol. 6, p. 172; Bayle, *The Dictionary Historical and Critical of Mr Peter Bayle*, vol. 3, F–L, 2nd edition (London, 1736), p. 453: s.v. Hierophilus. On the dictionary, at its most popular between 1720 and 1740, see Pierre Rétat, *Le Dictionnaire de Bayle et la lutte philosophiqie au xVIIIe siècle* (Paris, 1971), p. 11 and p. 62; it continued the success of the *Nouvelles de la Republique des Lettres*, which Bayle edited. See also Sally L. Jenkinson, *Bayle: Political Writings* (Cambridge, 2000), 'Introduction', p. xviii; Hubert Bost, *Pierre Bayle historien, critique et moraliste* (Turnhout, 2006), p. 43.

[50] See Aesch. *Eumenides*, 1128–1132. I owe this link to Nicole Loraux. Kenneth J. Dover, 'The Political Aspects of *Aeschylus' Eumenides*', *Journal of Hellenic Studies*, 77 (1957), pp. 230–37 provides a discussion of the extent to which Aeschylus was using the play to comment on the role of the Areopagus court in Athenian life, and the relevance of the radical democratic government in Athens when the play was staged.

[51] John Potter, *Archaeologia Graeca*, vol. II (London, 1722), p. 324. Agnodice appears in Book 4, Chapter 14, 'Of their Customs in Child-bearing, and managing Infants'; the previous chapter covers 'Of the Confinement, and Employments, of their Women'. Ancient Greek customs surrounding women remained of interest in eighteenth-century England. On Potter, see L.W. Barnard, *John Potter. An Eighteenth Century Archbishop* (Ilfracombe, 1989); pp. 22–5 discuss the *Archaeologia Graeca*.

for John Keats as for John Henry Newman.[52] What readers would take away was this suggestion that men-midwives had, until Agnodice, managed all types of birth in classical Athens. Bayle's historical dictionary also argued for previous use of men-midwives in childbirth:

> One might conclude from [Hyginus'] discourse, that from the time that Agnodice laid the women, they no longer imployed the Physicians in that affair, which would prove against this author's own observation, that they made use of their assistance in it before.[53]

A 1759 discussion of whether women should be allowed to practise medicine, by Jean Paul Rome d'Ardène, presented what the Athenians did, not as a desirable model, but as the exception to the normal pattern of human history. As *only* the Athenians had banned women from medicine, with the story of Agnodice showing that even they had soon been forced to change that law, the logical conclusion for d'Ardène was that custom and history support women in the role.[54] So Athens becomes the anomaly, not the ideal. A variation on this was to stress the very short period in which women were banned from practising midwifery; as the physician-historian Jules Rouyer put it in 1859, 'this law was only in operation for a very short time'.[55] D'Ardène did not even mention midwifery; for him, the story was entirely about medicine. Agnodice's first patient is simply 'une femme malade': it is their exclusion from treating any women's diseases ('les malades du sexe') at all that annoys the physicians, and they spread rumours damaging to the reputation of both Agnodice and her patients, accusing her of leading 'une vie licencieuse'.[56] For d'Ardène, Agnodice is just one of a long historical line of successful women

---

[52]   Walter J. Bate, *Keats: A Collection of Critical Essays* (Englewood Cliffs, NJ, 1964), p. 29; Ian Turnbull Ker (ed.), *Letters and Diaries of John Henry Newman*, vol. 18: *New Beginnings in England, April 1857–December 1858* (London and New York, 1968), p. 193, a letter of 1857 to J.B. Morris, asking him 'at what age a Jew (the first born) was formally registered in the family pedigree; – at circumcision? at five years old? on his father's death? – e.g. I turn to Potter, and find at once that Athenian boys were registered at *five* – but I can get no information any where about Jewish'. The footnote identifies this as the 1804 edition of Potter.

[53]   Bayle, *Dictionnaire Historique et Critique*, p. 83: 'car on pourroit conclure de son discours, que depuis qu'Agnodice accouchoit les femmes, elles n'employoient plus à cela les Medecins, ce qui prouveroit contre la proper Remarque de cet Auteur, qu'elles se servoient de leurs bons offices auparavant'. Translation in main text is that given in Bayle, *A General Dictionary*, p. 172; *The Dictionary Historical and Critical of Mr Peter Bayle*, vol. 3, p. 453.

[54]   Jean-Paul Rome d'Ardène, *Lettres interessantes pour les médecins de profession*, vol. 2 (Avignon, 1759), pp. 16–19.

[55]   Jules Rouyer, *Études médicales sur l'ancienne Rome* (Paris, 1859), p. 151: 'cette loi ne fut en vigueur que pendant peu de temps'.

[56]   D'Ardène, *Lettres interessantes*, pp. 17 and 18.

physicians, and the exclusion with which Hyginus' account opens is a 'capricious law, one specific to this state'.[57] The omission of any reference to midwifery is noteworthy, since the story as first told by Hyginus mixed midwifery and medicine, being introduced with 'the ancients had no midwives' but otherwise concerning medicine more generally. In François Gayot de Pitaval's 1732 compilation of anecdotes and sayings, *Bibliotheque des gens de cour, ou mêlange curieux*, the story opens with Hyginus' 'Les Anciens n'avoient point *d'Accoucheurs* (my italics)' but then stresses the midwifery context even more by saying that women were dying specifically 'dans l'accouchement'.[58] But he then went on to say that Athenian law prevented women practising *medicine*. Agnodice (here, Agdonice) felt attracted to that science.[59] After she had learned medicine, she heard women who were giving birth, and after letting them know her true sex she delivered them.[60] The next section starts by saying that, in the past, women's modesty prevented them from giving birth with the assistance of an accoucheur, but nowadays they sacrifice their modesty to fashion. This comment makes this very much an eighteenth-century reading, in which the story of Agnodice is used to attack the lack of modesty of 'modern' women who choose male birth attendants, as well as attacking the male midwives/accoucheurs of that period.

Over the history of the reception of Agnodice, those who wanted to see this story as historically accurate could focus on the alleged absence of midwives as praiseworthy, an anomaly, a short-lived aberration, or a reaction against the excesses of even earlier midwives. In addition, the story could become entirely about childbirth, or could lose all connection with midwifery, and become a story about women physicians. Scholars are still surprisingly reluctant to abandon it altogether as a historical source: for example, in 1997, while concluding that 'the dubious source and fantastic setting make it unwise to place any reliance on the anecdote's veracity', Holt Parker still insisted that 'there may be some remembrance here of a historical character, perhaps indeed a woman doctor'.[61]

In the world outside the narrow group of medical texts used by Laqueur, engagement with the two stories that are my focus here has been extensive. I think that it is precisely because Agnodice's story is impossible to place in any genre of writing that it has remained so open to interpretation, and has been retold for so long. Phaethousa dies: Agnodice lives. She is presented as an active agent, in control of

---

[57] D'Ardène, *Lettres interessantes*, p. 19: 'Loi capricieuse, particulière à cette république'.

[58] François Gayot de Pitaval, *Bibliotheque des gens de cour, ou mêlange curieux* (Paris, 1732), vol. 4, pp. 146–7.

[59] Ibid., p. 146: 'se sentant de l'inclination pour cette Science'.

[60] Ibid.

[61] Holt Parker, 'Women Doctors in Greece, Rome, and the Byzantine Empire', in Lilian R. Furst (ed.) *Women Healers and Physicians: Climbing a Long Hill* (Lexington, KY, 1997), p. 146; Dean-Jones, '*Autopsia, Historia* and What Women Know', p. 47 n. 23, however, finds the story 'without doubt apocryphal'.

her own destiny. She chooses her direction in life and travels to achieve her goals, achieving success as a healer. Unlike the heroine of Susanna and the Elders, her decision to reveal her body to an audience is entirely her own. Even when she is in the power of others, summoned before the court, she takes back control, lifting up her clothes to reveal that she is not a man. At the beginning of the story, Agnodice '*desired* to learn medicine' (Lat. *concupivit medicinam discere*). The strength of the verb, picked up for example in the surgeon Guillemeau's treatise on childbirth, where the English version of 1612 uses 'verie desirous', again recalls the Greek novel, and its interest in the inner emotional lives of its characters.[62] Such is her obvious agency in the story that she has also remained as a role model, not just for La Barbe but also for a contemporary Swiss group promoting understanding of transsexual, transgender and intersexual people. Fondation Agnodice includes on its website a page on 'Who was Agnodice?' in which they give a variation on the standard story of her disguise, trial and acquittal.[63] In this version, Agnodice was encouraged by her father to study medicine; she came top in the medical examinations of 350 BC;[64] her supporters assembled in front of the temple [*sic*] and threatened to die with her; and the law was only changed to allow other women to study medicine in the year after her trial.

In the next two chapters I shall be exploring further the story of Agnodice, both in an ancient and an early modern context. In a Hippocratic model of the body, the predominance of blood in the wet and spongy flesh of a woman, and the role of the womb in containing and then releasing that blood, are central to establishing a 'two-sex' model, or at least one that foregrounds the differences between men and women. In addition, the womb is consistently the organ that fails to fit neatly into an inside/outside, 'one-sex' model. It is my contention that the negotiations and conflicts surrounding the sex of those helping in childbirth are crucial to the way that difference between men and women is represented.

---

[62]   Guillemeau, *Child-Birth*, p. 79 has 'verie desirous to studie therein'.

[63]   <http://www.agnodice.ch/Qui-etait-Agnodice-350-av-JC> accessed 7 January 2011. This is taken from a 2005 version, <http://www.voltairenet.org/spip.php?page=reche rche&lang=fr&recherche=agnodice&x=0&y=0> accessed 16 June 2011.

[64]   This (consciously?) recalls Philippa Fawcett's 1890 achievement in achieving the highest marks in the Mathematical Tripos in Cambridge, at a time when women could not be awarded degrees; she was ranked 'above the Senior Wrangler'. See <http://www. diverse.cam.ac.uk/stories/fawcett/> accessed 12 November 2011.

Chapter 6
Educating Agnodice

Novel or historical account, echoing hagiography or explaining material culture; whatever Agnodice is, this is not a work by a well-known author from the canon of ancient literature. Nor, unlike the sources used by Laqueur, does it come from natural philosophy or medicine. Instead, it is a story that is hard to pin down, not only in its genre but also in its content, which shifted over the period of its popularity, from the sixteenth to the nineteenth century, in particular on whether Agnodice was regarded as midwife, or as physician. As the previous chapter has already indicated, the uncertain genre of the story made Agnodice's uncertain gender no less appealing to its users, male and female alike. In its various versions, the 'true sex' of the central character is generally very easily disguised by changes to her clothing and hair; Hyginus makes this seem simple, as all she had to do was cut her hair and wear male clothing (Lat. *demptis capillis habitu virili*). But, as we have seen, this challenges Galen's comment in *On Seed*, quoted in Chapter 1, that 'We also distinguish man from woman ... not undressing them first so that we may examine the difference in their parts, but viewing them with their clothes on.'[1] For Galen here, sexual difference is obvious without uncovering the body itself: for Hyginus, as in the tradition of the ancient novel, disguise can confuse the audience. However, in later versions the simple uncovering of Agnodice's lower body no longer features as the only way in which her 'true sex' is ultimately revealed.

In the previous chapter, I ended by considering the story as 'history'. The impression of historical accuracy largely depends on the inclusion of Herophilus as Agnodice's teacher; as the only other named character, and as a real figure famous for his work on the female body, he appears to give it a historical context. However, that context would be third-century BC Alexandria, which is problematic when the opening statement that 'The Athenians had no midwives' and the later reference to the Areopagus court both set the story in Athens, and suggest an earlier date.

But Herophilus is significant in another way: as a champion of the one-sex body, who discovered the 'female testes' because he was expecting to find the same organs on the inside of a woman as were present on the outside of a man. In this chapter I shall explore how the various versions of Agnodice's time with Herophilus reflect changing ideas about women's roles, and show that a focus on the two sexes as different, rather than mirror images of each other, accompanies an insistence on a separate branch of medicine for women. First, however, an overview of some users of the story will give a sense of the changing contexts

---

[1] *On Seed* II 5. 8–12, pp. 181–3; see above, p. 38.

in which Agnodice featured during the period when one- and two-sex ideas of the body coexisted. The popularity of Agnodice grew in the period in which the *Gynaeciorum* – a substantial printed collection of ancient, Arabic and contemporary texts on the diseases of women – was compiled, expanded and reprinted; sixteenth-century Europe saw a high level of interest in how medicine should treat women, both within and outside childbirth.[2] But it became even more popular in the seventeenth and eighteenth centuries, when it interacted with changing ideas about midwifery, female modesty, and the appropriate sex for those treating women both in childbirth, and beyond.

'That famous maiden'

I shall begin by illustrating women's own engagement with Agnodice, and the types of text in which they encountered her. The theme of education features strongly in one of the earliest retellings of Agnodice's story after it was printed in 1535; that written by Catherine Des Roches. Cast as an attack on men's envy of educated women, this narrative poem was first printed in 1579, when a collection of writings by Catherine and her mother Madeleine was published after the death of Madeleine's second husband. Madeleine and Catherine hosted a salon in Poitiers, and the principles of humanist education had been applied to Catherine's upbringing; Madeleine was admired by the humanist Scaliger as 'the most learned person in Europe, among those who knew only one language'. This presumably means Latin; as Tilde Sankovich has observed, knowing one's native language would hardly count.[3] In appropriately classicising style, the two women were hailed as the Muses, with their salon as Parnassus.[4] Born in 1542, Catherine never married; unlike her mother, she also learned Greek and probably Italian, and could have met the story of Agnodice in an edition of Hyginus or in the work of Tiraqueau, who retold the story in print when Catherine was seven.[5] The appeal of the strong and educated virgin Agnodice to this unmarried Renaissance woman seems obvious. In Catherine's version, the character of a personified 'Envy' enters the story, and prevents women from receiving an education; the poem as a whole

---

[2]   A table showing the gynaecological and obstetrical treatises included in these collections is given in King, *Midwifery, Obstetrics and the Rise of Gynaecology*, pp. 4–5. On the significance of this period in terms of the wider history of male involvement in gynaecology and obstetrics, see M.H. Green, *Making Women's Medicine Masculine*.

[3]   Sankovitch, *French Women Writers and the Book*, p. 44.

[4]   Jean-François Dreux du Radier, *Bibliothèque historique et critique du Poitou*, vol. 2 (Paris, 1754), p. 429.

[5]   See above, p. 132; André Tiraqueau, *De nobilitate*; Charles Tiraqueau, who I assume is the grandson of André, was a visitor to the Des Roches salon; see Sankovitch, *French Women Writers and the Book*, p. 44.

is presented as one of Catherine's textual 'progeny'.[6] The theme of education also features in Louise Bourgeois (Boursier), born in 1563, and midwife to Marie de Medici between 1601 and 1609, when she published the first volume of her own work; the second followed in 1617. Her husband was a surgeon who – like Jacques Guillemeau – had been trained by Ambroise Paré, and Bourgeois read Paré's publications, but also other surgical books perhaps owned by her husband, such as the work of Paul of Aegina.[7] In *Instruction à ma fille*, she comments to her daughter that, due to her having a brother-in-law who is a physician, a husband training to be one, a brother who is a pharmacist and a father who is a surgeon, together with a mother who is a midwife, 'the body of medicine is a single whole in our household'.[8] In her own particular identification with classical antiquity, Bourgeois regarded not Agnodice, but Phaenarete, the midwife who is named as the mother of Socrates in Plato's *Theaetetus* (149a1–2), as her adviser and her adoptive mother.[9]

---

[6]   Kirk D. Read, 'Touching and Telling: Gendered Variations on a Gynaecological Theme', in Kathleen P. Long (ed.), *Gender and Scientific Discourse in Early Modern Culture* (Aldershot, 2010), pp. 269–70.

[7]   On Paré, mentioned as having trained her husband (who lived in Paré's house for 20 years) and as a source for her own knowledge, see Bourgeois, *Observations diverses*, vol. 2, p. 108; see also M.H. Green, *Making Women's Medicine Masculine*, p. 308; Alison Klairmont Lingo, 'Causes and Cures for Female Infertility, Premature Delivery, and Uterine Disease in the Work of Ambroise Paré and Louise Bourgeois', in Denis Buican and Denis Thieffry (eds), *Biological and Medical Sciences, Proceedings of the XXth International Congress of History of Science* (Liège, 20–26 July 1997) (Turnhout, 2002), pp. 33–8 and ibid., 'Une femme parmi les obstétriciens du XVIIe siècle', <http://www.societe-histoire-naissance.fr/spip.php?article4>, 2008, accessed 16 May 2012; on Bourgeois (1563–1636) in general see Wendy Perkins, *Midwifery and Medicine in Early Modern France: Louise Bourgeois* (Exeter, 1996); Colette H. Winn, 'De sage (-) femme à sage (-) fille: Louise Boursier, Instructions à ma fille (1626)', *Papers on French Seventeenth-Century Literature*, 24 (1997); François Rouget, 'De la sage-femme à la femme sage: réflexion et réflexivité dans les Observations de Louise Boursier', *Papers on French Seventeenth-Century Literature*, 25 (1998); Bridgette Sheridan, 'Whither Childbearing: Gender, Status, and the Professionalization of Medicine in Early Modern France', in Long (ed.), *Gender and Scientific Discourse in Early Modern Culture*, pp. 248–54. The reference to Paul of Aegina comes in Louise Bourgeois (Boursier), *Fidelle Relation de l'accouchement, maladie et ouverture du corps de feu Madame* (1627), p. 16 (= Rouget and Winn, p. 107): 'J'ay leu dans Paul Aeginate.'

[8]   *Instruction à ma fille*, in Bourgeois, *Observations diverses*, vol. 2, pp. 201–202 (= Rouget and Winn, p. 124): 'le corps de la medecine est entier dans notre maison'.

[9]   Ibid., pp. 200–201 (= Rouget and Winn, pp. 123–4; Perkins, *Midwifery and Medicine in Early Modern France*, pp. 26–7): 'La Sage Phanerote mere de ce grand Philosophe Socrate prit pitié de moy, me consola, & conseilla d'embrasser ses sciences … à cause d'elle, dont je serois fille adoptive, tous les disciples de son fils Socrate me seroyent favorables.' She then states her identity again as 'petite fille de Phanerote'.

Seventeenth-century readers encountered Agnodice through a wider range of sources. First was the midwifery manual aimed at an audience of surgeons written by Jacques Guillemeau, published in French in 1609 and in English in 1612.[10] Although writing about midwifery, Guillemeau did not present the story to his male audience as one about childbirth; Agnodice 'became the scholler of Herophylus the Physition' and learned from him not midwifery but 'Physicke'. Agnodice's first patient was a woman who was suffering from a gynaecological disorder; she was 'troubled in her naturall parts', and Agnodice went on to 'cure' – not deliver – many other women.[11] Nicolas Culpeper's *Directory for Midwives*, first published in 1651, also told the story, as did William Sermon's *The Ladies Companion or the English Midwife*, the history of midwifery chapter of which was heavily dependent on Guillemeau, although unlike him Sermon did not give a full version of Agnodice's story, only referring in passing to 'that famous Maiden ... Agnodicea'.[12] Like Guillemeau, Sermon focused on the proper 'government' of the pregnant woman's body; he took other parts of his book from *The Complete Midwives Practice*, a work of 1656 attributed to four midwives.[13]

But Agnodice was not only found in Tiraqueau's defence of women, or in midwifery texts. She also featured in early modern dictionaries in Latin; more like what we would think of as encyclopaedias, these transmitted Agnodice's story to wider audiences across Europe. Charles Estienne's *Dictionarium historicum ac poeticum* went into nine editions between 1553 and 1600, with a further eleven in the seventeenth century.[14] Only in the 1590 edition was Agnodice added, in an

---

[10]   Guillemeau, *De l'heureux accouchement*, 1620 edition, pp. 154–6; ibid., *Child-Birth*, pp. 79–80.

[11]   Ibid., pp. 79–80; in the 1620 French edition, p. 155, the first patient is 'malade en ses parties honteuses'. See further below, p. 200.

[12]   William Sermon, *The Ladies Companion or the English Midwife* (London, 1671), p. 2.

[13]   Rebecca Kukla, *Mass Hysteria: Medicine, Culture, and Mothers' Bodies* (Lanham, MD, 2005), p. 20. On Guillemeau and Sermon: see for example King, *Hippocrates' Woman*, p. 183; Caroline Bicks, *Midwiving Subjects in Shakespeare's England* (Aldershot, 2003), p. 49; Elaine Hobby, 'Gender, Science and Midwifery: Jane Sharp, The Midwives Book (1671)', in Claire Jowitt and Diane Watt (eds), *The Arts of Seventeenth-Century Science: Representations of the Natural World in European and North American Culture* (Aldershot, 2002), p. 157; Hobby, 'Yarhound, Horrion, and the Horse-Headed Tartar', p. 40. On the relationship between Sermon's *The Ladies Companion* of 1671 and *The Complete Midwives Practice* (London, 1656), see Doreen Evenden, *The Midwives of Seventeenth-Century London* (Cambridge, 2000), pp. 8–10.

[14]   After Estienne's death in 1559 it is not known who carried out the editorial work, but changes were based on Natale Conti, *Mythologiae* (1568) and Vincenzo Cartari, *Imagines Deorum* (1581); DeWitt T. Starnes and Ernest William Talbert, *Classical Myth and Legend in Renaissance Dictionaries: A Study of Renaissance Dictionaries in their Relation to the Classical Learning of Contemporary English Writers* (Chapel Hill, NC, 1955), pp. 8–9 and pp. 213–25, esp. pp. 218 and 222; John Mulryan, 'Translations and Adaptations of

abridged version of Hyginus' text, missing out the appeal on her behalf by the leading women of Athens.[15] This was, as we have seen, the period in which any 'one-sex' approach to the body was being rejected as 'absurd' and a Hippocratic model of 'difference' was becoming more significant. In 1624, Thomas Heywood used Estienne's dictionary as the basis of the version of Agnodice he presented in his 1624 *Gynaeikeion: or, Nine bookes of various history concerning women*; it was included in the section 'Of such as have died in child-birth'.[16]

Literary versions of the story, like that written by Catherine Des Roches, were rare, but in 1688 another woman, Elizabeth Cellier, retold the story at some length. Cellier, known to history as 'the Popish midwife', identified very strongly with Agnodice, and her work is also significant because it was through it that Sophia Jex-Blake later encountered the tale. In her pamphlet *To Dr ... An Answer to his Queries, concerning the Colledg of Midwives*, Cellier added many details, and even another character: Agesilea, wife of a member of the Areopagus, whom Dr Agnodice was supposed to have seduced.

In her own words 'born and brought up under Protestant Parents' in the 1640s, Cellier converted to Catholicism during the Civil War after seeing how her parents were persecuted for their loyalty to the King.[17] She lived through, and participated in, a period in which English women were engaging with print culture, but in

---

Vicenzo Cartari's *Imagini* and Natale Conti's *Mythologiae*: The Mythographic Tradition in the Renaissance', *Canadian Review of Comparative Literature*, 8 (1981), p. 274 notes that Conti went into 27 editions, in Latin and in French translation. Estienne's dictionary was based on the *Elucidarius carminum et historiarum seu Vocabularius poeticus* (1498) of Herman Torrentinus (Van Beeck); the final edition I have been able to find of this is 1550 (BL). Both Thomas Heywood's *Gynaikeion: or, Nine bookes of various history concerning women* (London, 1624) and Lemprière's *Classical Dictionary* (1788) were based on Estienne's dictionary.

[15]   Estienne, *Dictionarium historicum ac poeticum* (1590). Agnodice is inserted between two entries, Agno and Agnonia (705 pp): *Agnodice, puella virgo medicinam discere cupiens, abscissa coma, habitu virili, se hierophilo cuidam tradidit in disciplinam, a quo probe edocta parturientem mulierum morbis medebatur, quas sexus sui clam certas faciebat. Tandem a medicis dolentibus se ad foeminas amplius non admittit (obstetrices enim antiqui non habuerunt) in iudicium pertracta quod discerent hunc esse illarum corruptorem: coram Areopagitis tunica alleuata se foeminam esse ostendit. Tunc Athenienses legem emendantes artem medicam discere mulieribus ingenuis permiserunt. Hyginus.*

[16]   Heywood, *Gynaikeion*, p. 203.

[17]   Elizabeth Cellier, *Malice Defeated, Or, a brief Relation of the Accusation and Deliverance of Elizabeth Cellier* (London, 1680), p. 1. On the dissemination of pamphlets in this period, see Mark Knights, *Politics and Opinion in Crisis, 1678–81* (Cambridge, 1994). All Cellier's publications and the responses to them have been reprinted with the original pagination as Volume 5 of *The Early Modern Englishwoman: A Facsimile Library of Essential Works*, Series II, *Printed Writings, 1641–1700: Part 3*, Mihoko Suzuki (ed.) (Aldershot, 2006).

many ways she remains a shadowy figure.[18] She enters the spotlight of history twice: first in 1679–1680, as a political figure, and then in 1687–1688, when she proposed organising the London midwives as a corporate body with an associated foundling hospital. This was designed to solve two problems at a stroke: deaths of mothers and children from 'Want of due Skill and Care, in those Women who practise the Art of Midwifry', and infanticide.[19] Cellier estimated that, in the area covered by the London Bills of Mortality, over 6,000 women had died giving birth in the preceding 20 years; the opening of Agnodice's story, with women dying rather than see a male physician, would immediately resonate with this. Cellier further suggested that 18,000 babies had died during labour or within a month of birth, the majority from errors made by midwives.[20] In her proposed college, midwives would pay membership fees, the income supporting unwanted children; £5 a year from each of the first 1000 midwives and, if more wanted to join, a further 1000 would be admitted at 50 shillings a year.[21] The college would be under female control, but with a monthly lecture being given by the 'principal Physician or Man-Midwife' of the college.[22] Midwives would train more junior ones; this was already happening in seventeenth-century London, but on an individual basis rather than within an institution.[23]

In her final work, *To Dr ...*, Cellier responded to criticism of her proposals, before again disappearing from the historical record, perhaps following into exile Mary of Modena, whom she says that she served professionally.[24] It is not clear whether her opponent 'Dr ...' was a specific individual or simply shorthand for

---

[18]   On women's writing in this period, see Hobby, *Virtue of Necessity*.

[19]   Cellier, *A Scheme for the Foundation of a Royal Hospital, and Raising a Revenue of Five or Six-thousand Pounds a Year, by, and for the Maintenance of a Corporation of skilful Midwifes, and such Foundlings, or exposed Children, as shall be admitted therein* (London, 1687), *Harleian Miscellany*, 1745, p. 243.

[20]   Ibid., p. 243; 'within the Space of twenty Years last past, above Six-thousand Women have died in Child-bed'. She estimates a total of 13,000 children dying 'abortive' and 5,000 'chrysome', with two-thirds of these being due to midwifery errors. 'Chrysome' or 'chrisom' deaths were within one month of birth; for the burials of these infants, the baptismal robe was used as a shroud.

[21]   Ibid., p. 244.

[22]   Ibid., p. 247. As Anne Barbeau Gardiner, 'Elizabeth Cellier in 1688 on Envious Doctors and Heroic Midwives Ancient and Modern', *Eighteenth Century Life*, 14 (1990), p. 25 points out, the amount of male involvement Cellier envisages in her college is minimal.

[23]   Ibid., p. 25 notes that this would be the effect of the scheme; in addition to 'that Person, who shall be found most able in the Arts, and most fit for that Employment' instructing the others 'by reading Lectures, and discoursing to them', a sum would be paid 'upon the Admitting any Woman to be Deputy to any Midwife' (Cellier, *Scheme for the Foundation of a Royal Hospital*, p. 245–6); Evenden, *The Midwives of Seventeenth-Century London* discusses the existing, less formal, 'deputy' system.

[24]   On Mary of Modena, see Elizabeth Cellier, *To Dr ... An Answer to his Queries, concerning the Colledg of Midwives* (London, 1688), pp. 7–8. Penny Richards, 'A Life in

physicians in general but in answering him – or them – Cellier argued for the historical primacy of midwives and for their organisation at a much earlier date than for any similar professional structure for physicians. She answered in the affirmative Dr ...'s question 'Whether ever there were a Colledge of Midwives in any part of the World?', and told the story of Agnodice as a key part of her answer. She may have known the 1647 work of Peter Chamberlen, *A Voice in Rhama*, in which he had written that some people were objecting to the college of midwives that he was then proposing, on the grounds that 'Because there never was any Order for instructing, and governing, of Midwives, therefore there never must be.'[25]

History was therefore essential to Cellier's defence of her proposal; for her, Agnodice provided both a historical precedent and a role model. She gave Hyginus' story a very personal spin, drawing on her own experiences in the London law courts of 1680 to change it so that it mirrored more closely her own life-story; Rachel Weil has singled out 'issues of modesty, cross-dressing, false sexual accusations, the perfidy of paid informers, and women's political action'.[26] As Ann Barbeau Gardiner observed, Cellier's version of Agnodice also uses Biblical rhetoric to tell the story as 'a romance of oppression and deliverance out of the Book of Judges'.[27] The level of identification of Cellier with the 'virgin girl' Agnodice may seem surprising, as Cellier had been married at least three times, but aligning herself with the virginal heroine could be seen as a strategy to counter her opponents' allegations. The rhetoric of modesty appears throughout the pamphlet war in which she was engaged in 1678–1680; midwife and bawd

---

Writing: Elizabeth Cellier and Print Culture', *Women's Writing*, 7 (2000), p. 414 has found evidence suggesting Cellier was in France from 1689.

[25]   Peter Chamberlen, *A Voice in Rhama: Or, The Crie of Women and Children* (London, 1647), p. 13. Her opponents alleged that the words of 'our Wonderful witty thing of a Mid-Wife' were in fact the product of 'a priest got into her Belly, and so speaking through her, as the Devil through the Heathen Oracles'; *The Scarlet Beast Stripped Naked, Being the Mistery of the Meal-Tub The second time unravelled* (London, 1680), p. 4; see also *The Tryal and Sentence of Elizabeth Cellier; for writing, printing, and publishing, a scandalous Libel, called Malice Defeated* (London, 1680), p. 24 in which Cellier's attackers accuse her of being 'an impudent lying Woman; or you had a Villanous lying Priest that instructed you to begin your Book with such a base Insinuation against the best of Religions'; Frances Dolan, *Whores of Babylon: Catholicism, Gender, and Seventeenth-Century Print Culture* (Ithaca, NY, 1999), p. 168. Whatever one thinks of this allegation – and Cellier appears to have been a highly articulate woman familiar with book culture – bearing in mind the Chamberlen family's previous record in proposing structures for the London midwives, it must be a possibility that one of them was associated with her 1687 proposal.

[26]   Rachel Weil, '"If I did say so, I lyed": Elizabeth Cellier and the Construction of Credibility in the Popish Plot Crisis', in Susan D. Amussen and Mark A. Kishlansky (eds), *Political Culture and Cultural Politics in Early Modern England: Essays Presented to David Underdown* (Manchester, 1995), p. 206.

[27]   Gardiner, 'Elizabeth Cellier in 1688', pp. 27–8.

were merged, and her enemies made use of all the midwifery stereotypes of their day, presenting her for example as a 'Brokeress of Buttocks', and accusing her of 'immodest practices'.[28] Her knowledge of female sexual anatomy must, logically, make her a supplier of sexual services, called in to use her 'moving Hand' to satisfy women's sexual desires:

> You're skill'd, what Nature's Fabrick is below,
> And all the secret Arts of Gropeing know,
> Sexes defect with D___do can supply ...[29]

Here, a woman uses her knowledge of the distinctive features of the female genitalia for the purposes of pleasure. In *To Dr* ... Cellier responded to such allegations by combining attacks on her unnamed doctor rival with defence of her own character, often based on the theme of feminine modesty. She mixed evidence of learning, both sacred and profane, with evidence that she was a reliable witness of events. As Rachel Weil's careful analysis has shown, Cellier constructed her credibility despite her identity as both a woman and a midwife; in addition, as a Catholic, she was assumed to be 'illiterate and deceitful'.[30] While the shadow of the Hippocratic Oath also fell on midwives, suggesting that they should not reveal what they learned in the course of their work, it was considered acceptable for them to lie if the aim was to help the woman in labour.[31] While her opponents insisted that midwifery was intrinsically incompatible with truth – as one pamphlet put it, 'Gossiping is so much the soul of Midwifery, that tis impossible for the Profession to subsist without it' – Cellier played with the rhetoric of women's secrets, suggesting that her midwife's experience of dealing with secrets made her testimony trustworthy.[32]

---

[28] *Modesty Triumphing over Impudence. Or, some Notes Upon a late Romance published by Elizabeth Cellier, Midwife and Lady Errant* (London, 1680), p. 11; *Mr Prance's Answer to Mrs Cellier's Libel. To which is Added the Adventure of the Bloody Bladder* (London, 1680), p. 17.

[29] *To the praise of Mrs. Cellier the popish midwife: On her incomparable book* (London, 1680).

[30] Weil, '"If I did say so, I lyed"', p. 194; Dolan, *Whores of Babylon*, pp. 164–5.

[31] Bicks, *Midwiving Subjects*, p. 46 on William Sermon's advice to midwives in *The Ladies Companion*, p. 6: 'able to flatter, and speak many fair words, to no other end, but only to deceive the apprehensive woman, which is a commendable deceipt, and allowed, when it is done for the good of the person in distress'. A similar approach is taken in *The Complete Midwife* of 1656; 'she ought to be prudent, wary and cunning, oft times to use faire and flattering words' (p. 76).

[32] *Thomas Dangerfield's Answer to a Certain Scandalous Lying Pamphlet, Entituled, Malice Defeated* (London: printed for the Author, 1680), p. 7: in full, 'all the World knows that Gossiping is so much the soul of Midwifery, that tis impossible for the Profession to subsist without it'.

In Cellier's version of the Athenian past, women were midwives from a very early date; she uses the godly midwives who saved Moses in *Exodus* 1 as evidence that they were professionally organised long before the physicians.[33] Establishing her knowledge of the Bible and her royalist credentials was part of creating herself as a credible witness, crucial in view of her enemies' attacks on her in 1679–1680.[34] It could also be read as an aspect of her Tory allegiance; as Ann Barbeau Gardiner noted, 'Like other Tories writing political works in the 1680s, Cellier asserts she is no innovator but is following good biblical and classical precedents by incorporating the midwives.'[35] Gardiner also pointed out that going back to an alleged college of midwives in Egypt has parallels with religious debates in this period, in which each side claimed that its faith was the 'primitive' one.[36]

Cellier attributed the ban on midwives in Athens, which she calls 'that Learned Idolatrous City', to two factors; 'some Physicians being gotten into the Government', and 'miscarriages happening to some Noble Women about that time'.[37] Mary Phillips has recently argued that 'Cellier's resistance to male incursion was a projection of alternative truths and an exercise of power through resistance.'[38] In 1687, the incursion took the form of the College of Physicians, supported by the government, gaining the right to control both the books and the personnel of medicine; by having the right to license medical books being published, and by prosecuting untrained practitioners within a seven-mile radius of London.[39] Hal Cook has linked the increasing powers of medical regulation by the College at this time to the need to police the boundaries of medicine in an era when different ideas about the body were flourishing alongside each other.[40] I would suggest that Cellier's 'Physicians being gotten into the Government' relates to this expansion of the College's control. As for the miscarriages, James II's second wife Mary of Modena had lost four babies and had four miscarriages before giving birth to a son – a Catholic heir – in 1688 in what became the 'warming-pan scandal'; issues

---

[33]   Cellier, *To Dr* ..., p. 3 based on Guillemeau, *Child-Birth*, p. 80; also picking up Guillemeau's use of Origen's eleventh homily on *Exodus* and the following sentence, which he relates not to the *Exodus* story, but to Agnodice: 'Beside this curiositie; necessitie, (the mistresse of Arts) hath contrained women, to learne and practise Physicke, one with another'. The issue of midwives appropriate to each faith community was a live one in Cellier's times, especially as she was a Catholic midwife apparently serving the Catholic community.

[34]   Weil, '"If I did say so, I lyed"', pp. 193–4.

[35]   Gardiner, 'Elizabeth Cellier in 1688', p. 24.

[36]   Ibid., pp. 26–7.

[37]   Cellier, *To Dr* ..., p. 5.

[38]   Mary Phillips, 'Midwives Versus Medics. A 17th Century Professional Turf War', *Management and Organizational History*, 2 (2007), 27–44.

[39]   Harold J. Cook, *The Decline of the Old Medical Regime in Stuart London* (Ithaca, NY and London, 1986), p. 204.

[40]   Ibid., p. 209.

of succession and concerns about royal fertility were widespread when Cellier was writing *To Dr* ....[41] A further shift in the story, although not this time one unique to her, occurs when Cellier expands the cause of death among women during the period when there were no midwives in Athens; it is 'both in Child bearing, and by private Diseases; their Modesty not permitting them to admit of men either to Deliver or Cure them'. When Agnodice wins a large clientele, in an echo of the traditional title of the physician St Luke, she 'became the Successful and Beloved Physician of the whole Sex, none but she being called to assist them'.[42]

But it is in the courtroom scene that Cellier, as befits a woman tried on two occasions for libel, most dramatically changes the story. She comments 'there being Witnesses to be found then (as of late Years, that would swear any thing for Money), [Agnodice] was upon their Testimony, condemned to death'.[43] These bribed witnesses are not in the original, nor in her sources; they come from Cellier's own experiences.[44] At her first trial, in June 1680, the jurors who acquitted her asked for payment (she refused this); at her second trial, in September, some of the witnesses for the defence changed their stories, or did not even turn up.[45] She also personalised the charge of adultery; rather than this being general, as in Hyginus, here it is a charge of 'committing Adultery with Agesilea one of the Areopagites Wives; it being easy to make Old Men, who had beautiful Wives, believe any thing of so young and handsome a Doctor'.[46] I have not found this character in any other version; possibly this is a reference to the accusations made against Cellier herself by her enemies, as her own chastity was called into question by her enemies many times.[47]

Cellier also developed the speech of the leading women of Athens; they do not simply condemn their husbands for their actions, but end their speech to the court

---

[41]   Despite the large number of witnesses to the birth, there was a rumour that the child had died and been replaced by an impostor smuggled into the birthing chamber in a warming-pan; Helen King, 'The Politick Midwife: Models of Midwifery in the Work of Elizabeth Cellier', in Hilary Marland (ed.), *The Art of Midwifery* (London, 1993), p. 119; Rachel Weil, *Political Passions: Gender, the Family and Political Argument in England 1680–1714* (Manchester, 1999), Chapter 3, 'The Politics of Legitimacy: Women and the Warming-Pan Scandal'.

[42]   Cellier, *To Dr* ..., p. 4.

[43]   Ibid.

[44]   Gardiner, 'Elizabeth Cellier in 1688', p. 28.

[45]   *The Tryal and Sentence of Elizabeth Cellier.*

[46]   Cellier, *To Dr* ..., p. 4.

[47]   Gardiner, 'Elizabeth Cellier in 1688', p. 28 states 'It is interesting that Cellier does not even consider the possibility that the midwives and noble women of Athens might have been inducing abortions'; however, there is no reason why she should, as this variant is not found at this historical period. Gardiner appears to be relying on Kate Hurd-Mead's version; see her n. 10, where she seems to believe Hurd-Mead's claim that there were other ancient versions of the story.

by 'protesting they would all die with her if she were put to Death'. Gardiner notes that this creates 'a veritable myth of female solidarity'; 'This romantic gesture seems to come out of Cellier's imagination.'[48] Finally, the story ends not just with free-born women (here, 'Gentlewomen') being free to 'Study and Practise all parts of Physick to their own Sex', but adds 'giving large Stipends to those that did it well and carefully, and imposing severe Penalties upon the unskilful and negligent', as well as claiming that thereafter there were 'many Noble Women who studied that Practise, and taught it publickly in their Schools as long as Athens flourished in Learning'.[49] The introduction of financial incentives is yet another of Cellier's additions to the story, and again recalls her proposed College.

Cellier's adaptation is interesting not only because of the ways in which she changes the story, but also for what her version shows about the books known to, and used by, midwives in this period. We can identify the published texts she used. Her Agnodice was mostly based on Guillemeau's 1612 *Child-Birth* which, as already noted, was focused not on midwifery but on physic; since Cellier was a midwife and was not making any claims for women's right to practise medicine more widely, this may seem odd.[50] In Cellier, as in Guillemeau, Agnodice 'found out a Woman that had long languish'd under private Diseases' and 'cured her perfectly'.[51] However, in keeping with her 1687 comments on high mortality rates, she extended Agnodice's story to cover deaths from both 'Child bearing' and 'private Diseases'.[52] She may also have read Heywood, in whose 1624 version of Agnodice a 'college' of physicians features; his version of the jealous doctors states that Agnodice is 'envied by the Colledge of the Physitians'.[53] Also, Heywood's stress on death – placing Agnodice in his section 'Of such as have died in child-birth', and noting that 'many' died as a result of refusing to let any man either 'be seen or known to come about them' – would have resonated with Cellier's own concerns.[54] Cellier would have met Agnodice in other books too; she was familiar with Culpeper's *Directory for Midwives*, and may have known Sermon's *The Ladies Companion or the English Midwife*.[55]

---

[48] Ibid., pp. 28–9. It does not feature in Guillemeau, *Child-Birth*, p. 81, where the leading women of Athens simply 'told them, that they did not account them, for their husbands, and friends, but for enemies; that they would condemne her, which restor'd them to their health'.

[49] Cellier, To Dr ..., p. 4. Gardiner, 'Elizabeth Cellier in 1688', p. 29 draws attention to Cellier's insistence on associating midwifery only with women at the higher end of the social scale.

[50] *To Dr* ..., p. 5 mentions Paré and Guillemeau.

[51] Cellier, To Dr ..., p. 3.

[52] Gardiner, 'Elizabeth Cellier in 1688', p. 28 notes that in Cellier's version women are dying 'both in Child bearing, and by private Diseases'.

[53] Heywood, *Gynaikeion*, p. 203.

[54] Ibid.

[55] Sermon, *The Ladies Companion*, p. 2.

After Cellier, knowledge of Agnodice continued to spread to the wider population, through male-authored midwifery treatises, dictionaries and encyclopaedic works. In 1694 *The Ladies Dictionary, being a general entertainment of the fair-sex. A work never attempted before in English* was published; a compilation from earlier sources, so some entries appear more than once. Agnodice features twice. In the first entry, she is simply listed as 'Agnodice, a Maid Physician'; not, interestingly, as a midwife.[56] The other entry gives a fuller account:

> Agnodice, a Virgin of Athens, who above all things, desired to study Physick, and became so famous therein that the Physicians envyed her, and accused her before the Areopagites or Judges, as an Ignorant Pretender; but she gave such Learned Demonstrations, that the Cause not only went for her, but an Order was made, That any free Woman of Athens, might practice Physick, and that the Men Physicians should no more meddle with Women in Childbirth, seeing the Women were as capable in all matters.[57]

It is interesting that, like the three-word version, this too focuses on Agnodice as *physician*. Agnodice is entirely at the centre of the story; Herophilus does not feature. Furthermore, in this version the ending is as much about banning men, as permitting women.

John Considine and Sylvia Brown have recently edited *The Ladies Dictionary*, and identified the sources for each entry in other works published in the 1690s. The short version of Agnodice comes from an edition of Elisha Coles' *A Dictionary, Latin and English*, where in the second part of the book Coles provides the entry 'Agnodice, who in mans apparel professed Physick, and so took the office of midwifery from men'.[58] The longer version is from Louis Moréri's *The Great Historical, Geographical and Poetical Dictionary*.[59] The French version had no separate reference to Agnodice, and the entry on Herophilus stated only that he was a famous physician who cured Phalaris of a dangerous disease.[60] The English version included more detail than *The Ladies Dictionary*; Moréri describes Agnodice's attendance at 'the School of Heropius [*sic*] in Man's Apparel; where having attain'd to perfection in the Theory, she fell to Practice the Cure of Diseases incident to child-bearing Women, whom she first acquainted with her Sex'. Neither

---

[56]   John Considine and Sylvia Brown (eds), N.H., *The Ladies Dictionary* (Aldershot and Burlington, VT, 2010), p. 32.

[57]   Ibid., pp. 4–5.

[58]   Elisha Coles, *A Dictionary, Latin and English* (London, 1679); *The Ladies Dictionary* uses the 1692 edition.

[59]   Louis Moréri, *The Great Historical, Geographical and Poetical Dictionary* (London, 1694).

[60]   Louis Moréri, *Le grand Dictionnaire historique* (Amsterdam and La Haye, 1702); Herophilus, vol. 3, p. 152.

the element of disguise nor that of revelation is repeated in *The Ladies Dictionary*. Moréri also repeats the original in having the accusation made against her being one of 'Debaucher[y]'. But he is the source for the ban on men in *The Ladies Dictionary*; the judges 'forbad the Men thenceforth to act the Midwife'.

Losing Control

Moréri's suggestion of theory as the sphere of men, practice as that of women, is a common one in this period. Readers of the story have continued to bring to it their expectations about how midwifery as a subject, or women as a group, should be taught, adding in their own speculations about the opening scenario; why were there 'no midwives' in Athens? Earlier writers, unable to countenance the absence of midwives from ancient Athens, and aware of references to them elsewhere in literature and epigraphy, have assumed that something had gone very wrong during Agnodice's lifetime. In 1760 the midwife Elizabeth Nihell, married to a surgeon-apothecary, suggested that

> the midwives themselves had perhaps occasioned the promulgation of so absurd a law. It is well known, that in those antient [*sic*] times, there were for female disorders women-physicians in form. Perhaps their encroachments on the province of the men, by exercising the art of physic in general, might make a restraint necessary, which was only so far faulty as that the remedy was in this, as it often is in other cases, carried into extremes.[61]

For her, separate spheres were not only the norm, but also natural. She presented the story as a 'feeble attempt' to thwart women's natural position as midwives, but she was as opposed to women physicians as she was to male midwives. Both were 'reprehensible' and 'dangerous', although for her the eighteenth-century phenomenon of 'men-midwives' was also 'ridiculous'.[62] While the label 'man-midwife' had been used sporadically in English since 1626,[63] in the seventeenth century it was normally applied to the man, in general a surgeon, who would intervene in difficult births to save the mother, sometimes by turning the child, sometimes by extracting a child who was already dead. By Nihell's time, it was used of those men who claimed the right to control all births, normal as well as difficult. This was not a straightforward 'takeover' of the sphere of the female midwife, but the last stage of a long struggle going back at least to the sixteenth century; our male sources tend to 'overestimate male

---

[61] Nihell, *A Treatise on the Art of Midwifery*, p. 220.

[62] Ibid., p. 3 and pp. 219–20. In the French version of 1771, too, these sentiments are expressed in identical wording to the English version.

[63] Lisa Forman Cody, *Birthing the Nation. Sex, Science, and the Conception of Eighteenth-Century Britons* (Oxford, 2005), p. 41.

prestige in the birthing room and underrate women's continuing ability to limit male practice, or refuse it altogether'.[64]

Agnodice also crossed the boundaries between male control of physic and women's control of childbirth in how she learned her skills. In her 1933 *A History of Women in Medicine* Kate Hurd-Mead included here activities that would have been the province of the surgeon in the early modern period. She stated that

> From [Herophilus] Agnodice must have learned how to perform embryotomy, using a boring and cutting instrument before crushing the child's head. She also performed Caesarian section on a dead mother and did other operations as taught by her master.[65]

Encouraged by Hurd-Mead's shift from assumption ('must have') to certainty ('She also performed'), more recent writers have taken up this addition to the story, and moved it even further. When Hurd-Mead addressed the issue of how women lost control of midwifery, she suggested that 'women doctors' *before* Agnodice 'were sometimes accused of immorality such as performing abortions, etc.'.[66] More specific than Nihell's proposition, this is a long-standing allegation; compare for example Augustus Gardner's 1851 elision of Agnodice with abortionists, mentioned in the Introduction, or Alexis Delacoux's retelling of 1834, in which women had lost their right to be midwives after going further than simply assisting in birth.[67] In a 1986 history of women in science, Margaret Alic wrote, 'In Athens in the fourth century BC women doctors were accused of performing abortions and were barred from the profession.'[68] Towler and Bramall's history of midwifery states 'Another charge against [Agnodice] was that she procured abortions. She is said to have successfully performed Caesarian sections'; we may note how the more cautious wording of the source, Hurd-Mead's 'on a dead mother', has been omitted here.[69]

---

[64]   Lianne McTavish, *Childbirth and the Display of Authority in Early Modern France* (Aldershot, 2005), p. 217. M.H. Green, *Making Women's Medicine Masculine* demonstrates the interest of male physicians in treating infertility, and thus coming closer to involvement in midwifery, before the fifteenth century.

[65]   Hurd-Mead, 'An Introduction to the History of Women in Medicine 1', p. 190.

[66]   Ibid.

[67]   For example, Alexis Delacoux, *Biographie des sages-femmes célèbres* (Paris, 1834), p. 3, 'S'il faut en croire Hyginus, les Athéniens eurent une loi qui défendait aux femmes d'exercer la médecine, ce qui tendrait à faire croire *qu'elles faisaient plus que des accouchemens*' (pp. 3–4, my italics). See also p. 25.

[68]   Margaret Alic, *Hypatia's Heritage: A History of Women in Science from Antiquity through the Nineteenth Century* (Boston, MA, 1986), p. 28.

[69]   Jean Towler and Joan Bramall, *Midwives in History and Society* (Beckenham: Croom Helm, 1986), p. 14.

The abortion references may go back to the dialogue *Theaetetus*, in which Plato's Socrates says that his own mother was a midwife, and that only those who have themselves given birth, but are past the age of childbearing, can take on this role. But does this reflect the historical Athenian midwife, or does it instead consciously play with the image of the midwife to make her better fit the 70-year-old Socrates, midwife of the soul?[70] Plato's Socrates suggests that a midwife 'can bring a difficult birth to a successful conclusion'; he adds that midwives have drugs to bring on labour or to calm labour pains, that they are enthusiastic matchmakers, and they know how to cut the umbilical cord and how to produce abortions. Again, this could relate to the Socratic midwifery of ideas; David Leitao has suggested that this relates to the view that false 'children' – ideas – should not be allowed to 'live'.[71] In the early modern period, there was concern about midwives and abortion in real life, sometimes taking this passage of Plato literally; Pierre Dionis, for example, insisted that midwives should avoid doing anything that could lead to an abortion. They should take care when giving remedies asked for by 'Maids or married Women' wanting to bring on a menstrual period, because this could be a sign of pregnancy; only when the midwife was certain that the reason for the absence of periods was an obstruction should she offer a remedy 'lest she cause an Abortion, or kill the Child in the Mother's Belly'.[72] As we shall see in the next chapter, the scope of a midwife's role in the past was far greater than it has been in modern times, and there is an element of projection here, with writers reading Hyginus' past in terms of their own situation.

For Hurd-Mead, the source of Agnodice's knowledge is Herophilus, but she also presented her education as taking place within the Hippocratic tradition; Hippocrates 'is frequently credited with establishing schools in these studies [that is, gynaecology and obstetrics] where women were received freely as pupils'.[73] There is no evidence for this. In a further embellishment, at the end of the Agnodice story, Hurd-Mead stated that 'a law was passed permitting women to study where

---

[70]   *Theaetetus* 149d–e. Diethard Nickel, 'Berufsvorstellungen über weibliche Medizinalpersonen in der Antike', *Klio*, 61 (1979), p. 516 regarded this passage as the best starting point for any study of the reality of women as providers of health care in antiquity. More recent scholarship has moved away from this position to see Plato's description of the midwife as 'tendentious and self-serving' (the words of David D. Leitao, *The Pregnant Male as Myth and Metaphor in Classical Greek Literature* (Cambridge, 2012), p. 232).

[71]   Ibid., p. 237.

[72]   *A General Treatise of Midwifery*, p. 336. The French original gives a more dynamic picture of women actively asking for remedies and deliberately keeping quiet about pregnancies; see *Traité general des accouchemens*, p. 419: 'Une Sage-femme doit être toujours en garde sur les remedes que des filles ou des femmes lui demandent pour leur procurer leurs ordinaires; car si c'est par une grossesse qu'elles sont arrêtées, ce qu'elles auront soin de lui taire, elle auroit grand tort de leur en donner avant que d'avoir bien examiné qu'elle est la cause qui les empêche d'être reglées.'

[73]   Hurd-Mead, 'An Introduction to the History of Women in Medicine 1', p. 192.

they pleased, and with whom they pleased, and to wear what suited their fancy'.[74] Another modernising and highly misleading version of the story, given in the entry for Agnodice in a recent *Encyclopedia of World Scientists*, is based on Hurd-Mead but goes even further in projecting a modern university system on to the ancient world, so that Hippocrates did not admit women to 'his primary medical school located on the island of Cos' but 'he did allow women to attend another of his schools in Asia Minor, where they could study gynecology and obstetrics'. This version suggests that after the death of Hippocrates women were forbidden to practise medicine 'possibly because Athenian rulers discovered that women gynaecologists were performing abortions'.[75] It then suggests that, growing up in the backlash from this, Agnodice went to study with 'the renowned Herophilus at the University of Alexandria'.[76]

Herophilus the Teacher

The narrative power of the story, and the ingenuity shown in filling in its gaps, has thus continued until the present day. Historically, one response to the naming of Herophilus in the story has been to reject any connection with the historical figure, taking as more significant the indicators of a fifth-century BC setting. In 1766 Jean Astruc commented that 'we are not to confound' Agnodice's teacher with 'the celebrated Herophilus, who lived soon after Hippocrates, as many have done'.[77] Writing in 1834, Alexis Delacoux too stated that this simply could not have been the historical Herophilus; the dates do not work, so it must be another one.[78] This view is based on Hyginus' wording, 'a certain Herophilus' which, as Heinrich von Staden put it, 'deprives Herophilus of his usual celebrity status'; would such a modifier be needed if this were the famous Herophilus?[79] With the exception of one character, who was either an eye-doctor or a horse-doctor, no other ancient medical practitioner with the name 'Herophilus' is known, but perhaps while his name was still very familiar in medical circles at the time Hyginus wrote, it was not known to a general audience, and thus not to Hyginus himself; hence 'a certain ...'.[80] Delacoux's collection of short biographies of historical midwives also noted that Herophilus worked in Egypt, while Agnodice practised in Athens; he did not entertain the possibility of Agnodice travelling to Egypt to study.[81]

---

74   Ibid., p. 191.

75   Elizabeth H. Oakes, *Encyclopedia of World Scientists* (New York, 2007), p. 6.

76   Ibid., p. 6.

77   Astruc, *A Short History of the Art of Midwifery*, p. xxiv.

78   Delacoux, *Biographie des sages-femmes*, p. 26.

79   Von Staden, *Herophilus*, p. 38.

80   A suggestion made by ibid., p. 38 and n. 7.

81   Delacoux, *Biographie des sages-femmes*, p. 26. The problem is also discussed by Diethard Nickel, 'Medizingeschlichtliches in den "Fabulae" des Hyginus', *International*

But if this were originally a novel, the plot could have involved the disguised Agnodice travelling to Alexandria to study; difficult journeys are a trope of ancient novels. Alternatively, it is feasible that the real Herophilus would at some time have travelled to Athens; Heinrich von Staden comments that 'the possibility that Herophilus at some point did practise and teach in Athens, and that an incident during his sojourn there somehow became fictionalized into this anecdote, cannot be excluded with absolute certainty'.[82] But, of course, as von Staden would be the first to admit, nor can it be included with absolute certainty.

As there was a historical Herophilus, I find it difficult to see the choice of this name (either by Hyginus or by his original source) as being anything other than deliberate. He is simply the most appropriate teacher possible for Agnodice because he wrote the earliest treatise on midwifery for which we have evidence: *Maiôtikon*, its reported title making it a book about what *maiai*, midwives, do, and *maia* is the Greek word behind Hyginus' *obstetrix*, as in 'The ancients had no midwives.' Von Staden, who has edited the surviving fragments of Herophilus' lost work, characterises the *Maiôtikon* as 'a wide-ranging work'. From the summaries of, and extracts from, Herophilus preserved in ancient writers including Soranus, Galen, Vindicianus and Paul of Aegina, it appears to have covered theoretical topics such as the material from which the womb is made, and the causes of disease in it, as well as embryology and the classification of the causes of difficult births, including discussion of various foetal positions.[83] While none of the surviving extracts concerns the practicalities of how to assist in childbirth, this does not mean that the original treatise did not cover this; it simply indicates the interests of the later (male) writers who preserved and discussed Herophilus' work. Nor is it always clear whether a reference in one of these later works should be assigned to the lost *Maiôtikon* or to another lost work of Herophilus, *On Anatomy*; von Staden provisionally suggests that some of the preserved material on the male and female reproductive organs was from this latter treatise, but this is based on assumptions about what we think about the level of theory that a midwife would have needed to know.[84]

In the ancient debate about whether gynaecology was necessary – or, to put it another way, about just how different from men women really were – Herophilus regarded the female body as suffering from the same disorders as the male body, made of the same materials, but with some 'affections' (Gk *pathoi*) specific to women. He considered that 'there is no affection peculiar to women, except conceiving, nourishing what has been conceived, giving birth, "ripening" the milk, and the opposites of these'.[85] As we saw in Chapter 1, Herophilus understood

---

Congress of the History of Medicine, 16 (1981), vol. II, pp. 171–2.

[82]   Von Staden, *Herophilus*, p. 39.

[83]   Ibid., p. 297.

[84]   Ibid.

[85]   Summarised in Soranus, *Gynaecology* 3.1 lines 49–52 (Budé, p. 4), tr. von Staden, *Herophilus*, p. 365. On the debates as to whether gynaecology was necessary, see King,

what he saw in his dissections of the female body by analogy with the male; von Staden notes that 'Even where he seems to have taken some halting steps away from the male model, he remains fundamentally enslaved to it.'[86] So, for example, he called the ovaries and the testicles the 'twins' (Gk *didymoi*), observing that women's 'twins' 'differ only a little from the testicles of the male'; he regarded the Fallopian tubes as 'spermatic ducts'. Von Staden also suggests that the assumption that the woman was modelled on the man may have had some benefit here, as it was working from this analogy that encouraged Herophilus to discover the ovaries, even though their function would not be understood for many centuries.[87] In terms of Laqueur's models of the body, this is clearly 'one-sex'; men and women have the same parts, and in this case men's parts move outside during early childhood. But there are still affections specific to women; while the organs may be analogous, what happens to them has no equivalent in the male body. So, does a one-sex model necessarily imply one medicine for both men and women, with a two-sex model suggesting that women need a separate branch of medicine? In Herophilus' version, who should treat the specific 'affections' to which women are subject? His authorship of a *Maiôtikon* would suggest that these are the responsibility of the *maia*, or midwife.

Not surprisingly, many commentators on Agnodice have agreed that Herophilus, as an expert on the reproductive female body, was an appropriate teacher for her; for example, Henry Carrington Bolton, who had been the Professor of Chemistry in the Woman's Medical College of the New York Infirmary from 1875–1877 and returned there in 1880 to deliver an address at the college's commencement exercises. His topic was 'The early practice of medicine by women', and he named Agnodice as 'the first female practitioner who received a medical education'. He dated her to 'about 300 B.C.' and stated that 'Herophilus, the greatest anatomist of antiquity and the first who dissected human subjects' was just one of her instructors.[88] For Bolton, then, writing within nineteenth-century discussions of whether women could learn medicine, Agnodice is a physician, not a midwife. In her 1977 study of the education of ancient women, Sarah Pomeroy commented that '(surely) Herophilus would have been the ideal teacher for the would-be obstetrician'.[89]

Midwifery, Obstetrics and the Rise of Gynaecology, pp. 8–16.

[86] Above, pp. 39–40; Von Staden, *Herophilus*, p. 167.

[87] Ibid., p. 168.

[88] Henry Carrington Bolton, 'The Early Practice of Medicine by Women', *Popular Science Monthly*, 18 (Dec. 1880), p. 192. On Bolton's career, see 'Sketch of Henry Carrington Bolton', *Popular Science Monthly*, 43 (Sept. 1893), pp. 688–95.

[89] Sarah B. Pomeroy, '*Technikai kai mousikai*: The Education of Women in the Fourth Century and in the Hellenistic Period', *American Journal of Ancient History*, 2 (1977), p. 59. The characterisation of Agnodice as a 'would-be obstetrician' assumes a distinction between midwife and obstetrician that is a modern one; in Hyginus, *obstetrix* simply means 'midwife'.

In some versions of the story, it is Herophilus rather than Agnodice who appears to take centre stage. In an early eighteenth-century list of ancient doctors, Agnodice's fame rested not just on being the 'first midwife', but on being a pupil of Herophilus.[90] An important source for later users was Bayle's *A General Dictionary, Historical and Critical*, first published in 1697, where in the later editions she featured not in her own right, but within the alphabetical entry on Herophilus. But although this implies that she was a supporting actor in *his* story, it was still her story that Bayle foregrounded, writing of Herophilus, 'a Physician of whom I can say nothing else but that he taught his art to a certain maid called Agnodice' before giving her story in full in an extensive footnote.[91]

Sometimes, as in Hyginus, Herophilus is Agnodice's only teacher: in later versions, where the story is read through the lens of modern medical education, she has many, but he is the one who has most influence on her. I have already noted that Henry Carrington Bolton used this multi-instructor model in 1880, and he may well have taken it from Alexis Delacoux's 1834 version, which was the standard reference point for the history of midwifery before Kate Hurd-Mead's work in the 1930s.[92] In Delacoux, Agnodice is taught by many knowledgeable physicians of her day, and learns midwifery from more than one person but 'in particular under Herophilus'.[93] Sometimes, within this imagined broad curriculum, Herophilus' lectures are even seen as being responsible for inspiring her interest in midwifery. This assumes that she arrived to learn medicine, but then 'specialised'; again, a modernising reading. For example, in Charles Clay's *A Cyclopaedia of Obstetrics*, published in 1848, Agnodice starts by learning medicine, and is taught midwifery – to which she becomes 'particularly partial' – by Herophilus. In this version, instead of the story ending with the law being changed to allow free-born women

---

[90] This is the list of ancient doctors in Johann Albert Fabricius, *Bibliothecae graecae*, vol. 13 (Hamburg, 1726), p. 42, where she is 'Agnodice, Hierophili discipula, obstetrix prima Athenis'.

[91] Bayle, *Dictionnaire Historique et Critique*, p. 83; 'Medecin, dont je ne saurois dire autre chose, si ce n'est qu'il enseigna la Medecine à une certaine fille nommée Agnodice'. See also ibid., *A General Dictionary* (1710), vol. 6, p. 172; ibid., *The Dictionary Historical and Critical*, vol. 3, F–L (1736), p. 453. In the English versions, Hierophilus is simply 'an Athenian physician remarkable only for instructing Agnodice, who though a Woman, in opposition to the Laws, learned of him the Art of Midwifry in Man's Apparel, and so practiced it; for which being accused, she gave so good reason for what she had done, that she escaped Punishment'. However, in the first edition there is a separate entry on Agnodice, 'An Athenian Virgin, who frequenting the School of Hierophilus in Man's Apparel, attain'd to the perfect Knowledge of Physick, and fell to practise the Cure of Diseases accident to Child-bearing Women, whom she first acquainted with her Sex. Being called in question by the Physicians, as a Debaucher of Women, she discovering her Sex before the Areopagites, not only clear'd herself, but occasioned an Order, whereby the Men were forbid to Act the Midwife.'

[92] Bolton, 'The Early Practice of Medicine by Women'; see above, p. 166.

[93] Delacoux, *Biographie des sages-femmes*, p. 26.

to study medicine, it is changed so that they can study only midwifery.[94] Clay was writing only three years before the foundation of the Woman's Medical College in Philadelphia, so any comment on women and a broader medical education carried a political charge.

In a recent history of midwifery in modern America, Judith Rooks retold the story so that Herophilus is affected by Agnodice, rather than the reverse: 'She was acquitted on the basis of supportive testimony by leading Athenian women. Hearing of this, Hierophilus wrote what is thought to be the first book on anatomy for midwives.'[95] This is an interesting reading because it implies a continuing relationship between pupil and teacher. But even to call the *Maiôtikon* a 'book on anatomy for midwives' is to beg a number of further questions; its audience is not known, and what sounds like a comparable work, Soranus' own book on gynaecology – which, unlike that of Herophilus, survives almost in full – was probably not written for a midwifery audience, despite its content including practical advice on birthing. Instead, a more likely audience for that book would be the Roman head of household looking for a good midwife or wet-nurse for the women under his care.[96]

An even more extreme recent version, in which she is the 'first female doctor and gynaecologist', goes so far as to give Agnodice a precise date: 'In the year 350 BC, on June 3rd, she obtained the highest marks in the medicine test.'[97] This imaginary dating is too early for Herophilus, whom von Staden placed at 330/320–

---

[94]   Charles Clay, *A Cyclopaedia of Obstetrics, Theoretical, Practical, Historical, Biographical, and Critical, Including the Diseases of Women and Children* (Manchester and London, 1848), p. 78.

[95]   Judith Rooks, *Midwifery and Childbirth in America* (Philadelphia, PA, 1999), p. 12. Based on misunderstanding of some weak secondary sources, this is a very unreliable version of the story in all particulars; for example, it has Hippocrates starting 'the first documented formal midwifery program'. For all these details Rooks relies on Maurine Withers, 'Agnodike. The First Midwife/Obstetrician', *Journal of Nurse-Midwifery*, 24 (1979), a poor article based on one encyclopaedia and the second edition of the *Oxford Classical Dictionary*. Withers, who sees Agnodice as a real and 'remarkable woman', does not even realise that there is only one ancient source for Agnodice, and insists on there being two 'descriptions' or 'versions' of her story.

[96]   Soranus 3.3.4 (*CMG* 4.95.17) and 4.1.4 (*CMG* 4.130.9). Von Staden, *Herophilus*, testimonia 193–202c, pp. 365–72. See Ann Ellis Hanson, 'A Division of Labor: Roles for Men in Greek and Roman Births', *Thamyris*, 1 (1994), p. 170 on Soranus Book 2 as 'a script for the midwife to follow when presiding over a normal birthing, yet it was also an assemblage of proper birthing procedures that enabled a Roman *pater familias* to judge competence in the midwives in the household over which he presided'.

[97]   <http://www.voltairenet.org/Agnodice-first-female-doctor-and> (dated 3 June 2005; accessed 16 June 2011). The point of the date is to make this an 'anniversary' story, it being posted on 3 June. The Voltaire Network describes itself as a 'web of non-aligned press groups dedicated to the analysis of international relations'; it is anti-American and right wing.

260/250 BC.[98] This 'medicine test' is not the only example of the projection on to Hyginus' story of a modern medical system. In 1912, when Gilbert McMaster gave a lecture on Agnodice, he went even further. He gave a date which would fit with what is known of Herophilus, but called him 'a famous physician and anatomist of *Athens*', and then claimed that:

> Right here, about 300 B.C. is an instance of a medical practice act, laws governing a license, a state board, and all that sort of thing, with the foreshadowing of the Woman's Medical College ... It is evident that there was a united body of medical men at that period, who were pioneers in organized opposition to illegal practices. There were no doubt exams, and statutes governing the practice of medicine.[99]

Herophilus, however, is not 'of Athens', but originally came from Chalcedon, and then worked in Alexandria. McMaster's reference to the Woman's Medical College brings in the suggestion that something in the story of Agnodice is relevant to a future women-only institution, but the only possible connection is that she was a woman; her own education was certainly not segregated, or there would have been no point in the disguise. His reference to the 'united body of medical men' with their 'organized opposition to illegal practices' recalls the College of Physicians in seventeenth-century London, prosecuting those who practised medicine without a licence; and those prosecuted certainly included women.[100]

The relationship between Agnodice and Herophilus has thus been understood in a range of ways. Sometimes he is her sole teacher, at other times just one of many. For Clay, it is Herophilus who leads to Agnodice's interest in midwifery: for Rooks, her trial is the stimulus for him to write the *Maiôtikon*. How do these responses to the story help us to understand the original? No other teacher is named there, and as I have already indicated it seems to me pointless to name Herophilus unless this is done to evoke the famous physician known for his work on midwifery and anatomy. To name him can be a further way of underlining the claim that knowledge of the female body was, at that time, in the hands of men. But the naming of Herophilus does not mean that Agnodice must have been a real person; anyone trying to make the story sound convincing could have chosen his name to insert here. If the medicine that Agnodice practises is thought to require anatomical knowledge, then he would indeed have been the ideal teacher.

98   Von Staden, *Herophilus*, p. 50.
99   Gilbert T. McMaster, 'The First Woman Practitioner of Midwifery and the Care of Infants in Athens, 300 BC', *American Medicine*, 7 (1912), pp. 202–5. On the Woman's Medical College, see above, p. 24. Extracts from McMaster's article, including Agnodice, were reprinted in the *British Journal of Nursing Supplement*, 49 (Dec. 14, 1912), pp. 486–8.
100   On the role of the College of Physicians in prosecuting irregulars, Cook, *The Decline of the Old Medical Regime in Stuart London*, Appendix 2, listing the regulatory activity of the College.

However, this brings us up against a major question in the history of midwifery education, one which I have touched on already; just what is a midwife supposed to know? This question depends on what her role is supposed to include: normal births? Difficult births? Diseases of women unrelated to childbirth? I shall return to this theme in the next chapter.

I have found just one version of the story that omits any reference to Herophilus: the one told by Elizabeth Nihell in the eighteenth century. The original English edition of Nihell contained no mention whatsoever of how Agnodice learned her craft; she was simply described as having 'dressed herself in mens cloaths, to elude the cognizance of the law'.[101] The French version of 1771 was fuller; Agnodice 'resolved to disguise herself, and in men's clothing, *went to learn* the art of midwifery in order to evade the pursuit of the Laws' (my italics).[102] This version is based on the 1708 work by Philippe Hecquet, *De l'indecence aux hommes d'accoucher les femmes*, which was also repeated ten years later when Pierre Dionis criticised it.[103] In Hecquet, not only midwifery but also medicine is mentioned, and Herophilus is named: Agnodice went to learn 'medicine, above all the art of midwifery, in the famous medical school of Herophilus'. Dionis, too, included this clause about Herophilus.[104] In Nihell's version, in contrast to her possible male sources, Herophilus has been removed; for Nihell, Agnodice still 'goes to learn ...' but there is no sense of where, how, or from whom, and this subtle omission (deliberately?) obscures the men who instruct women.

Nihell is thus performing precisely the opposite manoeuvre to that of her predecessor and rival, the prominent man-midwife William Smellie. Summarising the history of midwifery in 1752, Smellie condensed the story into 'Hyginus relates, that in Athens a law was made, prohibiting women and slaves from practising physick in any shape: but the mistaken modesty of the sex rendered it afterwards absolutely necessary to allow free women the privileges of *sharing this art with the men*' (my italics); for him, men's attendance in childbirth is constant

---

[101]   *A Treatise on the Art of Midwifery*, p. 220.

[102]   *La Cause de l'humanité*, p. 184 n. (a): 'prit le parti de se déguiser, et sous l'habit d'un homme, *alla s'instruire* de l'art d'accoucher pour se dérober à la poursuite des Loix'.

[103]   Philippe Hecquet, *De l'indecence aux hommes d'accoucher les femmes* (Paris, 1708); I am using here the pagination of the edition published by Trevoux: l'Imprimerie de S.A.S. and Paris: chez la Veuve Ganeau, 1744. For his versions of Agnodice, see Dionis, *Traité general*, pp. 439–40, translated as *A General Treatise of Midwifery*, pp. 353–4.

[104]   Hecquet, *De l'indecence aux hommes*, p. 32, 'prit le parti de se déguiser, et sous l'habit d'un homme, alla s'instruire de la Médecine, sur tout l'art d'accoucher, dans la fameuse école de Médecine d'Hierophile' = Dionis, *Traité general*, p. 440. The other place in the story at which it is clear that Nihell has Hecquet's text in front of her is the reference to fashion; in Hecquet, Agnodice 'entra en pratique avec tant de succès et de vogue, que la jalousie en prit aux médecins. Ils attaquent le prétendu Accoucheur ...' (p. 32) while in Nihell, she 'entra en pratique avec tant de succès et de vogue, que la jalousie en prit à ceux qu'on avoit chargé de suppléer aux Sage-Femmes. Ils accuserent ce prétendu Accoucheur ...' (p. 184).

before and after Agnodice's story.[105] Unlike Nihell, who made this a story about midwifery, Smellie was – perhaps deliberately – ambiguous as to whether the 'art' here is midwifery or medicine more broadly, but the context favours midwifery.[106] Here, although the story still needed to be told, being by then an expected part of the history of medicine, it was not Herophilus but Agnodice who was left out. For Smellie, it was not her, but Hippocrates, who founded midwifery; he was 'Father of Midwifery as well as medicine'.[107]

Agnodice the Pupil

In the late seventeenth century, writing to advise a minimalist approach to normal childbirth, Percival Willughby criticised midwives who used 'too much officious doings' and suggested that 'A woman is not borne a midwife; It is education, with practice, that teacheth her experience.'[108] In Willughby's period, the focus was on working with an experienced senior midwife, rather than on learning from books; he praised the London system in which 'The young midwives ... bee trained seven years first under the old midwives, before they bee allowed to practice for themselves.'[109] A similar model was used elsewhere in Europe at this time.[110] The different models at which this hints – natural ability, education, practice, books, apprenticeship – raise questions of what Agnodice is thought to have learned in her time with Herophilus, and how she learned it. Are there any hints in the earliest version of this story in Hyginus as to what sort of knowledge or skill Agnodice was supposed to have gained from her teacher, and whether it would have been classified as medicine or as midwifery?

I have already mentioned Kate Hurd-Mead's suggestion that Agnodice learned from Herophilus 'how to perform embryotomy' as well as how to carry out

---

[105]   William Smellie, *A Treatise on the Theory and Practice of Midwifery*, 2nd edition, corrected (London, 1752), p. ii, picked up by [Philip Thicknesse], *Man-midwifery Analysed: and the Tendency of that Practice Detected and Exposed* (London, 1764), p. 15. The first edition of Smellie even omitted the name of Hyginus; it starts 'In Athens a law was made ...' while the second edition has 'Hyginus relates, that in Athens a law was made ...'.

[106]   Smellie, *Theory and Practice of Midwifery*, p. ii.

[107]   Ibid., p. iv; King, *Midwifery, Obstetrics and the Rise of Gynaecology*, p. 92.

[108]   Percival Willughby, *Observations in Midwifery*, ed. Henry Blenkinsop (Warwick, 1863), p. 209 and p. 73; see also p. 206. Born in 1596, Willughby practised midwifery himself and also had midwives in his family. He lived in London from 1656–60, so would have been familiar with the London midwifery system from this period.

[109]   Ibid., p. 73.

[110]   For the French evidence, see McTavish, *Childbirth and the Display of Authority*, p. 30 and pp. 50–51, n. 39.

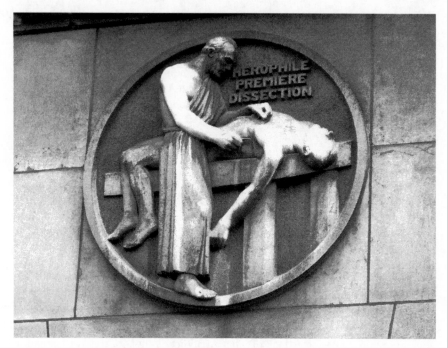

Figure. 6.1   Herophilus is represented as 'dissector' on the Paris Faculty
               of Medicine medallions; to the right of the main entrance, this
               image is used, with Agnodice two medallions further to the right.
               Courtesy of Ralph Shephard

Caesarean section and other procedures.[111] Herophilus is best known to medical
history for performing human dissection (Figure 6.1);[112] so would Agnodice, too,
have needed to examine cadavers? The answer given to this question is heavily
dependent on when it is produced. Hal Cook has drawn attention to a Mrs Nokes,
a midwife in the first half of the seventeenth century, who had apparently dissected
at least one body, and who taught one man anatomy.[113] But she was an exception: in
early modern Europe anatomy was more commonly seen as irrelevant for women,
with no value for a midwife. For example, in the 1670s Percival Willughby said
that for midwives lower down the scale of literacy, 'it would do no good to speak
to them of the anatomizing of the womb, or to tell them of the learned works of

---

[111]   Hurd-Mead, 'An Introduction to the History of Women in Medicine 1', p. 190;
above, p. 162.

[112]   Although Hurd-Mead has no evidence for her statement that he 'dissected many
hundreds of human bodies'.

[113]   Cook, *Decline of the Old Medical Regime*, p. 33, citing the Annals of the Royal
College of Physicians, vol. 3, folio 188b.

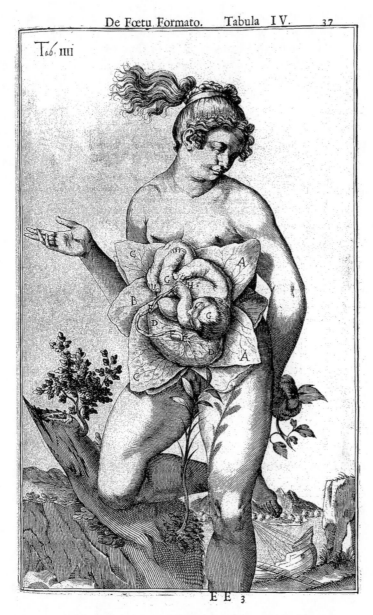

De Fœtu Formato.   Tabula IV.   37

Tab. IIII

E E 3

Figure 6.2   Spigelius, 'De formato foetu liber singularis aeneis figuris exornatus' in *Opera quae extant omnia* (Amsterdam: Johannes Blaue, 1645), table 4

Mercatus, or Sennertus, or Spigelius'.[114] Even *telling* midwives about anatomy was seen as irrelevant to what they did; they were certainly not expected to find it beneficial to see bodies for themselves. On the limited value of books showing anatomy, even the well-known illustrations in the editions of Spigelius, one of which is reproduced here (Figure 6.2), striking as they are, would do nothing to help a midwife understand the birthing process.

The question of whether a midwife needed to know anatomy and, if so, whether she needed to attend dissections, became more prominent as a result of eighteenth-century changes in the training of men for midwifery which concentrated on knowledge of the mechanics of birth, so that understanding pelvic anatomy became central. *The Midwife Rightly Instructed* (1736) is a dialogue between a surgeon and a young woman called 'Lucina' – the name of a Roman goddess of childbirth – who comes to a surgeon for 'Lectures' after having two years with an 'Instructress' that had proved less than satisfactory.[115] Its author, the Cambridgeshire surgeon Thomas Dawkes, suggested that men's superiority came from their knowledge of anatomy based on dissection; where contemporary authors disagreed, it was to dissection that he appealed for the truth. Although he thought that midwives should at least see a skeleton, he did not think that they needed experience of dissection.[116]

By the mid-eighteenth century there is also evidence that the models of, or based on, the female pelvis, which were used to train men-midwives, were also employed to train some women. William Clark wrote in 1751 of women in London having access to 'the anatomical Wax-work, with suitable Lectures', and noted that some male tutors 'instruct both sexes by mechanical Demonstrations'.[117] But even if anatomy was now considered relevant to midwives, this did not mean that they were thought to need to attend dissections. In the nineteenth century, resistance to dissection for women remained strong; this was a period in which a

---

[114] Willughby, *Observations in Midwifery*, p. 2.

[115] Thomas Dawkes, *The Midwife Rightly Instructed* (London, 1736), pp. xxv–xxvi; reprinted in Stephen Freeman, *The Ladies Friend* (London, 1787), pp. 291 ff, where the pupil is renamed 'Sophia'. Lisa Forman Cody, 'The Politics of Reproduction: From Midwives' Alternative Public Sphere to the Public Spectacle of Man-Midwifery', *Eighteenth-Century Studies*, 32 (1999), p. 487 and n. 44 does not seem to realise that Freeman is copying Dawkes. Adrian Wilson, *The Making of Man-Midwifery. Childbirth in England, 1660–1770* (Cambridge, MA, 1995), p. 116 notes that Dawkes was one of the provincial practitioners of the 1730s who 'bridged the divide' between the different views of pro- and anti-forceps London men-midwives.

[116] Dawkes, *The Midwife Rightly Instructed*, pp. xii–xv and p. 24 on the surgeon's reference to 'my own Experience' of dissecting women who die in late pregnancy.

[117] William Clark, *The Province of Midwives in the Practice of their Art* (London, 1751), p. 2. This may be a reference to lectures given in conjunction with one of the waxworks on display in this period; see for example *A Catalogue and Particular Description of the Human Anatomy in Wax-Work, and several other preparations to be seen at the Royal-Exchange* (London, 1736).

widespread argument against allowing women to enter medical schools was that it would in some way damage their femininity, causing, in Laura Kelly's words, 'a loss of womanliness'.[118] Male physicians stated that they were unable to 'imagine any decent woman wishing to study medicine'.[119] Even at the end of the nineteenth century, when women were allowed to train as physicians, the dissecting-room remained a male preserve; women, if they were allowed to dissect, had to do it without men present.[120] Yet, despite this long history of separating women from dissection, in some versions of the Agnodice story, the association of Herophilus with dissection is so strong that Agnodice's medical education simply has to include this; for example, in the apothecary Richard Walker's *Memoirs of Medicine*, published in 1799, Agnodice's 'passion for the art induced her to attend anatomical dissections, disguised in man's attire'.[121]

The Latin used for Agnodice's purpose in going to Herophilus is quite open; she *tradidit in disciplinam*. Grant translates this by saying that Agnodice went 'to a certain Herophilus *for training*' while Smith and Trzaskoma have 'became the student of a certain Herophilus *for formal instruction*'.[122] The translations carry their own assumptions about what Agnodice learned; 'training' implies a craft, while 'formal instruction' suggests theoretical learning. Neither English term is really appropriate here. A comparable passage from a similar date would perhaps be the description in Suetonius' life of Nero of him being 'consigned to the training' (Lat. *in disciplinam traditus*) of the philosopher Seneca the Younger, when he was ten years old.[123] The Latin verb *disco* means to learn, and can have the sense either of acquiring knowledge or of learning a skill; Hyginus' representation of what Agnodice learns from Herophilus as a *disciplina* is thus indeterminate, and cannot be used to support any arguments about whether the story was originally about midwifery or medicine, craft or science. The distinction is in any case

---

[118] Laura Kelly, '"Fascinating Scalpel-Wielders and Fair Dissectors": Women's Experience of Irish Medical Education, *c*.1880s–1920s', *Medical History*, 54 (2010), p. 499; p. 498 mentions the use of segregated dissecting rooms in Irish medical education; Catriona Blake, *The Charge of the Parasols: Women's Entry to the Medical Profession* (London, 1994).

[119] Carol-Ann Farkas, 'Aesculapius Victrix: Fiction about Women Doctors, 1870–1900' (PhD thesis, University of Alberta, Edmonton, Alberta, 2000), p. 45, quoting Jex-Blake, *Medical Women*, p. 72 on Professor Laycock. Farkas also describes the mob throwing mud at women who tried to attend extramural anatomy lectures in Edinburgh in 1870.

[120] In Dublin a century later, men and women were usually taught together, but Kelly, '"Fascinating Scalpel-Wielders and Fair Dissectors"', pp. 509–10 points out that the one area where segregation was insisted upon was dissection.

[121] Richard Walker, *Memoirs of Medicine, Including a Sketch of Medical History*, Book 1 (London, 1799), p. 56.

[122] Grant, <http://www.theoi.com/Text/HyginusFabulae5.html#274> accessed 4 July 2011; R.S. Smith and Trzaskoma, p. 180.

[123] Suetonius, *Nero*, 7.1.

inappropriate in the ancient world; the original Greek word used would almost certainly have been *technê*, a term meaning art, craft or science. It has been defined as any 'practical activity that required intellectual competence *as well as* manual dexterity, was based on scientific knowledge, produced results that it was possible to verify, and was governed by well-defined rules that could be transmitted by teaching' (my italics). To avoid reading this definition in too modernising a way, we should remember that among these 'arts', 'crafts' or 'sciences' the Greeks included subjects as diverse as shoe-making and divination.[124]

In contrast to the early modern history of midwifery, where practice was gendered female and theory male, the ancient Greek art of medicine thus involved manual as well as intellectual skills. In his *Republic*, set in around 421 BC, Plato observes that the minds of a male or a female healer have the same nature, providing direct evidence that both sexes could be engaged in the medical *technê*; in Latin, the *ars medicina*, as in the opening statement of Agnodice's story, that the Athenians forbade any slave or woman from learning the *ars medicina*.[125] In his analysis of the Hippocratic *Oath*, Heinrich von Staden has also suggested that one of the characteristics of a *technê* is that it creates a sense of belonging to a group stretching across the generations.[126] In this sense, teaching a woman a craft/science would be a significant move, not an individual transaction but rather an initiation into a group.[127]

This chapter has underlined just how open to interpretation the story of Agnodice is. While we know of midwives in the Greek and Roman worlds, and have some evidence for them being involved in difficult births as well as in areas

---

[124]   Gian A. Ferrari and Mario Vegetti, 'Science, Technology and Medicine in the Classical Tradition', in Pietro Corsi and Paul Weindling (eds), *Information Sources in the History of Science and Medicine* (London and Boston, MA, 1983), p. 202; in *Technology and Culture in Greek and Roman Antiquity* (Cambridge, 2007), p. 9, Serafina Cuomo examines ancient discussions of *technê* in relation to the features of 'great usefulness, moral ambiguity, [and] strong political resonance'.

[125]   ... *nam Athenienses cauerunt ne quis seruus aut femina artem medicinam discere*; Sarah B. Pomeroy, 'Plato and the Female Physician (*Republic* 454d2)', *American Journal of Philology*, 99 (1978), p. 497 notes that one Renaissance manuscript, Vind. Bon. Sc., omitted the reference to a female medical nature; Gerard Boter, *The Textual Tradition of Plato's Republic* (Leiden, 1989), p. 215 notes that this omission 'must be deliberate, but cannot possibly be correct'.

[126]   Heinrich von Staden, '"In a Pure and Holy Way": Personal and Professional Conduct in the Hippocratic Oath?', *Journal of the History of Medicine and Allied Sciences*, 51 (1996), pp. 412 and 416. On the social status of the ancient physician see also H.F.J. Horstmanshoff, 'The Ancient Physician: Craftsman or Scientist?', *Journal of the History of Medicine and Allied Sciences*, 45 (1990), pp. 176–97.

[127]   Lesley Dean-Jones, *Women's Bodies in Classical Greek Science* (Oxford, 1994), p. 32 argues that, in the Hippocratic Oath, the statement that the swearer will regard his teacher's children as equal to his male siblings could be taken to mean that his teacher's daughters, too, could be taught medicine by him.

that are not narrowly confined to the birthing process, we also know of female physicians; early modern readers of the story knew of these women, too. Does evidence exist outside Hyginus for the gendering of medical practice? Where should Agnodice be placed in the structure of ancient health care? We have seen that the story was retold with very specific purposes as part of early modern and modern debates about who should practice both medicine, and midwifery. In the next chapter, we shall continue to reflect on the relationship between these two areas, and consider what Agnodice's patients are supposed to be suffering from; how broad is the scope of her practice in Hyginus, and how has this subsequently been interpreted by her readers?

Chapter 7
Agnodice's First Patient

In the previous chapters we have reflected on the possible origins of the story of Agnodice. In many ways reminiscent of a Greek novel, with what may appear to be 'natural' – sex, midwifery – being presented as something that needs to be taught, the story has elements that make it sound like a historical account. However, it resolutely refuses to be tied to any point in reality; the name of Herophilus suggests a third-century BC date, but it is difficult to do much with a name, and the Athenian setting of the story does not correspond with what little is known of the real Herophilus' movements. The inclusion of Herophilus may invite us to read the story in a 'one-sex' way, but nobody in the story suspects that Agnodice is a woman in whom the inside organs have moved outside; instead, everything she does underlines the complete difference between the sexes. Where Phaethousa's 'outside' is at two levels, the public and the private, with the public suggesting that she is a man, but her genitalia confirming that she is a woman, Agnodice's chosen disguise projects a public image that is so persuasive that only her display of her lower body can counter it. As we have seen, for her later readers, Agnodice has oscillated between being read as a 'midwifery' story and being understood as a 'women physicians' story: the opening sentence about the absence of midwives does not seem to fit with the rest of the framing of the story, nor with its ending in which women are permitted to practise 'medicine'.

In this chapter I want to use these varied readings and their historical contexts to discuss further Hyginus' version, its possible original context, and its subsequent uses. After reflecting on the issue of the contrasting emphases on medicine, or on midwifery, in different adaptations of the story, I shall focus on two key passages, both of which are important when considering Laqueur's models of the 'one-sex' versus the 'two-sex' body. The first of these is the reference to shame that forms part of the opening of Hyginus' story: *antiqui obstetrices non habuerunt, unde mulieres verecundia ductae interierant*, literally 'The ancients had no midwives; because of this,[1] women perished, misled by shame.' This sentence was omitted entirely from Tiraqueau's sixteenth-century version. How does shame relate to the differences between the male and the female body, and the sex of those caring for each, and how does Agnodice's display of her body to her first patient and to the court fit in here? What is she supposed to be proving? With the identical gesture of lifting up her tunic (*tunica sublata/tunicam alleuauit*), in both cases she 'showed herself to be a woman' (*ostendit se feminam esse*). To her patients, this is a gesture

---

[1]   Literally 'from where'; 'because of this' is the translation of R.S. Smith and Trzaskoma, *Apollodorus' Library and Hyginus' Fabulae*, p. 180. Grant similarly has 'as a result'.

of solidarity, but to the court it carries a rather different message. In both cases, she is showing the absence of a penis; for her patients, this makes her someone in front of whom shame is unnecessary, but to the court this absence proves that she is unable to have seduced her patients. The second passage is that in which Agnodice treats her first patient. How have different readers understood what is wrong with this woman in particular? This will help to answer certain questions implicit in the story: namely, for what conditions are women in general thought to be unwilling to consult men, and can a woman be effectively treated by a man? Is the difference between men and women, focused on childbirth, such that they require their own sex to treat them, and if this is true in childbirth, then does it also apply to medical conditions? I shall be arguing that the different versions of Agnodice's story owe very little to Laqueur's assumptions about the history of the body, and much more to the changing sexual politics of medicine that may, or may not, choose to play up the factor of 'difference'. The story not only moves us into an area of knowledge far from the mainstream medical and scientific sources favoured by Laqueur, and told over a long period from his 'one-sex' into his 'two-sex' era; it also demonstrates the importance of reading each version in detail, and shows how irrelevant the notions of 'one- and two-sex' are to understanding the body as represented here.

Defining Terms

Why are there no midwives at the start of the story? Are we to assume that birth was simply seen as something separate from disease, with midwives being in charge of birth and male healers treating women's diseases? But what if birth did not proceed normally, due to some underlying or acute condition? Furthermore, early modern writers could present pregnancy *as* a disease; Guillemeau wrote that 'the greatest disease that women can have is that of the nine Moneths, the Crisis and cure whereof consists in their safe deliverie'.[2] Guillemeau went on to note that women have always been midwives but, in contrast to many early modern writers, recent scholarship has responded to Hyginus not by accepting his opening scenario as historically accurate, but by assuming that midwives were barely visible to the Hippocratic writers, and indeed the *maia*, or midwife, does not appear at all in the earliest Greek medical texts, the *Diseases of Women* treatises of the Hippocratic corpus; Ann Hanson has proposed that this silence is responsible for Hyginus' 'the ancients had no midwives'.[3] Nancy Demand argued that in ancient Greece midwifery was 'a female activity that in general was taken for granted', with Hippocratic physicians 'only called in if special difficulties were being

---

[2]   Guillemeau, *Child-Birth*, p. 81; ibid., *De l'heureux accouchement*, 1620 edition, p. 156, 'la plus grande maladie que les femmes puissent avoir, est celle des neuf mois, dont la crise & guarison ne fait par leur accouchement'.

[3]   Hanson, 'A Division of Labor', p. 181.

experienced'.[4] Sue Blundell stated that 'Female wisdom concerning childbirth was doubtless handed down by word of mouth. Consequently, we possess very little information about normal deliveries.'[5] All this is problematic; the argument from silence could be reversed, and we could instead argue that it is precisely because we have so little information about normal deliveries that we assume they must have been controlled by women. In other historical periods, the scope of the role of the midwife has been far wider than it is now. In the eighteenth century, midwives could also practise some medicine and surgery, including bloodletting, so that Adrian Wilson proposed that 'The midwife was the women's doctor, and perhaps the women's confidante, of early-modern England.'[6] It is therefore possible that the Hippocratic writers were deliberately excluding any reference to midwives due to professional rivalry.

To make matters more complicated, *Diseases of Women* does include isolated references to women whose identities cannot easily be mapped either on to the category of 'midwife' or that of 'female physician', and scholarly response to their presence is instructive. In the Hippocratic corpus, for example, in the final chapter of the treatise *On Fleshes* we meet *akestrides*. Like the Greek word commonly translated as 'physician' – *iatros* – the male form of this noun simply means 'healer'. It comes from the verb *akeomai*, 'to heal' or 'to mend'; the verb, and words based on it, can also be used in other craft contexts, being applied to mending clothes or shoes. The writer states that anyone wanting proof that a child born in the seventh month survives, while one born in the eighth month never does, should 'go to the *akestrides* who are present at birth and ask them'.[7] 'Female physicians' would perhaps seem a better translation here than 'midwives', and the great nineteenth-century translator of the Hippocratic corpus, Emile Littré, indeed called them 'the female healers who helped women in childbed': Paul Potter, however, recently translated the word as 'midwives', presumably influenced by the context here.[8]

Another character who is hard to place is *hê omphalêtomos*, the 'cord-cutter'; the feminine form of the definite article means that this is a woman, which would otherwise not be clear.[9] Like the *akestrides*, she features only once in the

---

4   Nancy Demand, *Birth, Death, and Motherhood in Classical Greece* (Baltimore, MD and London, 1994), p. 66; Sue Blundell, *Women in Ancient Greece* (London, 1995), p. 110.

5   Ibid., p. 111.

6   A. Wilson, *The Making of Man-Midwifery*, p. 38.

7   *Fleshes* 19, L 8. 614. Jacques Jouanna, *Hippocrate* (Paris, 1992), p. 175 makes a lot of this passage, which also states that all the author knows on this topic is what women have told him (Littré 8.610); for Jouanna, this single reference is evidence that 'Les accoucheuses étaient appréciées pour leur expérience même par les médecins.'

8   Littré 8. 615, 'les guérisseuses qui assistent les femmes en couche'; cp. Potter, Loeb VIII, p. 165.

9   Plato, *Theaetetus* 149e uses the nominal form, 'cord-cutting', as one of the roles of the midwife.

Hippocratic corpus, where she is criticised for cutting the cord too soon.[10] Is this a fixed and limited role? Is she a midwife or female healer to whom the role of cutting the cord is specifically allocated? Or is this something that can be done by any woman present, rather than a specific identity? In another Hippocratic treatise, *Superfetation*, concern is expressed about tearing the cord.[11] In Plato, Aristotle and later Soranus, cutting the umbilical cord is one of the roles of a midwife; Soranus described how midwives were unhappy about using iron to cut it, as this was seen as bad luck.[12] Early modern medicine also saw cutting the cord as one of the roles of the midwife, requiring much skill; writing in 1671, Jane Sharp mentioned the midwives' belief that cutting it short was supposed to make a girl's vagina narrow and ensure she would be 'modest', while for boys it should be cut long so that they would have a longer penis.[13] Once again, we meet the problem of how to use this patchy, *longue durée*, evidence. Does the midwife always fill the role of cord-cutter?

A further Hippocratic reference, once again an isolated one, is to the *iêtreousa*, who features in a description of a difficult delivery in which the child, who appears to be dead, is too large to come out or is presenting in an oblique position. If the child is presenting head first, the woman should be shaken on her bed at each contraction, with a man taking each of her feet.[14] The *iêtreousa*'s role is to open the mouth of the womb gently, then to pull on the umbilical cord. This suggests that the context of *Superfetation*'s comment on someone tearing the cord refers to a manoeuvre of this kind, and that it was one that could be – or that was always? – performed by a woman. Like Potter translating *akestrides*, Littré here gave 'sage-femme', based on the midwifery context: Ann Hanson, however, translated as 'the woman who doctors', arguing that the choice of this word – like *akestrides*, and *iatrinê*, a female form of the male noun for a healer – means that she 'possessed medical ability or training'.[15]

In the sources, women who may have more general medical training are a little easier to find and to identify than midwives, mostly due to the evidence of inscriptions, but again the terminology is not straightforward. Epigraphically, women are identified either as *medica*, or as what sounds like the Greek equivalent, *iatrinê*. But without fuller accounts in other types of source material we cannot say what their role was; specifically, would they treat men as well as women, and

---

[10]   *Diseases of Women* 1.46, Littré 8. 106.

[11]   *Superfetation* 8, Littré 8.482; Loeb IX, p. 324–6.

[12]   Aristotle, *History of Animals*, 587a9–24; Plato, *Theaetetus* 149e; Soranus, *Gynaecology* 2.6.7–11, Budé p. 17.

[13]   'A Midwives skill is seen much if she can perform this rightly', Sharp, *The Midwives Book* (ed. Hobby), pp. 164–5.

[14]   *Diseases of Women* 1.68, Littré 8. 145. Hanson, 'A Division of Labor', p. 173, n. 59 notes that *trôsmôn*, translated by Littré as 'dans un avortement', could be either an abortion or a miscarriage; in any case, it means that the child is already dead.

[15]   Hanson, 'A Division of Labor', p. 175.

how would their roles differ from those of midwives?[16] Holt Parker extended the positive evaluation of silence to women physicians as well; what is important, he argued, is precisely the absence of any surviving discussion of these women, or any list of their names, because it shows that women in healing roles, although 'undoubtedly only a small percentage of the medical personnel', were considered unremarkable.[17]

A further twist is that modern scholars have tried to distinguish between midwives, with limited theoretical knowledge or training, and a practice restricted to childbirth: and 'obstetricians', with a higher level of education. Modern translations of Hyginus reflect assumptions about this hypothetical two-tier model. In 1960, Mary Grant translated the opening Latin as 'The ancients didn't have obstetricians', but R. Scott Smith and Stephen Trzaskoma have recently rendered this more accurately as 'The ancients did not have midwives.'[18] In her influential 1977 article on the education of women in the ancient world, Sarah Pomeroy followed Grant's 'obstetrician' translation.[19] For her, Agnodice 'wanted to become an obstetrician', and 'The career of obstetrician is to be distinguished from that of a midwife as requiring more formal education.'[20] But, while it gets over the historical problem of imagining an Athens without any midwives at all, translating *obstetrices* as 'obstetricians' and then inserting into Hyginus' story a distinction between 'obstetricians' (new, formally educated) and 'midwives' (always in existence, but not educated), is highly misleading. The Latin *obstetrix* did not originally suggest a male operator, nor a higher level of education; its etymology,

---

[16] Flemming, 'Women, Writing and Medicine in the Classical World', *Classical Quarterly*, 57 (2007), p. 257. Flemming developed the earlier study of Nickel, 'Berufsvorstellungen über weibliche Medizinalpersonen in der Antike', which in turn built on Hurd-Mead, 'An Introduction to the History of Women in Medicine' and Paul Diepgen, *Die Frauenheilkunde der Alten Welt*, Handbuch der Gynäkologie 12, 1, Geschichte der Frauenheilkunde 1 (Munich, 1937). The evidence from the Greek world to the Latin West is conveniently listed in H. Parker, 'Women Doctors in Greece, Rome, and the Byzantine Empire', pp. 140–46, who updates the epigraphic listing of Louis Robert, 'Femmes médecins' (s.v. *Mousa Agathokleos iatreinê*) in Nezih Firatli and Louis Robert, *Les Stèles funéraires de Byzance grécoromaine* (Paris, 1964), pp. 175–8.

[17] H. Parker, 'Women Doctors in Greece, Rome, and the Byzantine Empire', p. 131. However, he does not have the data from which to calculate the percentages.

[18] R.S. Smith and Trzaskoma, *Apollodorus' Library and Hyginus' Fabulae*, p. 180. It is not clear where their 'many' comes from. Grant's translation still dominates; for example, <http://zagria.blogspot.co.uk/2012/06/hagnodike-3rd-century-bce-physician. html> accessed 14 November 2012, wrongly attributed to 'Mary Beard'.

[19] Above, p. 166; Pomeroy, '*Technikai kai mousikai*', p. 59. She does not cite Grant, or indeed any edition of Hyginus, but I assume from the similarities that she was in fact using Grant's translation.

[20] Pomeroy, '*Technikai kai mousikai*', pp. 59 and 58. She even criticised Peter M. Fraser for 'mistakenly' referring to Agnodice as 'the first midwife' in his *Ptolemaic Alexandria* (Oxford, 1972), vol. II, pp. 503–4, n. 57.

from the Latin verb *obsto*, is simply 'to stand before', or 'to meet face-to-face'. Comparable to the Anglo-Saxon 'midwife' meaning to stand 'with a woman', it is thus simply the standard Latin word for 'midwife', and here presumably translates the Greek *maia*. To translate it in any other way is to impose a distinction taken from the nineteenth- and twentieth-century American situation, in which the medical profession's opposition to female midwives has been far more complete than in Britain.[21]

Scholars have also proposed that status distinctions between female healers increased over time. Fridolf Kudlien argued that the term *iatrinê*, 'woman physician', emerged in the Hellenistic period, and he saw her as someone who was both a midwife and a 'gynaecologist'.[22] He proposed that this meant 'a greater and greater jurisdiction' for such women, citing the treatise which the first century BC physician Heracleides of Taras addressed to the *iatrinê* Antiochis as evidence of the high regard in which they could be held, and the high status they could reach.[23] Holt Parker suggested that the *iatromaia*, an identity found in some funerary inscriptions, was a midwife with some extra medical training, located halfway between midwife and physician.[24] But in the lexicon of the fifth or sixth century AD writer, Hesychius, the entry for midwife, *maia*, opens: 'Grandmother, nurse, and the physician (Gk *iatros*) attending women in labour'. The text of Hesychius is complex, the result of abridgements and interpolations; it survives in only one manuscript, dated to the fifteenth century.[25] But, even bearing in mind all these cautions, this source suggests that a midwife *is* a physician. Here, as in a much better-known source, the funerary inscription of the Athenian woman Phanostrate, dated to the second half of the fourth century BC, a woman is not called anything that sounds like 'female physician', but is simply a 'physician'. Phanostrate, both midwife (*maia*) and physician (*iatros*), 'caused pain to none'; for those trying to find a historical location for her fellow Athenian, Agnodice, she can be a useful

---

[21]   On the differences between the British and the American history of midwifery from the nineteenth century onwards, see Judy Barrett Litoff, *The American Midwife Debate: A Sourcebook on its Modern Origins* (Westport, CT and London, 1986), a collection of primary sources with commentary. See also Richard and Dorothy Wertz, *Lying In: A History of Childbirth in America* (New York, 1977). Hanson, 'A Division of Labor', p. 174 observed that the American situation has affected our reading of Hippocratic treatises in which men appear to be attending normal births.

[22]   Fridolf Kudlien, 'Medical Education in Classical Antiquity', in Charles D. O'Malley (ed.), *The History of Medical Education*, UCLA Forum in Medical Sciences, no. 12 (Berkeley and Los Angeles, CA, 1970), p. 17; see also Valentina Gazzaniga, 'Phanostrate, Metrodora, Lais and the Others. Women in the Medical Profession', *Medicina nei Secoli, Arte e Scienza*, 9 (1997), p. 282.

[23]   Kudlien, 'Medical Education in Classical Antiquity', p. 18.

[24]   H. Parker, 'Women Doctors in Greece, Rome, and the Byzantine Empire', p. 132.

[25]   ... *kai peri tas tiktousas iatros*; Hesychius, s.v. *maia*; on Hesychius see Eleanor Dickey, *Ancient Scholarship* (Oxford, 2007), pp. 88–90.

dating aid, suggesting that the change in the law after Agnodice's court appearance must have predated her own dual role.[26] The problem with that interpretation is of course that it does not fit with the mention of the third-century BC Herophilus.

A further question concerns whether the *iatrinê* is a woman who is simply a physician like any other, or a woman who only treats other women. Rebecca Flemming has noted that some inscriptions that do not use any term for 'midwife' or 'woman physician' claim universality for the woman they honour – 'saviour of all', 'protector of her fatherland from disease' – which may suggest that some women were indeed treating men as well as women.[27] Gillian Clark has drawn attention to Aemilia, a woman in Gaul in the late fourth century AD, who – perhaps in an echo of Agnodice? – chose virginity and 'practised the arts of medicine in the way men do'.[28]

The evidence for different female roles in midwifery and/or medicine in antiquity is thus highly fragmentary, spread over a millennium, and offering a poor base on which to build a chronology arguing for the expansion of women's roles in healing. Yet this has not prevented further speculation about how such expansion could have taken place. Nancy Demand believed that 'female physicians' in fifth- and fourth-century BC Greece were midwives who had gained extra experience and reputation by learning from, or working alongside, Hippocratic (male) physicians.[29] She observed that craftspeople were the most literate in antiquity, and that this was the social stratum from which midwives seem to have come; she also speculated that, as books in antiquity were read aloud, midwives could have been 'auditors in a medical course or read medical treatises themselves'.[30] In her earlier work on women physicians in ancient Greece, Sarah Pomeroy went further in suggesting that they would have had what she calls 'advanced formal education'; they would have 'successfully completed the studies necessary to become physicians'.[31] This scenario sounds very modern, and it is misleading, projecting a much later model of medical training on to the ancient world.

In addition to arguing from silence and making assumptions about the terminology used for healers, modern scholarship tends to project back a model originating in early modern Europe, in which midwives were responsible for

---

[26] IG II/III, 3² 6873. Holt Parker, 'Women and Medicine', in Sharon L. James and Shelia Dillon (eds), *A Companion to Women in the Ancient World* (Oxford: Blackwell, 2012), p. 122 argues that 'and' (*kai*) on the inscription is 'making a clear distinction between the two roles'. However, this is pushing the reading of a basic conjunction.

[27] Flemming, 'Women, Writing and Medicine', pp. 259–60. H. Parker, 'Women Doctors in Greece, Rome, and the Byzantine Empire', p. 137 also suggests that women physicians treated men.

[28] G. Clark, *Women in Late Antiquity*, p. 68 citing Ausonius, *Parentalia* 1.13–14: *more virum medicis artibus experiens.*

[29] Demand, *Birth, Death, and Motherhood in Classical Greece*, pp. 67–8.

[30] Ibid., p. 67.

[31] Pomeroy, 'Plato and the Female Physician', p. 500.

normal births, and male surgeons for difficult births. But it is misleading to suggest that, in the ancient Greco-Roman world, normal birth was the concern only of midwives. Male physicians certainly did not regard it as outside their area of expertise. For example, in the Hippocratic treatise *Diseases* 1, in a description of the *kairoi*, the 'opportune moments' when action must be taken at precisely the right time for a successful outcome, we read that the most acute moments include 'when you must deliver a woman that is giving birth or miscarrying'.[32] There are numerous other examples in the Hippocratic texts of physicians attending pregnant women, including being present at births. For example, in *Diseases of Women*, the author notes that when a woman is giving birth she breathes rapidly, and the speed increases as the moment of birth draws near; he goes on to list a number of other symptoms of approaching birth, and gives remedies to ameliorate them. Some of these are for 'difficult' births – such as a dry labour – but the general observations apply to all births.[33] In *Epidemics*, Ann Hanson identified 33 such case histories, in 19 of which there was information on the births; only five of these were identified by the writers as 'difficult', while in another seven we can find some evidence of complications.[34] From this material, Antoine Thivel and Lesley Dean-Jones have both argued that Hippocratic physicians must have attended normal births.[35] Furthermore, these men considered that remedies to promote conception, signs of pregnancy and care during pregnancy came into their sphere of control.[36]

Medicine or Midwifery?

Returning now to the story of Agnodice, in its original context, was this intended to be a story about medicine, or about midwifery? Being located in a list of discoverers/inventors, Agnodice is immediately set up to be 'the first' at something, and in line with this it opens with a situation in which 'the ancients had no midwives'. Yet, as we have seen, what she desires to learn is stated as 'medicine' and when the law

---

[32]   *Diseases* 1.5, Littré 6. 146.

[33]   *Diseases of Women* 1.34, Littré 8. 78–80.

[34]   Hanson, 'A Division of Labor', pp. 171–3.

[35]   Dean-Jones, *Women's Bodies in Classical Greek Science*, p. 212 going rather further than Antoine Thivel, *Cnide et Cos? Essai sur les doctrines médicales dans la Collection Hippocratique* (Paris, 1981), p. 137, as Hanson, 'A Division of Labor', p. 173 n. 53 observes. *Nature of the Child* 30 (Littré 7. 530–40; renumbered as 19 in Loeb X, pp. 80–90 because the latest editor, Paul Potter, discounts the tradition by which this was the second part of a longer treatise that started with the treatise *On Generation*) opens 'Whenever a woman is about to give birth', which implies that medical men were present at this point.

[36]   Ibid., discussed in Hanson, 'A Division of Labor', pp. 176–8; *Superfetation* 12–13 (Littré 8.484; Loeb IX, p. 326); *Superfetation* 18 (Littré 8.486; Loeb IX, p. 330); *Superfetation* 26 (Littré 8.488–90; Loeb IX, 332–4); the topic of the best way of ensuring pregnancy is repeated in *Superfetation* 30 (Littré 8.498–500; Loeb IX, pp. 342–4).

is changed at the end of the story, it is not so that free-born women can practise as midwives, but so that they can learn the art of medicine.

Is this a casual elision of the two fields, or an indication that the story was originally about medicine, but was given its opening line in order to make it fit into 'who invented/discovered what'? Often, as we have already seen, later versions mix the two professional fields, with midwifery presented as a subdivision of medicine. For example, as I noted in Chapter 6, the early nineteenth-century Agnodice of Alexis Delacoux has a rounded medical education and then specialises in midwifery; other versions, too, imagine her learning general medicine, then choosing to concentrate on this branch.[37] A less well-thought-out statement, but one which also seems to assume that midwifery is part of medicine or physic, features in the 1679 dictionary which summarises the plot simply as: 'Agnodice, who in mans apparel professed Physick, and so took the office of midwifery from men'.[38] This already assumes that the absence of female midwives means the presence of male midwives. This is not an obvious move (as it could simply mean no midwives at all) but it is encouraged by the phrase about 'shame', to which I shall return in the next section of this chapter, and also by the presence in the story of the jealous doctors who find they are not wanted once Agnodice appears on the medical scene; while nothing is explicit here, this suggests that they had formerly seen these patients. But, historically, was midwifery part of 'medicine'/'Physick', or was it something existing independently, practised by different people? For Delacoux, it is the physicians, wanting to take over control of childbirth, who deliberately extend the boundaries of 'medicine' so that it will encompass 'midwifery'.[39] The range of possibilities in existing translations, as well as in the different renditions of the story given by subsequent readers, allow us to think about the different options, and also their implications. As I have already suggested, Agnodice is 'good to think with' precisely because of the contradictions in Hyginus' text that make these different readings possible.

After 1535, the date when Hyginus' work began to circulate in print, the story of Agnodice spread and evolved, as we have seen. But in her early modern afterlife, Agnodice began as a woman physician, rather than a midwife. It seems to have been so obvious that midwifery was a woman's role that the opening statement of Hyginus could be dropped entirely. Shorn of its opening scenario, the story became one about medicine. So, in the 1550s, Agnodice featured in Tiraqueau's list of '*Foeminae medicae*', 'Women physicians', which began with the goddess Diana (in her Greek form, Artemis); this was part of a work on 'nobility' and the

---

[37]   Delacoux, *Biographie des sages-femmes*, p. 26.

[38]   Coles, *A Dictionary, Latin and English*, n.p.

[39]   Delacoux, *Biographie des sages-femmes*, p. 25: 'ils prétendirent en même temps que les accouchemens, formant une branche de la médecine, devaient être exclusivement exercés par eux'.

aim was to show that practising medicine is not incompatible with nobility.[40] This was an issue because, from the Roman Empire onwards, to work with the hand was considered ignoble. Tiraqueau repeated the text of Hyginus almost word-for-word, but completely omitted the opening statements that 'the ancients had no midwives', and that this was leading to women dying from shame.[41] He also referred to the story in the 1554 edition of his *De legibus connubialibus*.[42] Furthermore, although the individuals referred to were goddesses and characters from Greek myth – for example, Helen of Troy, Agamede, and Cleopatra – it was common knowledge that there had been women in healing roles in the ancient world; as we saw in Chapter 6, Elizabeth Nihell commented that 'It is well known, that in those antient [*sic*] times, there were for female disorders women-physicians in form', possibly based on the 1612 English translation of Guillemeau: '… Antiquity telleth us, that there have beene Mid-wives even from the beginning: yea, that divers of that sexe have practised Physicke'.[43]

Giving a list of women doctors from the ancient world did not mean that the compiler thought that women should be able to attend universities with men, and subsequently qualify alongside them. The powerful physiques of statues from antiquity suggested to sixteenth-century people that ancient bodies were more impressive than their own: perhaps this superiority meant that the women of the

---

[40]   Tiraqueau, *De nobilitate et iure primogeniorum*, 5th edition, Chapter 31, p. 410. The first edition was in 1549 (Paris) with a second undated, then a third in 1559 and a fourth in 1560.

[41]   The other changes he makes are minor; giving '*aegritudinem*' for Hyginus' '*imbecillitatem*' and then in the final line, where Hyginus has the Athenians changing the law so that free-born women could learn the *ars medicina*, inserting *caveruntque*, making this 'and stipulated that freeborn women could learn medicine'. The theme of shame will be explored further below.

[42]   Tiraqueau, *De legibus connubialibus* (Venice, 1576), Book 3, no. 69; p. 57a; there was no reference to Agnodice, in either the very short 1513 first edition, or the 1524 400-page edition, because Micyllus' edition of Hyginus did not appear until 1535. The 1546 fourth edition is considerably expanded. Agnodice entered the 1554 edition of 720 pp. (Lyons), for which material was added to Book 3. This became the final form of this book, nothing further being added for the 1576 edition; see Jacques Bréjon, *André Tiraqueau (1488–1558): un jurisconsulte de la Renaissance* (Paris, 1937), p. 54 and 381.

[43]   Nihell, *A Treatise on the Art of Midwifery*, p. 220; Guillemeau, *Child-Birth*, p. 79; ibid., *De l'heureux accouchement*, 1620 edition, pp. 153–4; above, p. 161. Helen of Troy uses a drug to cure grief and anger given to her by Polydamna of Egypt (Homer, *Iliad*, 4.222–6); Agamede understands all the drugs of the earth (*Iliad* 11.741). See Matthew Dickie, *Magic and Magicians in the Greco-Roman World* (London, 2001), pp. 22–3, who points out that Agamede was seen as a sorceress in the Hellenistic period but, in her Homeric context, was originally more like a root-cutter, a group which combined medical uses of drugs with ritual collection of the materials from which to make them.

classical world were more capable of study.[44] It may be from Tiraqueau's work that Catherine Des Roches, whose narrative poem *Agnodice* has already been discussed, took the story and, for her too, this was not a midwifery story, but concerned educated women confronting men's envy. For her, Agnodice was a herbalist, healing women with 'the special virtues of flowers, leaves, and roots, / especially with a herb picked on the very spot / where Glaucus from a man became a god after eating it'.[45] Glaucus was an accidental 'discoverer' of the healing properties of a plant; he discovered that this herb conveyed immortality after watching a fish he had caught come back to life when it fell on to it. Catherine Des Roches merged this story with that of Agnodice, showing her ability to play creatively with the classical tradition.

In sixteenth-century Europe, women's roles as the only midwives appeared to be secure. Men assisted only with difficult births, and a past with 'no midwives' was unimaginable. Only as the right of women to be midwives in normal births started to be challenged did the story of Agnodice become primarily a midwifery story. This challenge peaked in the eighteenth century but built on a gradual shift of professional boundaries that had started much earlier. Scholars used to argue that, in the early modern world, before the rise of the man-midwife in the seventeenth and eighteenth centuries, 'women's health was women's business'. Monica Green has convincingly demonstrated the inadequacy of this traditional view, and shown that the scope of the midwife's role has changed over time.[46] Green summarised the early history of midwifery by suggesting that late antique and early medieval midwives had a significant role; they 'were expected to be the main caretakers of *all* of women's particular health concerns – that is, gynaecology (which demanded knowledge of the internal workings of the body and the causes of disease) as well

---

[44] On Sylvius (Jacques du Bois), a Galenist who argued that the human body had declined since antiquity, see for example Cunningham, *The Anatomical Renaissance*, p. 133. Not only are we smaller than them, with a shorter life-span, but even 'the internal parts differ in size, number, and shape in different parts of the world, and both the writing of the ancients and our bodies abundantly testify that the same things that the ancients observed are not still found in all our bodies'. Sylvius, *In Hippocratis et Galeni physiologiae partem anatomicam Isagoge* (Paris, 1555), p. 11 translated by Siraisi, *History, Medicine, and the Traditions of Renaissance Learning*, p. 25.

[45] 'Agnodice', in *Les Oeuvres des Mes-dames des Roches de Poetiers mere et fille* (Paris, 1578). Written with her mother Madeleine, the poem is reprinted in full in Anne R. Larsen, *From Mother to Daughter: Poems, dialogues and letters of les dames Des Roches* (Chicago IL, 2006), pp. 122–31. The reference here is to lines 96–9 (Larsen, *From Mother to Daughter*, pp. 126–7); in the original, 'Par la vertu des fleurs, des feuilles et racines, / D'une herbe mesmement qui fut cueillie au lieu / Où Glauque la mengeant d'homme devint un Dieu'. The reference to Glaucus is to Ovid, *Metamorphoses* 13. 904–65.

[46] Monica H. Green, 'Women's Medical Practice and Health Care in Medieval Europe', in Judith Bennett et al. (eds), *Sisters and Workers in the Middle Ages* (Chicago, IL, 1989), pp. 39–78.

as obstetrics'.[47] In the Latin West, during the late antique period, 'gynaecological material was more often found in separate, specialized texts ... usually addressed either explicitly or implicitly to women, especially midwives (*obstetrices* or *medicae*)'.[48] This would suggest that the elision between 'midwife' and 'medicine' in Hyginus reflects a real situation in which women cared for other women both within and beyond birthing. But these professional and literate midwives had disappeared by around the thirteenth century; while women continued to assist other women giving birth, none of these was a 'midwife' in any formal sense.[49]

In early modern Europe, the situation was far more complicated, so that by the fifteenth and sixteenth centuries, medical men were not only assisting in difficult births, but also – and increasingly – taking over the treatment of gynaecological conditions, thus leaving midwives with little to do except assist in normal births.[50] Of course, while this was the ideal, in practice midwives, especially outside major towns, would probably have done far more. Green has shown that physicians entered the domain of women's healthcare by presenting themselves as experts on curing infertility, using this as a way of asserting superiority over female healers in other areas of women's health. Only at the end of the fifteenth century did the expectation of literacy in midwives, and the production of handbooks for them, begin to resurface again. To some extent, this coincided with the development of licensing for midwives, a practice which suggests concern over their proficiency, but in fact was focused more on their personal qualities within the community than on what they knew. It is not clear when Church licensing of midwives began in England; the date of 1512 is often given, but Doreen Evenden has shown that the picture is more complicated.[51] In Germany, midwives were regulated from 1450; in France, in the Paris region at least, from around 1560.[52]

When the story of Agnodice became more widely known in the second half of the sixteenth century, this occurred at a time when men were underlining their claim to be the proper practitioners of women's medicine by co-opting the Father of Medicine himself – Hippocrates – as a gynaecologist. The context in which Micyllus' 1535 edition of Hyginus appeared was thus one in which men were doing far more women's medicine than they had been for some centuries, and where women's role as midwives – untrained, and unlicensed – was beginning to be an area of concern to the church or the state. The story of Agnodice started to take on a new significance. Was it evidence that midwifery had not always been

---

[47]   M.H. Green, *Making Women's Medicine Masculine*, p. 35. G. Clark, *Women in Late Antiquity*, p. 69 on some less well-known examples from this period.

[48]   Ibid., p. 16.

[49]   Ibid., pp. 135–6.

[50]   Ibid., p. 262.

[51]   Evenden, *Midwives of Seventeenth-Century London*, p. 25.

[52]   Richard L. Petrelli, 'The Regulation of French Midwifery during the *Ancien Régime*', *Journal of the History of Medicine and Allied Sciences*, 26 (1971), pp. 276–92, 277.

in the hands of women? Alternatively, could it provide a model of an educated midwife: one who appeared to be most unlike the image of the 'ignorant' midwife constructed in order to assist male takeover of this field in the early modern period?[53]

In the eighteenth century in particular, the age of the *man*-midwife, translations of the opening scenario, 'The ancients had no midwives; because of this, women perished, misled by shame', included a very explicit childbirth connection; for example, stating not just that women 'perished' but that they 'were perishing *in childbirth*', or expanding on the reference to shame to state that women preferred to die rather than have men *deliver them*. For example, as we saw in Chapter 5, de Pitaval's 1732 version stated that women were dying specifically in childbirth.[54] This could have been taken from Le Clerc's 1723 influential history of medicine, where the emphasis was on how women preferred to die rather than have men assist them.[55] But Le Clerc also stated that there had been a long history of women going to other women for treatment for 'certaines maladies secretes' – rather than birthing itself – due to feeling uncomfortable with male doctors. This, for him, is the normative situation; indeed, he insisted, it is women's right to consult other women for such conditions.[56] In a later French work, the 1761 *Le Contre-Poison, ou la nation vengée*, we find the story told with '*many* women dying in childbirth' (my italics).[57] In 1766, for Astruc it is again specifically in giving birth that women 'through modesty, rather chuse to run the risque of death, than make use of men on this occasion'.[58] All these versions obscure the fact that the Latin original does not

---

[53]   In an important article, David Harley examined how the image of the 'ignorant midwife' was a construct of her opponents; see his 'Ignorant Midwives – A Persistent Stereotype', *Society for the Social History of Medicine Bulletin*, 28 (1981), pp. 6–9. An early example of the construct features in Chamberlen, *A Voice in Rhama*, p. 13: after taking the midwife's oath 'with the testimonie of two or three Gossips, any may have leave to be as ignorant, if not as cruel, as themselves'.

[54]   Above, p. 147.

[55]   Daniel Le Clerc originally wrote *Histoire de la médecine ou on voit l'origine et le progress de cet art* (Geneva, 1696), translated as *The History of Physick, or, an account of the rise and progress of the art* (London, 1699). A longer version was published in French in 1723, including a history of medicine (*Histoire de la médecine*, Amsterdam), and it was here that he told the story of Agnodice, p. 432. On contemporary criticisms of Le Clerc, see King, *Midwifery, Obstetrics and the Rise of Gynaecology*, pp. 86–8. Le Clerc, *Histoire de la médecine*, p. 432, 'des hommes les accchouchassent'.

[56]   He refers to it as 'ce droit' and 'cet établissement'; *Histoire de la médecine*, p. 432.

[57]   *Le Contre-Poison, ou la nation vengée* (Amsterdam, 1761), p. 17, 'plusieurs Dames mouroient en travail d'enfant'. Like R.S. Smith and Trzaskoma, the author inserts 'many' here.

[58]   From the English translation, Astruc, *Art of Midwifery*, p. xxiii. His wording, for example the initial law forbidding 'women and slaves to study physic, that is, the art of midwifry' (p. xxiv) recalls that of Le Clerc, who in 1732 also made physic and 'l'art d'accoucher' equivalent: Le Clerc, *Histoire de la médecine*, p. 432.

actually mention childbirth here. It may be significant that they are all published in French, and it was France that led the way in Europe as regards the male-midwife, or *accoucheur*. Jacques Guillemeau's *De l'heureux accouchement des femmes* was published in 1609, although the English translation was printed only three years later.[59]

But, one could respond, does Hyginus need to mention dying 'in childbirth' when he has already said there were 'no midwives'? Surely what midwives do is to assist in childbirth, so if there were no midwives then it is obvious that women were dying because they refused to see male medical practitioners when in labour? But if, when he wrote, the role of midwife encompassed far more than birthing, then saying there were 'no midwives' implies no female assistants in any form of medicine.

Early modern treatises on midwifery endorse a wide role for women in medicine to their own sex. They often have surprisingly little to say about the details of a normal delivery, but – whether written by women or by men – they deal with encouraging conception, treating a range of diseases of women, swaddling the baby, and treating cosmetic problems and childhood conditions. For example, in 1671 the midwife Jane Sharp noted that 'Whoever rightly considers it will presently find, that the Female sex are subject to more diseases by odds than the Male kind are, and therefore it is reason [*sic*] that great care should be had for the cure of that sex which is the weaker and more subject to infirmities in some respects above the other.' She went on to list 'the white Feaver, or green Sickness, fits of the Mother, strangling of the Womb, rage of the Matrix, extreme Melancholly, Falling-sickness, Head-ach, beating of the arteries in the back and sides, great palpitations of the heart, Hypochondriacal diseases from the Spleen, stoppings of the Liver, and ill affections of the stomach by consent from the womb', going on to discuss some of these in more detail.[60] All the disorders listed here could, to a significant degree, be accounted for in terms of menstrual suppression or other

---

[59]   The characterisation of the French as the main users of men-midwives is made in contemporary sources, such as Bayle's historical dictionary; in the 1736 English second edition (p. 453), he adds that since the first edition he has read in a Leipzig journal that French women, even the newly married, are not concerned about showing their bodies to surgeons when they are about to give birth. But other nations are quite different; there, he says, women would only involve a man if 'the pain is so strong as to overcome their repugnance'. He cites, and quotes from, *Acta Eruditorum Lips. Supplem.* vol. 2 section 1 p. 470. [Thicknesse], *Man-Midwifery Analysed*, p. 18 similarly attacks the women of Genoa as lacking virtue. While McTavish, *Childbirth and the Display of Authority*, p. 27 rightly warns against over-emphasising national difference in this area ('The international exchange of books and prevalence of translations means that treatises produced in different countries were often in dialogue with each other'), it is nevertheless clear that contemporary sources did stress such differences.

[60]   Sharp, *The Midwives Book*, opening of Book 5, Chapter 5; ed. Hobby, pp. 190–91. On white fever/green sickness see King, *The Disease of Virgins*.

conditions of the womb; because the midwife was concerned with the womb, she could be seen as the best person to deal with them.

Is it possible to correlate the role of the midwife with the dominant model of female/male difference? In the second century AD, Soranus' full discussion of the question of previous writers' views as to whether women have diseases that only they suffer makes it clear that opinion in ancient medical writers was divided. Soranus noted that one current approach to medicine – the empirical approach – focused on the difference between men and women, on the grounds that people will call in midwives when women are suffering from 'something unique to them, which they do not have in common with men'.[61] This suggests that using midwives (or, bearing in mind the difficulty of defining our terms here, female physicians) for all conditions unique to women is, in Laqueur's terms, 'two-sex'. But another ancient model, that of the Hippocratic treatise *Diseases of Women* 1.62 in which 'the healing of the diseases of women differs greatly from the healing of the diseases of men', suggests a more extreme 'two-sex' model, one in which absolutely any symptom a woman experiences may need to be seen differently just because it occurs in a female body.[62] Looking at this in terms only of 'one-sex' or 'two-sex' glosses over the different possibilities present within what Laqueur presents as a single model.

Several possibilities thus arise from considering the relationship between midwifery and medicine in Hyginus' story of Agnodice. While seventeenth- and eighteenth-century readers were more likely to add extra details to make this even more firmly a story about midwifery, others continued to see it as a story about women and medicine. How did Hyginus see it? Perhaps the original Greek story he inherited was one about a woman learning medicine, but in order to make it fit into his list of 'Who invented/discovered what' he added in the sentence about the ancients having no midwives. Perhaps, in the Roman context in which he wrote, a world without female physicians seemed highly improbable; maybe it was simply impossible to say that 'The ancients had no women physicians (*medicae*)' because everyone knew the names of women with healing roles. However, another possibility is that he saw *obstetrices* and *medicae* as the same thing, and did not separate out a role of childbirth assistant from a role of female physician to women; only later in the history of reception of the story did the terms cease to be interchangeable. As we continue to ask how the different readings of this story in later centuries raise questions about how it is told in Hyginus, we now need to examine more closely Agnodice's encounter with her first patient. What was wrong with this woman, and how did Agnodice help?

---

[61] Soranus, *Gynaecology* 3.1 lines 33–6 (Budé, p. 3).

[62] Hippocrates, *Diseases of Women* 1.62 (Littré 8.126).

Misled by Shame

For some users of Agnodice, although the story in Hyginus starts and ends with medicine, the introductory sentence about the absence of midwives still took precedence, and so this was a story about childbirth; women died giving birth, because they refused to see male practitioners. As I have already noted, the Latin does not in fact say this explicitly: instead, it says that they died because they were 'misled by shame'. Later in the story, we read of male practitioners losing business, suggesting that there would have been assistance available from men, but the women were not willing to consult them.

Does the use of 'shame', in Latin *verecundia*, as the reason why women were dying help us to understand this story? To use E.R. Dodds' famous distinction between the world of Homer as a shame-culture, as opposed to fifth-century Greek culture and Christianity as guilt-cultures, the concept of shame is linked to being discussed; in shame-cultures one's behaviour is based on making sure one is not talked about by others, the issue being 'loss of face'.[63] Agnodice's story is very much about reputation and rumour; it hints at the possible damage to a woman's reputation if she allows a man to see her 'shameful parts', and of course Agnodice herself suffers later in the story when the rumour mill insists that she is only being chosen by her patients for sexual gratification, both theirs and hers. For a 'one-sex' model, women's parts are identical to those of men, only in different locations. In 'one-sex' terms, Agnodice does not display the shameful presence of a penis – as does Heraïs – but rather the entirely correct 'interiority' of her penis. Her patients feel *verecundia* if a man sees their genitalia; Agnodice feels no such reaction when she shows her own to her patients, and when she shows her genitalia to the men of the Areopagus, this is not about shame, but about her innocence on the charge that brought her there. A 'one-sex' model does not help us to understand how this story works.

The trope of women's modesty features strongly in the history of Western medicine, in both 'medicine' and 'midwifery' contexts. In *Diseases of Women* 1, which dates to the fourth century BC but may represent oral traditions from the fifth century, a physician wrote that 'women are ashamed to tell [what is wrong with them] even if they know, and they suppose it to be a disgrace, because of their inexperience and lack of knowledge'.[64] This, however, was not a reference to childbirth, but to gynaecology. The scenario is so close to that which opens the Agnodice story that it may have been known to whoever wrote the latter; this would add support to the suggestion that the story was originally about gynaecology,

---

[63]   E.R. Dodds, *The Greeks and the Irrational* (Berkeley, CA and London, 1951), p. 18. Dodds' thinking was clearly influenced by the perceived irrationality of the Second World War, and also by the thinking of the anthropologist Ruth Benedict.

[64]   *Diseases of Women* 1.62 (Littré 8.126), tr. Ann Ellis Hanson, 'Hippocrates: *Diseases of Women* 1', *Signs: Journal of Women in Culture and Society*, 1 (1975), p. 582; 'for they are ashamed to tell' is *kai gar aideontai phrazein*.

with the 'no midwives' sentence being added later to make it fit into a list of 'who invented what'. The term for 'being ashamed' in this Hippocratic passage is *aideontai*, from *aidôs*, meaning respect or awe, as well as shame: failing to maintain *aidôs* leads to 'disgrace', *aischron*, from a related noun for shame or dishonour, *aischynê*.[65] A common Greek term for the genitalia of either a man or a woman is *ta aidoia*, 'the shameful parts', but also having the sense of 'the parts deserving respect'. While in some contexts 'shame' seems to be the best English translation of *aidôs*, in others 'modesty' would be a better fit. The ideas of 'decorum' and 'appropriate behaviour' also contribute.[66] As we saw at the beginning of Chapter 5, other ancient medical writers repeated the Hippocratic theme of women's modesty/shame making them difficult to treat, as in Caelius Aurelianus' claim that female physicians were necessary so that the diseases affecting the female pudenda would not need to be exposed to the eyes of men; shame-culture is often linked to the sense of sight, and to the gaze.[67] Like the Hippocratic writer, here he is not talking about a midwifery context, but rather one of 'women's diseases', treated by *medicae*, women physicians.[68] Similar comments appear in medieval works, such as the twelfth-century *On the Conditions of Women* (*Liber de sinthomatibus mulierum*):

> ... women, from the condition of their fragility, out of shame and embarrassment
> do not dare reveal their anguish over their diseases (which happen in such a
> private place) to a physician.[69]

Sounding like another echo of the Hippocratic passage, this comment too is not restricted to childbirth. Elsewhere in this medieval treatise, shame does feature specifically in that narrower context; women feel shame when men look at

---

[65]   On these terms, and the suggestion that *aidôs* can be inhibitory, *aischynê* more retrospective, see the discussion by David Konstan, *The Emotions of the Ancient Greeks: Studies in Aristotle and Classical Literature* (Toronto, 2006), pp. 93–5.

[66]   On the complexity of these terms, see Douglas Cairns, *Aidos. The Psychology and Ethics of Honour and Shame in Ancient Greek Literature* (Oxford, 1993). Cairns does not discuss medicine, for which see Danielle Gourevitch, 'Pudeur et pratique médicale dans l'Antiquité classique', *La Presse médicale*, 3 (1968).

[67]   See for example Shadi Bartsch, *The Mirror of the Self: Sexuality, Self-Knowledge and the Gaze in the Early Roman Empire* (Chicago, IL, 2006), pp. 132–4.

[68]   Caelius Aurelianus, *Gynaecia*, p. 1 (above, p. 129); note the phrase *virilibus oculis*, 'to the eyes of men'.

[69]   *On the Conditions of Women* 2, tr. Monica H. Green, *The Trotula. A Medieval Compendium of Women's Medicine* (Philadelphia, PA, 2001), p. 71. Green notes that the Latin term *medicus* used here *may* mean that women are unwilling to show their bodies to a healer of either sex, although she suggests that the sense here is of a male healer (p. 249, n. 3 and p. 37).

them during and after giving birth.[70] In *On the Conditions of Women* shame thus combines being seen – as in Caelius Aurelianus – and speaking to a man, as in the Hippocratic passage.[71] Both references use the same term for shame; *verecundia*, the same word that Hyginus used for the emotion causing women to avoid seeking treatment, until Agnodice offered them her services. In the original Greek lying behind our text of Hyginus, *verecundia* would have been *aidôs*, the same word used in the Hippocratic *Diseases of Women*.

The Hippocratic observation that modesty/shame makes women unwilling to tell men about the disorders of their reproductive organs features widely not only in medieval but also in early modern medicine. For example, in 1636 John Sadler introduced the *Sick Woman's Private Looking-Glass* – a book restricted to diseases of the womb – as based on Galen and Hippocrates. In an echo of the Hippocratic *Places in Man* 47, 'the womb is the cause of all diseases of women', he stated that the womb is responsible for the most serious diseases of the body, and then echoed *Diseases of Women* 1.62 by saying that women endanger their health not only by being ignorant of their own bodies but also by their reluctance to speak to a physician about them.[72] A woman, 'through her modestie, being loth to divulge and publish the same unto the Physitian to implore his aide, shee conceals her griefe and so encreaseth her sorrow'.[73]

Early modern writers who tell Agnodice's story, or allude to it, make explicit the logical connection between unwillingness to talk to male physicians, and the development of women as healers to their own sex. In the 1612 English translation of Guillemeau's treatise on childbirth, the story of Agnodice is introduced with the scene-setting statement that

> necessitie, (the mistress of Arts) hath constrained women, to learne and practise Physicke, one with an other. For finding themselves afflicted, and troubled with divers diseases in their naturall parts, and being destitute of all remedies, (for

---

[70]   *On the Conditions of Women* 92; M.H. Green, *The Trotula*, p. 100. See also M.H. Green, *Making Women's Medicine Masculine*, p. 52, on how some manuscripts of this treatise specify that *women* attendants at a birth should also avoid looking directly at a woman in labour.

[71]   In Caelius Aurelianus, *oculis perscrutanda* (above, p. 129).

[72]   *Places in Man* 47; see Elizabeth Craik (ed.), *Hippocrates, Places in Man* (Oxford, 1988), p. 86. King, *Midwifery, Obstetrics and the Rise of Gynaecology*, p. 11 discusses a few of the uses of this passage in sixteenth-century writing on the female body.

[73]   Sadler, *Sick Woman's Private Looking-Glass*, 'Epistle Dedicatory'. This is an interesting book because of its merger of ancient medicine and claims from dissection; for example the seven-celled uterus is denied on the basis of dissection, but the Hippocratic idea of a right and left chamber of the womb, with male children being formed in the right, female in the left, is reported as being *proven* for 'those that have seene Anatomies'; see pp. 7–8.

want whereof many perished, and died miserably) they durst not discover, and lay open their infirmities, to any but themselves.[74]

He then goes on to give the full story of Agnodice from Hyginus. When William Sermon copied this passage in the 1671 *The Ladies Companion, or the English Midwife*, in a section on the antiquity of midwives, it became

> Sometimes necessity (the Mistress of Arts) hath forced women to practise Physick, especially one with the other; for finding themselves much afflicted, and sorely troubled with many distempers in their natural parts, being ashamed to discover their infirmities to any but themselves, maketh many of them to study and practice Physick, as that famous Maiden did, called *Agnodicea*.[75]

Unlike Guillemeau, Sermon stopped his rendition of the Agnodice story here. While he added some emphasis to the remarks on women's suffering – they are 'much' afflicted, 'sorely' troubled – he also omitted Guillemeau's reference (taken from Hyginus) to women's deaths. In addition, he brought back 'shame' to the passage: 'being ashamed to discover their infirmities'. In Guillemeau, part of the problem was the absence of 'remedies': in Sermon, 'many' women study and practise physic, making the reader wonder whether Sermon has stopped copying Guillemeau not because Agnodice was so familiar by the 1670s that he needed to say nothing more, but instead due to a reluctance to see her – 'famous' as she is – as a pioneer.

Not long after Sermon wrote, suggestions started to be made that women's new willingness to use men to supervise childbirth hinted at a serious *lack* of such modesty in those who employed them, and so was to be deplored. The 1735 edition of Pierre Bayle's historical dictionary cited *Nouvelles de la Republique des Lettres*, January 1686, pp. 28–30, writing that

> Time has been that it was the fashion to be ashamed to make use of a Man-Midwife, and we read in Louise Bourgeois a very dexterous Midwife, that Henry IV charged her to do her duty so well with queen Mary de Medicis, that it might not be necessary to have recourse to a man; for her modesty, added he, would suffer too much by it. At present it is à la mode to be void of that shame: our age is much more enlightened than the preceding.

The editor added that

> This raillery against the present age is not well grounded; for if on one hand there is now less shame in some respects, impudence on the other hand is less

---

[74] Guillemeau, *Child-Birth*, p. 80; ibid., *De l'heureux accouchement*, 1620 edition, p. 155, 'estans destitutees de tous remedes'.

[75] Sermon, *Ladies Companion*, p. 2.

than it was at Athens. Are there any virtuous women at present, who would have
the assurance in a full auditory to take up their peticoats, and demonstrate to the
judges that they are women? Agnodice did so in the Areopagus, the gravest and
most venerable tribunal that was in the world.[76]

This turns around the theme of shame; it is not the women who employ men-
midwives who lack it, but Agnodice, who displayed her sex to a male audience.
Another use of Agnodice in this debate featured in Philip Thicknesse's *Man-
Midwifery Analysed* of 1764. Thicknesse was opposed to the man-midwife,
arguing that for 'many generations' it was 'women only' who had been birth
attendants.[77] He condemned the 'indecent and destructive practices'[78] of men-
midwives, particularly 'touching'; the insertion of one or two fingers into the
vagina to determine the stage of pregnancy. He regarded fashion – 'my Lady Betty
Modish' – as the main reason why women preferred a man to attend them.[79] He
played on the ending of Agnodice's story, with 'free women' being able to practise
midwifery, saying that it is 'free' – that is, loose – women who encourage man-
midwifery today.[80]

So, where the Agnodice story presented modesty as leading to women's deaths,
some eighteenth-century writers suggested that the lack of modesty of the women
who entrusted themselves to male care in childbirth risked a fatal outcome. In her
attack on William Smellie and his fellow men-midwives, Elizabeth Nihell stated
that 'It may however with more reason and truth be averred, that the admittance
of men to that function by women, would be in the women a most egregiously
MISTAKEN MODESTY. Since, surely the virtue or grace of female modesty is
not an object to be held so cheap, as to be sacrificed for worse than nothing, for
nothing better, in short, than the purchace with it of danger or perdition to both the
mother and child.'[81] Women's shame/modesty could be condemned by men who
wanted access to their bodies: those who opposed male attendants in childbirth
could then attack women who used such men as lacking in shame/modesty.

---

[76]   Bayle, *The Dictionary Historical and Critical* (1736), p. 653; Bayle died in 1706,
and the first English edition of 1703, in two volumes (London: J. Hartley), does not give
this full account from Hyginus with Bayle's own additions.

[77]   [Thicknesse], *Man-Midwifery Analysed*, p. 11.

[78]   Ibid., p. 1.

[79]   Ibid., p. 4.

[80]   Ibid., p. 15.

[81]   Nihell, *A Treatise on the Art of Midwifery*, pp. 220–21. See Laura Gowing,
Common Bodies. Women, Touch and Power in Seventeenth-Century England (New Haven,
CT, 2003), p. 40 on the eighteenth-century construction of female modesty.

Trouble Down Below

In terms of the use of the story to address concerns about midwifery or about women's role in medicine more widely, the final aspect that needs to be discussed is whether Agnodice's first patient was giving birth. As we have already seen in other instances, modern translations into English help to uncover the difficulties the Latin poses. In Mary Grant's translation, Agnodice 'heard that a woman was in labor'; this was repeated for a wider ancient history audience in Sarah Pomeroy's article on the education of ancient women, published in 1977, where she went to help 'a woman in labor'.[82] But in Smith and Trzaskoma's translation this becomes the rather coy 'whenever she heard a woman was having trouble below her waist'.

So is the first patient giving birth, or is something else wrong with her? The Latin is *et feminam laborantem audisset ab inferiore parte*. Taking first the use of the verb *laboro*, the context of a story about 'the ancients having no midwives' may encourage the reader to take this as concerning 'labour', and this is how I myself understood it in an earlier discussion of Hyginus.[83] Reading the different versions given by early modern readers of the story has, however, convinced me that this is the wrong interpretation. While the Latin *labor* can mean the labour of childbirth, the verb *laboro* has a range of meanings from 'to perform physical work', to 'to be distressed physically' and 'to suffer from pain or disease', and there is no reason to narrow down its meaning here.[84]

As we have already seen, for sixteenth-century readers this was more likely to be a story about women physicians than about midwives. In Tiraqueau, Agnodice learns 'the art of medicine', and he repeated Hyginus' words about the *femina laborans* precisely. In Catherine Des Roches' Agnodice poem of 1579, the women do not suffer from problems in childbirth at all, but rather from 'fevers, faintness and other illnesses'.[85] Yet in some early modern texts, such as the retelling of the story of Agnodice in the entry for Herophilus in Pierre Bayle's 1697 *Dictionary*, Agnodice first treats 'a woman, in labour'. Subsequently the women 'finding themselves eased in their labour by Agnodice, would no longer employ any other but her, in their other distempers, in which they had no reason to be ashamed to send for a Physician'.[86] Here, then, Agnodice starts with childbirth and then extends into treating all conditions of women, not just those for which they would

---

[82]   Pomeroy, '*Technikai kai mousikai*', p. 59.

[83]   King, 'Agnodike and the Profession of Medicine', p. 54.

[84]   *Oxford Latin Dictionary*, s.v. *laboro*. In a recent discussion of the myth, Kirk Read, *Birthing Bodies in Early Modern France: Stories of Gender and Reproduction* (Aldershot, 2011), p. 85, correctly notes that this does not have to be about childbirth; the verb *parturire* could have been used instead.

[85]   Des Roches, *Agnodice*, lines 73–7: 'Les dames aussitost se trouverent suivies / De fiebvres, de langueur, et d'autres maladies'; Larsen, *From Mother to Daughter*, pp. 126–7.

[86]   Bayle, *A General Dictionary, Historical and Critical* (1710), p. 172; Bayle, *The Dictionary Historical and Critical* (1736), p. 453.

feel shame if they revealed them to a man. This insertion of 'a woman, in labour' into the story may have originated a decade after Catherine Des Roches' version, with Charles Estienne's *Dictionarium historicum ac poeticum* of 1590, where the word *parturientem*, 'being in labour', was substituted for Hyginus' less specific *laborantem*.[87]

Thomas Heywood, in probably the most familiar version of Agnodice for an English-speaking audience in this period, used Estienne's dictionary in his 1624 *Gynaeikeion*, and therefore he too made the first patient into a birthing case. Agnodice's first patient was 'a noble ladie ... in child-birth, in the middest of her painfull throwes'; 'throws' here are labour pains. This embellishment makes Agnodice even more emphatically about midwifery. Indeed, at the end of Heywood's version, instead of the Athenians changing the law so that women could study medicine, Athens becomes the first Greek city 'that freely admitted of Mid-wives'.[88]

But, even at the time when Heywood was writing, early modern writers did not exclusively understand Agnodice's first patient as a woman giving birth. For example, in 1609 Guillemeau has her first patient as 'malade en ses parties honteuses', that is, 'sick in her shameful parts' in French, and 'troubled in her naturall parts' in the 1612 English translation.[89] In his description of Agnodice's treatment of this patient, again there is no suggestion that she was giving birth: 'the woman committed her selfe, into her hands, who drest, and cured her perfectly: and with the like care and industrie she looked to many others, and cured them'.[90] As we saw in Chapter 6, the 1688 retelling by the midwife Elizabeth Cellier, who used Guillemeau, similarly gave 'she found out a Woman that had long languish'd under private Diseases' and 'cured her perfectly' (precisely Guillemeau's words).[91] Reading these different early modern versions convinces me that the Latin leaves the meaning open, but that the preferred translation would be that Agnodice heard a woman 'suffering', without any sense of giving birth. In this case, it becomes a story about medicine, not midwifery, in our sense of the words.

A related phrase, *ab inferiore parte*, is also relevant here. Some later versions of the text of Hyginus insert a comma before this phrase, thus trying to separate

---

[87] Estienne, *Dictionarium historicum ac poeticum*: Agnodicea is inserted between two entries, Agno and Agnonia, and the story begins *Agnodice, puella virgo medicinam discere cupiens, abscissa coma, habitu virili, se hierophilo cuidam tradidit in disciplinam, a quo probe edocta* parturientem *mulierum morbis medebatur*.

[88] Heywood, *Gynaeikeion*, pp. 203–4; reprinted in 1657, pp. 285–6.

[89] Guillemeau, *De l'heureux accouchement*, 1620 edition, p. 155. Read, *Birthing Bodies*, p. 85 suggests that Guillemeau's 'ses parties honteuses' is projecting *his own* embarrassment on to the woman, rather than this being present in the Latin. If so, this is lost in the English.

[90] Guillemeau, *Child-Birth or, the Happy Deliverie of Women*, p. 79.

[91] Cellier, *To Dr ...*, p. 3. Gardiner, 'Elizabeth Cellier in 1688', p. 28 notes that in Cellier's version women are dying 'both in Child bearing, and by private Diseases'.

it from *laborantem*.[92] Without the comma, one is inclined to translate literally as 'heard a woman suffering from the lower part'; with the comma, making this *feminam laborantem audisset, ab inferiore parte, veniebat ad eam*, we could translate as 'she heard a woman suffering; she came from the lower part to her', suggesting that Agnodice was on the lower floor of a house and heard the woman crying out upstairs. This could be supported by evidence of the living arrangements of classical Athenians, as it is assumed by scholars – although on the basis of what is now acknowledged to be very flimsy data – that in a two-storey house the women's quarters would have been upstairs.[93] Smith and Trzaskoma's broader reading, 'whenever she heard a woman was having trouble below her waist', interprets the 'lower parts' as an anatomical term. Looking at Latin writers from roughly the same period as Hyginus, the term *inferior pars*, literally, 'lower part', is attested in the writer Celsus, whose first century AD encyclopaedia included an extensive section on medicine.[94] In a chapter on a violent disorder arising 'from the womb' (Lat. *ex vulva*), he used *inferior pars* to mean the female genitalia. Because the term appears in a discussion of menstrual blood bursting out from the nose at a time when it should instead come out 'from the lower part', *ex inferiore parte*, the focus here is on the lower position in the body, rather than on the other sense of the word *inferior*, namely lower in status, or 'unworthy'.

Does this help us to understand Hyginus? I would suggest that the Greek original here would have been *hysteron*; literally 'the lower parts', this is also used to mean 'the womb'. Indeed, often found in the plural, *hystera* is one of the most common of the various Greek terms for the womb; Galen noted that Hippocrates and Plato used it in the plural, and explained this usage as being valid because, he said, the womb contains two chambers, with a single 'neck'.[95] Soranus linked the term to *hysteron*, 'after', which he interpreted as meaning that the womb 'demonstrates its own activity later' and that it 'lies behind the viscera'.[96] In terms

---

[92] For example, the translations given in C. Iulii Hygini, Augusti Liberti, *Fabularum Liber* (Lyons, 1608), p. 52r; *Hygini. Quae hodie extant, adcurante Joanne Scheffero ... Accedunt et Thomae Munceri In Fabulas Hygini Annotationes* (Hamburg, 1674).

[93] Susan Walker, 'Women and Housing in Classical Greece: The Archaeological Evidence', in Averil Cameron and Amélie Kuhrt (eds), *Images of Women in Antiquity*, 2nd edition (London, 1993), p. 83; this evidence has been revisited by Marilyn Y. Goldberg, 'Spatial and Behavioural Negotiation in Classical Athenian City Houses', in Penelope M. Allison, *The Archaeology of Household Activities* (London and New York, 1999), p. 143. The main literary evidence is Lysias 1.9.3, where Euphiletos' wife moves down from her normal room when she needs to care for the baby, thus conveniently meaning that she can admit her lover to the house without her husband noticing.

[94] Celsus, *De medicina* 4.27.1D. On this term and other euphemisms of the 'female parts' kind, see James N. Adams, *The Latin Sexual Vocabulary* (London, 1982), p. 95.

[95] Galen, *On Anatomical Procedures* 12.2 (Duckworth, *Galen On Anatomical Procedures*, pp. 113–14), written in around 200 AD.

[96] *Gynaecology* 1.4, Budé p. 8. See Véronique Dasen and Sandrine Ducaté-Paarmann, 'Hysteria and Metaphors of the Uterus in Classical Antiquity', in Silvia Schroer (ed.),

of the actual etymology of the term, it may be linked to a Sanskrit word meaning 'upper part' or 'back part' and that the Latin *uterus* may in turn be connected with the Greek *hyderos* meaning 'dropsy' or 'swollen belly'.[97]

The related Greek word *hysteros* means that which is spatially 'behind', or temporally 'afterwards'.[98] There is a joke told by Athenaeus, who lived from the end of the second century to the beginning of the third century AD, and thus may have been contemporary with Hyginus, about a prostitute called Leontion ('Lion', a typical courtesan name). Leontion was upset because her lover was paying more attention to Glykera ('Sweetie') who had arrived later than she had done, and when asked what was the matter replied *hê hystera me lypei*, which means both 'my womb hurts' and 'the woman who arrived after me hurts me'.[99] Prostitutes were often represented using jokes and double entrendres, and the witty Leontion is elsewhere described as having become 'a philosopher'.[100] In his treatise *On Seed* Galen wrote 'of the so-called later parts', *tôn hysterôn onomazomenôn moriôn*, some of which females lack entirely, while others that they have are of a different kind. Here, however, he clearly meant what we would think of as the secondary sex characteristics.[101] Both the Latin *inferior pars* and the Greek *hysteron* have a strong sense of 'trouble down below', suggesting that the first patient was not in labour, but suffering from a disorder associated with the womb.[102]

In this chapter I have suggested that the story of Agnodice was originally about women as physicians, but was transformed into a midwifery story by Hyginus, perhaps to make it fit into a list of 'firsts'. In terms of dating the first version, this would mean finding a time when women physicians were common; however, as we have seen, the evidence does not allow us to do this. While it was understood as a 'women physicians' story in the sixteenth century, as men moved into gynaecology and then into midwifery it started to be read with a renewed emphasis on midwifery, including interpreting the first patient as a woman in labour. Later models of the role of the midwife, and of professional distinctions

---

Images and Gender. Contributions to the Hermeneutics of Reading Ancient Art, Orbis Biblicus et Orientalis 220 (Fribourg, 2006), p. 240.

[97] LSJ; Pierre Chantraine, *Dictionnaire étymologique de la langue grecque* (Paris: Klincksieck, 1999), p. 1151.

[98] Ibid., pp. 1162–3.

[99] Athenaeus 585d. On the context of prostitution in antiquity, see for example Christopher A. Faraone and Laura McClure (eds), *Prostitutes and Courtesans in the Ancient World* (Madison, WI, 2006); Alison Glazebrook and Madeleine M. Henry (eds), *Greek Prostitutes in the Ancient Mediterranean, 800 BC–200 CE* (Madison, WI, 2011); on courtesans in Athenaeus, McClure, *Courtesans at Table* gives many references to Glykera and discusses the wit of the courtesan.

[100] Athenaeus 588b; McClure, *Courtesans at Table*, pp. 80–83 and p. 104.

[101] *On Seed* II 5.10, *CMG* V 3, 1, p. 182.

[102] 'Down below' remains a euphemism today, as in the deliberately dual meaning of the title of William Golding's 1989 novel *Fire Down Below* (London: Faber & Faber).

based on training, have also been projected on to it. I have already suggested in this book that the womb is the organ that most challenges any inside/outside, 'one-sex' interpretation of the body; it is important both as a container and as a conduit for menstruation – the phenomenon that demonstrates the totally different, 'two-sex' flesh of the female body – and as the place where the child grows and from which it is expelled. Agnodice's gesture of self-revelation shows total difference; in 'two-sex' terms, it could also give her the right to treat women for whatever affects them 'down below'.

Lesley Dean-Jones identified Agnodice as 'the supposed first female physician of antiquity', who returned to Athens where she treated 'many women suffering from gynaecological ailments'.[103] If we read Agnodice in the context of a medical world in which the women who assist in childbirth also deal with other forms of 'trouble down below', this makes sense of the later section of the story in which the jealous doctors find that they are not wanted by women, without us having to assume that they had previously been acting as midwives in addition to treating the diseases of women. Agnodice's story contained the potential to become a step on the way to the complete rejection of male healers.

Possible origins for the story of Agnodice have also been identified in this chapter; the Hippocratic *Diseases of Women* 1.62, where women are reluctant to speak to a male physician about their diseases, and Caelius Aurelianus' claim that female physicians are needed so that women do not have to expose their genitalia to men. But we have also seen her echoes across time, in the virgin Aemilia who 'practised the arts of medicine in the way men do', or the medieval *On the Conditions of Women* where women 'out of shame and embarrassment' do not speak to a physician. Agnodice has interacted with the classical medical texts as well as being used and reused by early modern texts.

In the final chapter, I shall bring together Phaethousa and Agnodice to explore the significance of different parts of the body in demonstrating the 'true sex'. How do their stories help us understand how sexual identity was understood in the early modern texts that used them?

---

[103]   Dean-Jones, *Women's Bodies in Classical Greek Science*, p. 32.

Chapter 8
Agnodice in Parts

In this chapter I want to draw together some of the conclusions that result from focusing on these two classical stories and the changes in how they were read and used over the period during which Laqueur's historical 'rupture' was supposed to be taking place. As we saw in the Introduction, he makes this supposed shift from the 'one-sex' to the 'two-sex' a far more hierarchical, one-way movement than did his main sources, Galen and *Aristotle's Masterpiece*, and his *Making Sex* has already been criticised for its focus simply on the genitals. In the classical and early modern worlds, as we have now seen, the body was sexed far more widely; models which Laqueur would label 'two-sex' existed throughout the period of his 'one-sex body', and in these sex could extend into every part of the flesh. In addition to considering the significance not only of the organs, but also of the fluids of the body, we need to look at the other parts of the body on which the fluids were thought to have an effect. In Chapter 1, I drew attention to Galen's comment in *On Seed* that 'A person who sees a bull from a distance recognizes it immediately as male, without examining its organs of generation … We also distinguish man from woman in this way, not undressing them first so that we may examine the difference in their parts, but viewing them with their clothes on.'[1] I also noted there Artemidorus' belief that a woman's dreams about growing a beard, having a penis, wearing men's clothing, having male body hair 'or something else virile' were interchangeable; the organs of generation were not privileged. In terms of the two stories I have been examining, looking at Phaethousa from the outside would suggest that she was a man, but undressing her would have solved the puzzle, although there is no reference to the physicians doing this. Perhaps, like Agnodice, this aspect of Phaethousa's case story should be read alongside Caelius Aurelianus' claim that 'it was finally decided by the ancients to institute female physicians, so that the diseases of a woman's private parts, when they needed to be examined, would not have to be exposed to male eyes'; it is possible that examining Phaethousa in this way was simply not an option for the physicians in the case story.[2] Agnodice, however, plays with Galen's formulation, changing her clothing so that those who cannot go beneath it assume that it must be telling the truth about her body, and only when she chooses does she reveal her normally hidden parts to prove her 'true sex'.

In the first sections of this chapter, I shall summarise the presentation of the various parts of the female body that feature in different versions of the

---

[1] *On Seed* II 5.8–12, *CMG* V 3, 1, pp. 181–3.

[2] Above, p. 129.

stories of both Phaethousa and Agnodice, and ask what these say to Laqueur and
to his emphasis on the one-sex body in which women 'are but Men turn'd Outside in'. I shall focus here on Agnodice, simply because more body parts were
involved in her story and its reception. Writing on the Greek novel – which I
suggested in Chapter 5 may be the genre behind Hyginus' version of Agnodice
– Helen Elsom suggested that the 'act of looking at a woman ... confirms the
manhood of the looker'.[3] In the story of Agnodice, however, those who look at her
are not just men: she first reveals her 'true sex' to the women she treats, for whom
the looking is an affirmation of shared identity, and only later to the men of the
Areopagus, who note her inability to have seduced patients, but also her violation
of the law forbidding women to have a medical role. Some early modern versions
omitted any description of precisely how she persuaded her patients to trust her,
or how she later avoided the charge of seducing them; for example, de Pitaval
simply stated that 'Agnodice proved her innocence in front of the members of the
Areopagus.'[4] By what means? Perhaps eighteenth-century readers were assumed
to know already what she did, so that there was no point in going into detail. In
other cases, however, it is clearer that early modern versions lose her gesture for
reasons of decency; in so doing, they start to explore other parts of the body and
their potential for showing sex, so that she may undress completely, show her
breasts, or 'reveal' her fluency or her intellect. Those who presented Agnodice as
a role model wanted to keep her decent: those who attacked what they believed
she stood for were, of course, more likely to focus on her act of self-revelation.
The reason why the story is being told affects how it is constructed. In this chapter
I shall first comment on the variations on this act given in the early modern and
later sources, and then go through the non-genital parts of the body featuring in the
different versions of Agnodice, in turn; where possible, I shall also compare them
with the story of Phaethousa.

'Lifting her tunic'

Laura Gowing has drawn our attention to a London midwife, Margaret Fookes,
who in 1620 was accused by a physician of mistreating her clients. In response,
she lifted her skirts, used 'base and contemptuous words' and said 'she would be
a midwife in despite of him'.[5] While there is no evidence that this was a conscious
re-enactment of Agnodice's gesture, the dating – eight years after Guillemeau's
Child-Birth brought the story to a wider English-speaking audience – means that
this must be a possibility. In any case, in this context the gesture would have

---

[3] Elsom, 'Callirhoe: Displaying the Phallic Woman', p. 228.

[4] Pitaval, *Bibliotheque des gens de cour*, p. 146: 'Agdonice [*sic*] prouva son innocence
devant les Aréopagites.'

[5] Gowing, *Common Bodies*, p. 35, using London Metropolitan Archives, WJ/SR
II/146.

been shocking. In Chapter 7, we saw that one variation on the theme of modesty that frames Agnodice's story was to complain about her own lack of it. In 1920, an alarmed Campbell Bonner described the gesture she used to the Areopagus as 'this unnecessarily immodest act'.[6] Earlier retellings of Agnodice had shared Bonner's shocked reaction. For example, in his *A General Dictionary, Historical and Critical*, Bayle criticised her for having taken up her petticoats in front of 'the gravest and most venerable tribunal that was in the world'.[7] He exclaimed indignantly 'Had she not already given before this sufficient proofs of her want of shame? Could she not discover her sex in a more modest manner than that she made use of with the women?'[8]

A further level of immodesty lay in having a 'virgin girl', young and inexperienced, in a midwifery role; although it was not unknown in the ancient world – the virgin goddess Artemis/Diana was midwife to her own brother – to an early modern audience it would have seemed unusual. Pierre Dionis, for example, discussed youth as a fault in a midwife, framing it in terms of a wider opposition between theory (male) and practice (female), observing that midwives gain their knowledge from experience, knowing 'little or nothing of the Theory of their Art'. The solution was to gain this experience in childhood; midwives, he wrote, can be 'bred up to the Business by their Mothers'.[9] But, even with such experience, Dionis considered that 'A Midwife ought to be a married Woman. It is very indecent for one who is suppos'd not to know the Way of a Man with a Maid, to undertake to do the Office of a Midwife.'[10] On this reading, Agnodice is by definition indecent, knowing more than any virgin should.

'Taking up her petticoats' is a fair rendition of the basic gesture found on both occasions in Hyginus, where Agnodice 'lifts up her tunic to show she is a woman (Lat. *femina*)'.[11] In ancient Greek terms, the gesture is one of *anasyrmos*, 'lifting up', and as I mentioned in Chapter 5 this appears in a variety of classical sources.[12] What, however, is Agnodice supposed to be revealing to her different audiences? In an earlier piece I wrote on her, I asked whether she was displaying absence – of

[6]   Bonner, 'The Trial of St Eugenia', p. 258.

[7]   Bayle, *The Dictionary Historical and Critical*, p. 453.

[8]   Bayle, *A General Dictionary*, vol. 6, p. 172; he calls Agnodice 'impudent'. The translation Bayle gives is referenced as being from *Nouvelles de la Republique des Lettres* 2 (Jan. 1686), pp. 28–30, which he also largely wrote: this was a review of the Dutch physician Theodoor Jansson ab Almeloveen's *Opuscula: sive Antiquitatum e sacris profanarum specimen* (Amsterdam, 1686), where the story of Agnodice was given on pp. 86–7.

[9]   Dionis, *Traité general des accouchemens*, pp. 416–7; *General Treatise of Midwifery*, pp. 335–6. The English version is not a straightforward translation; for example, as one may expect, the French version has far more praise of the Hôtel-Dieu and its training on p. 418.

[10] Dionis, *Traité general des accouchemens*, p. 417; ibid., *General Treatise of Midwifery*, p. 336.

[11] R.S. Smith and Trzaskoma, *Apollodorus' Library and Hyginus' Fabulae*, p. 180.

[12] Above, p. 139–41.

the male genitalia – or presence – of the female genitalia, or even of the as-yet unproductive womb that is hinted at beneath her presumably flat stomach. There, I linked her *anasyrmos* to a set of stories in a group of ancient sources dating from the third century BC to the fifth century AD, in which mature women confront their menfolk – sons, or sons and husbands – as the men run away from a battle.[13] In these stories, like Agnodice, the women speak, as well as lifting their clothes: they challenge the masculinity of the men and ask them if they would like to crawl back inside the wombs from which they had once emerged. Classical scholars of the twentieth century found the 'fine speeches' of the women 'incompatible with such a primitive act' and suggested that the former had entered these stories only when the meaning of the gesture had been forgotten; however, in the sources it is 'both sight and hearing' that affect the men.[14] In these 'war stories', the speeches make it clear that *anasyrmos* should not be read simply as the display of the external genitalia; it also evokes the womb. In this particular context, the gesture seems to infantilise the male audience, with the women suggesting that the role of a mature man is to fight, and that of a mature woman is to give birth. The gesture evokes in the male audience a feeling of *aidôs* or of *aischynê*; the same sensation that, in the story of Agnodice, prevented the women from revealing their bodies to male healers. For Agnodice, however, the aspects of speech and gesture are divided up. It is the collective of 'noble women' that makes the speech to accompany her gesture, and they do not invite the men of the Areopagus to return to the womb, but tell them 'You are not husbands but enemies, for you condemn to death she who discovered health (Lat. *salus*) for us.'

The meaning of the gesture of *anasyrmos* varies according to who performs it. In the war stories, it not only occurs as part of a group action, but also changes its significance because it is being performed by mature women, rather than an individual 'virgin girl'. As a gesture by an individual, *anasyrmos* also features in the myth of Baubo, who tries to make the goddess Demeter laugh when her daughter Persephone has been taken by Hades to the underworld. In the versions of this myth, it is unclear whether Baubo simply shows her genitals, or has painted a face on her belly.[15] Here, as performed by an old woman, the gesture is funny; while there is an element of humour in the war stories, particularly in the words used by the women to recall their men to their proper roles, nobody laughs. In the war stories, normal gender boundaries are threatened by men who

---

[13]   King, 'Agnodike and the Profession of Medicine', pp. 63, 65–6.

[14]   Salomon Reinach, 'Le Rire rituel', in ibid., *Cultes, mythes et religions* vol. IV (Paris, 1912), p. 117, n. 2; Jacques Moreau, 'Les Guerriers et les femmes impudiques', *Annuaire de l'Institut de Philologie et d'Histoire orientales et slaves*, 11 (1951), pp. 286 and 290 similarly saw the gesture as 'primitive' but also speculated that the words only entered the story after the meaning of *anasyrmos* had almost been forgotten. On 'sight and hearing', King, 'Agnodike and the Profession of Medicine', p. 66.

[15]   Above, p. 140.

are not living up to their assigned roles. The gesture becomes one of restoring normality, using the sexed body to imply gender roles, showing that these women are 'in place' and recalling the men to their own proper place in society, as warriors. In Hyginus, instead, the boundaries have been put up in the wrong place, so that men are doing what women should do.

Other than Hyginus' story of Agnodice, I know of no classical stories in which a 'virgin girl' performs *anasyrmos*. Yet some early modern versions foreground Agnodice's identity as a 'virgin girl' or 'maid' rather than having her show herself to be a 'woman', *femina*, as in Hyginus' version. They also use variations on the verb 'to discover', thus avoiding being entirely explicit about precisely how Agnodice showed herself to be a 'maid'. In the 1612 English translation of Guillemeau, this verb featured in the demonstration of sex to the first patient: 'But when Agnodicea had assured her (by discovering of her selfe) that she was a maide ...' (in the French original, 'fille'). Elizabeth Cellier who, as we saw in Chapter 6, based her 1688 version of the story on Guillemeau, picked up his wording here for *both* audiences: Agnodice 'had discovered that she was a Maid' to her patients and was then forced 'to discover her Sex to save her Life' in court.[16] In Dionis too, 'Elle fut découverte' (in the English translation, she was 'discover'd').[17] In Potter's influential history of Greece, she 'revealed herself to her own sex' and then before the court 'discovered what sex she was made of'. Potter's wording seems to tone down the action a little, so that the verb 'to discover' shifts slightly from the earlier 'to reveal', with 'discovering one's sex' sounding closer to 'announcing one's sex'.[18] Sometimes, Agnodice is just 'convincing', without spelling out what convinces her audience. In the 1766 English version of Jean Astruc, the women accepted Agnodice's attention 'when she had convinced them that she was a woman'.[19] To the men, however, 'Agnodice shewed them that she was a woman.' However, in the French version of this treatise, published in 1768, both occasions became visual displays: the women accept her 'when she had made them see that she was a maid', while to the men she 'made them see that she was a woman'.[20] The language of the

---

[16]   Cellier, *To Dr* ... p. 4.

[17]   Dionis, *Traité general des accouchemens*, p. 354; ibid., *General Treatise of Midwifery*, p. 440.

[18]   The OED gives the meanings (1) 'To remove the covering from', (3a) 'To disclose or expose to view (anything covered up, hidden, or previously unseen) ... Now *rare*' and (4a) 'To divulge, reveal, disclose to knowledge (anything secret or unknown) ... *arch.*' The quotations given show that, at the time when Potter was writing, 3a and 4a coexisted.

[19]   Astruc, *Elements of Midwifery*, p. xxiv; French *L'Art d'accoucher réduit à ses principes* (Paris, 1768), p. xxxiv.

[20]   Astruc, *Elements of Midwifery*, p. xxiv; *L'Art d'accoucher réduit à ses principes*, p. xxxiv: 'quand elle leur eut fait *voir* qu'elle était une fille' and 'leur fît *voir* qu'elle étoit une femme' (my italics).

various versions can conceal the visual nature of what Agnodice does, and discover/convince are ambiguous, perhaps deliberately so.

'Putting aside her garment'

In the version that entered Estienne's *Dictionary* in 1590, Agnodice revealed her sex 'in secret' (Lat. *clam*) to her fellow patients – precisely how is not specified – but lifted her tunic to the court.[21] The English translation of Guillemeau, used by Cellier, took up this distinction, and used the safer 'discover' for the first patient, but was far more explicit for the second display, to the court. Here, it specified that Agnodice again 'made it evident that she was a maide', but this time by what seems to be a fuller revelation: 'putting aside her garments'.[22] In the original French of Guillemeau, however, her gesture was explicit for both audiences, as she 'lifted her robe' to her patient, but 'removed her robe' to the court.[23] Grant's translation, derivative here as elsewhere, renders the gesture which Agnodice performs to show her true sex in both instances as 'she removed her garment', but that does not seem to be what Hyginus meant.[24] On the twentieth-century medallions that adorn the exterior of the Paris Medical Faculty in rue des Saints-Pères, where she is labelled as a woman physician rather than a midwife, Agnodice has not just removed an outer garment, but stands before her accusers completely naked (Figure 8.1), more like the anatomical figure in Chapter 5 (Figure 5.2). Where does this total nudity come from? Possibly, from Guillemeau's 'removal'/'putting aside' of her robe to the male court, but that could have been understood as an outer garment rather than all her clothing. A very casual reading of the 1771 French translation of the midwife Elizabeth Nihell's version of the story may also suggest complete 'derobing'; following Hecquet, she has Agnodice 'sous l'habit d'un homme, alla s'instruire de l'Art d'accoucher pour se dérober à la poursuite des Loix'. But this means instead that she 'in male attire, went to learn the art of birthing to evade the pursuit of the laws'. In the French version of Nihell, there is no revelation of Agnodice's body, at any point in the story; when she meets her patients, there is no suggestion of how she reassures them, and when she is before the Areopagus she only 'declares' her sex.[25] This accurately renders the English original of 1760, where Agnodice had disguised herself 'to elude the cognizance

---

[21]   To the patients, *quas sexus sui clam certas faciebat*: to the court, *tunica alleuata se foeminam esse ostendit*; Estienne, *Dictionarium historicum ac poeticum*.

[22]   Guillemeau, *Child-Birth*, p. 81.

[23]   Guillemeau, *De l'heureux accouchement*, 1620 edition, p. 155, 'levant sa soutane / ayant osté sa soutane'.

[24]   Grant, *The Myths of Hyginus*. On the problems of this translation, R.S. Smith and Trzaskoma, *Apollodorus' Library and Hyginus' Fabulae*, p. lv.

[25]   Nihell, *La Cause de l'humanité*, p. 184 n. (a) : '… par la déclaration qu'elle fit de son sexe elle se justifia pleinement'.

of the law'; she was then accused in court 'against which she easily defended herself by a declaration of her sex'.[26] Rather than lifting her tunic, in nineteenth-century versions she could simply 'open' it; for example, in Jules Rouyer's study of ancient Roman medicine, published in 1859, 'she opened her tunic' to the

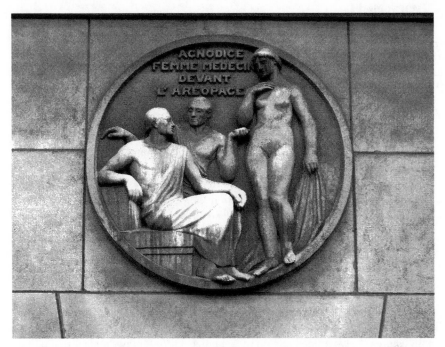

Figure 8.1   Agnodice 'the woman physician' before the Areopagus on the Paris Faculty of Medicine. Courtesy of Ralph Shephard

potential patients, then 'again lifted up her tunic' to the court.[27] This wording was repeated in Gustav Joseph Witkowski's biography of Agnodice published in his *Accoucheurs et sages-femmes célèbres* of 1891.[28]

Thomas Heywood's 1624 version similarly differentiated the gestures, but he had a more dramatic gesture than *anasyrmos* for the first patient, and a more discreet one for the court; for him Agnodice 'was forced to strip her selfe before the women, and to give evident signes of her woman-hood' to them, and then when 'the Judges were readie to proceed to sentence against her; when shee opening her brest before

---

[26]   Nihell, *A Treatise on the Art of Midwifery*, p. 220.

[27]   Rouyer, *Études médicales sur l'ancienne Rome*, p. 157: 'elle ouvrait son tunique' followed by 'relevant alors sa tunique'.

[28]   Gustav Joseph Witkowski, *Accoucheurs et sages-femmes célèbres: esquisses biographiques* (Paris, 1891), p. 2.

the Senat, gave manifest testimonie that she was no other then a woman'.[29] To an audience of women, he sees complete self-revelation as appropriate, but to an all-male audience it is her breasts rather than her genitals that are displayed.

'Twin apples'

In Chapter 6, we encountered the earliest engagement with Agnodice by a woman, the 1579 narrative poem by Catherine Des Roches. In *Agnodice*, the heroine, who is presented as using herbal remedies, hides her 'twin apples' in order to learn medicine.[30] Later, in front of her potential patients, she 'uncover[ed] her breasts' round white apples, and the beautiful blond tresses of her golden head' (which in this version of the story was not cut, but only hidden).[31] These women admired 'the little twin mounts of adorable breast'[32] and 'kissed her mouth and her breast a thousand times, while receiving help from her happy hands. Soon, one could see women and girls recover their fresh skin, and become more beautiful.'[33] This is a homoerotic Agnodice, with the final reference to skin recalling the later healer 'Agnodice' mentioned in the Introduction; her advertised remedies included 'a Liquid, which adds to the Face a Fresh and Lively Lustre and Colour, by stirring up the Blood to a quicker Circulation, proper for all those that look as Pale as Death'.[34] At the end of the story, in front of the men of the court, and condemned to die, Agnodice 'quickly uncovered the gold of her blond hair, and, showing them her beautiful breasts, pleasant dwelling places of the Muses, of virtue, of grace, of love, she lowered her eyes, filled with shame'.[35]

In the seventeenth century, too, exposing the breasts was regarded as 'acceptable, if immodest', and contrasted strongly with lifting one's skirts, normally associated with whores.[36] This milder version of Agnodice's lifting of her tunic was modified even further in a nineteenth-century drawing of her, found in Delacoux's collection

---

[29]   *Gynaikeion*, pp. 203–4.

[30]   Sankovitch, *French Women Writers and the Book*, p. 61; *Les Oeuvres des Mesdames des Roches de Poetiers mere et fille*, line 88, 'Les voulant secourir couvrit sa double pomme'; Larsen, *From Mother to Daughter*, pp. 122–31.

[31]   Lines 108–9, 'Lors descouvrant du sein les blanches pommes rondes, / Et de son chef doré les belles tresses blondes'.

[32]   Line 114, 'Et de son sein poupin le petit mont jumeau'.

[33]   Lines 118–21, 'Baiserent mille fois et sa bouche et son sein, / Recevant le secours de son heureuse main. / On voit en peu de temps les femmes et pucelles / Reprendre leurs teins frais, et devenir plus belles.'

[34]   'Agnodice; the WOMAN physician', British Library 551.a.32 (199).

[35]   Tr. Sankovitch, *French Women Writers and the Book*, p. 62; lines 145–8, '… Descouvrit promptement l'or de sa blonde teste, / Et monstrant son sein beau, aggreable sejour / Des Muses, des vertus, des graces, de l'amour, / Elle baissa les yeux pleins d'honneur et de honte.'

[36]   Gowing, *Common Bodies*, p. 35 and pp. 36–7.

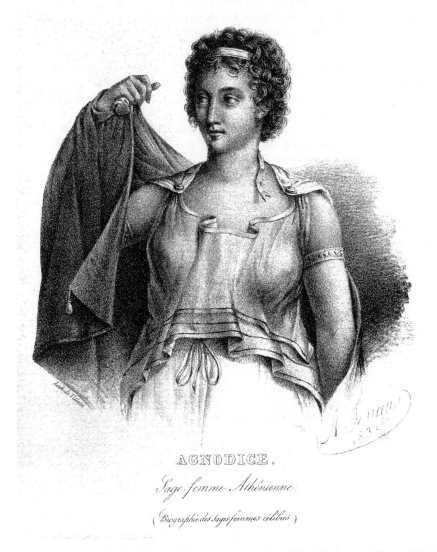

AGNODICE.

Sage-femme Athénienne.

(*Biographie des sages-femmes célèbres.*)

Figure 8.2   Agnodice: Delacoux, *Biographie des sages-femmes celebres* (1934), facing p. 25

on famous midwives, where she simply undoes her mantle to show her chiton, with just the shape of her breasts being visible (Figure 8.2). Here, then, it is considered perfectly acceptable to show one's external genitalia to fellow women, but not to men; while in other versions of the story, such as that of Catherine Des Roches, both displays are censored. Kendall Tarte has described Des Roches' *Agnodice* as a 'poem that dramatizes the power of female coyness'.[37] Certainly, the Dames Des Roches believed in the combination of chastity and intelligence, personified in Catherine herself. Although Agnodice reveals her body to men, she is represented as blushing when she does this.

Catherine Des Roches takes the presence of female parts, rather than the absence of male parts, as the important feature in proving sex. When Agnodice uncovers her body to the women to gain their trust, it is noteworthy that she does this as a series of body parts: breasts, hair, complexion, eyes, mouth and hand, and also 'sweet words'.[38] But not, however, genitalia. Showing the breasts to demonstrate one's female sex conclusively is, as I noted in Chapter 5, also found in classical sources, such as Aristophanes' *Lysistrata*, where one of the female characters refers to Menelaus who, at the sight of Helen of Troy's 'two little apples bare', dropped his sword, unable to go through with killing her.[39] However, as with the meaning of *anasyrmos* shifting according to the person performing it, different breasts give different messages. Ann Hanson and David Armstrong drew attention to a passage in Nonnus' *Dionysiaca*, dating to the early fifth century AD, in which one of Artemis' nymphs falls into disfavour after contrasting her own breasts – 'unripe grapes', thus little, like those of Des Roches' Agnodice – with the more womanly breasts of the (virgin) goddess.[40] The size of Agnodice's breasts is part of her identity as a 'virgin girl', not a fully grown woman. In the Hippocratic case story, Phaethousa's breasts never feature; the only parts of her body that are mentioned are those visible without adjusting the clothing.

Eloquence and Intellect

In her recent chapter on Elizabeth Cellier's phrase 'discover her Sex', Anne Barbeau Gardiner did not appreciate the visual sense of 'discovery' that was present in Cellier's sources, and so presented Agnodice as having 'told the women her secret'.[41] But in other engagements with the story, both in the early modern period and later, it is indeed Agnodice's eloquence, sometimes combined with the experience of hearing her voice itself, that persuades the court of her innocence.

---

[37]   Kendall B. Tarte, *Writing Places: Sixteenth-Century City Culture and the Des Roches Salon* (Newark, DE, 2007), p. 56.

[38]   Lines 113–17, 'ses doux propos'; Tarte, *Writing Places*, p. 57.

[39]   Aristophanes, *Lysistrata*, 115–16.

[40]   Ann Hanson and David Armstrong, 'Two Notes on Greek Tragedy. The Virgin's Voice and Neck: Aeschylus, *Agamemnon* 245 and Other Texts', *Bulletin of the Institute of Classical Studies,* 33 (1986), pp. 98–9; Nonnus, *Dionysiaca*, 48.531–3, 362–9. For comments on the 'fetishisation' of the breast in Nonnus, see Ronald F. Newbold, 'Fear of Sex in Nonnus' Dionysiaca', *Electronic Antiquity*, 4.2 (1988), <http://scholar.lib.vt.edu/ejournals/ElAnt/V4N2/newbold.html> accessed 12 September 2012.

[41]   *To Dr* ... p. 4; Gardiner, 'Elizabeth Cellier in 1688', p. 28.

Catherine Des Roches' Agnodice used 'sweet words' to persuade women to let them treat her, while in Bayle's *Dictionary*, when Agnodice is accused, it is her explanation of why she disguised herself to help women that wins the day: 'she gave so good reason for what she had done, that she escaped Punishment'.[42] Rather than representing her as revealing her body, the eighteenth-century anti-Caesarean doctor Jean-François Sacombe ('the Juvenal of French physicians') has her summarising the situation to the court in a mere three words:

On la traîne au Sénat, mais grâce à la nature,
Agnodice en trois mots confondit l'imposture:
Je suis femme, dit-elle ...[43]

The sheer brevity of Agnodice's answer in Sacombe's version contrasts with the traditional image of the gossiping midwife, a good representation of whom occurs in Pierre Dionis' treatise on midwifery, published in French in 1718 and in English translation in 1719. Here, Dionis states that the midwife should 'leave off several Vices proper to their Sex and Profession', including gossiping about other cases, and also telling 'of a great many extraordinary Cases as true'.[44] With her laconic speech Agnodice, in contrast, becomes a model of the correct use of words.

Sacombe's reference to 'la nature' may suggest that not only the three words, but also the way in which she says them, have the power to change the situation: her voice itself is feminine. One may wonder why nobody had suspected that she was a woman before this event, simply by her voice. The answer is simply that here there was a spectrum of possibilities, as in the range of genital possibilities of a 'one-sex' body. In the Introduction, I noted that the presence of a shrill voice in a man could be taken to mean that he had been female in the womb, but had changed sex there. In 1986, Ann Hanson and David Armstrong collaborated on an article on the voice of the virgin in ancient Greek sources; they showed that, based on an analogy between the top and the bottom of the channel believed to go from the mouth to the vulva, defloration was thought to affect the voice, making it deeper.[45] Of course, it does not deepen to the level of Phaethousa's voice, which is part of her masculine appearance; there is a spectrum from the girl, through the mature woman, and to the man. All this would suggest that the 'virgin girl' Agnodice would have a very high voice, but this could have been read as evidence of a sex change before birth. Physiognomic literature of the

[42]   *The Dictionary Historical and Critical*, p. 653.

[43]   Jean-François Sacombe, *La Luciniade ou l'art des accouchements, poème didactique* (Paris, 1792), chant 3, 26–7; Delacoux, *Biographie des sages-femmes célèbres*, p. 26; see Martial Dumont, 'La délirante "Luciniade" de l'anticésarien Jean-François Sacombe', *Revue Française de Gynécologie et d'Obstétrique* 66 (1971), pp. 199–204.

[44]   Dionis, *Traité general des accouchemens*, pp. 416–17; ibid., *A General Treatise of Midwifery*, p. 335. On midwives and gossip, see above, p. 156.

[45]   Hanson and Armstrong, 'Two Notes on Greek Tragedy', *pp. 97–8*.

Roman Empire – another genre not addressed by Laqueur – listed the features by which a masculine or a feminine body could be identified, and suggested that a high voice was part of the identity of the androgyne, the effeminate male.[46] Possibly, then, we are to assume that Agnodice passed as a man because she was assumed to be an effeminate one; or, by emphasising her youth, perhaps she passed as a very young man. In a 1912 version of Agnodice, her voice is represented very differently, as a source of her authority; when she was taken before the court in her masculine clothing, she announced that she could 'in three simple words' refute the charges against her, and spoke to answer them in 'a voice whose full, rich, swelling tones were like unto an organ's'.[47] On this reading, she passed as a man more easily because she sounded like one.

In some versions of the story, Agnodice's body ceases to be of interest, and instead the focus is on her mind. In *The Ladies Dictionary* of 1694, the motif of exposure was completely obliterated, so that it is Agnodice's intellect that persuades the court; 'she gave such Learned Demonstrations, that the Cause not only went for her, but an Order was made, that any free Woman of Athens might practice Physick, and that the Men physicians should no more meddle with Women in Childbirth, seeing the Women were as capable in all matters'.[48] Is this, however, a knowing joke, with the reader expected to understand exactly what it was that Agnodice 'demonstrated'? In 1769, when Elisabetta Caminer Turra told the story in 'On Exceptional Women', picking it up from a dictionary of historical women published in the same year, it was in a section on 'our sex's desire for knowledge'.[49] The famous French midwife Marie Anne Victoire Boivin (1774–1841) was addressed in an elegy by Daniel Wyttenbach, the Professor of Greek Literature at Leyden, as 'The French Agnodice': during her lifetime, Alexis Delacoux singled out as Boivin's main quality her 'mérite scientifique'.[50] In Sophia Jex-Blake's nineteenth-century version, it was purely Agnodice's 'skill

---

[46]   Simon Swain (ed.), *Seeing the Face, Seeing the Soul: Philemon's Physiognomy from Classical Antiquity to Medieval Islam* (Oxford, 2007), pp. 187–9 on the voice of the *androgynos*; p. 559 for the fourth-century AD treatise, *Anonymus Latinus*, where Chapter 5 lists the qualities of the masculine body, Chapter 6 those of the feminine.

[47]   James S. Sprague, 'Agnodice', *Dominion Monthly and Ontario Medical Journal* 38 (1912), p. 11. In fact she takes more than the three words given in Sacombe, saying 'I am but a woman, and my name Agnodice.'

[48]   N.H., *The Ladies Dictionary*, pp. 4–5.

[49]   Catherine M. Sama (ed. and tr.), *Elisabetta Caminer Turra: Selected Writings of an Eighteenth-Century Venetian Woman of Letters* (Chicago, IL, 2003), p. 170; the dictionary was Jean-François Delacroix, *Dictionnaire historique portatif des femmes célèbres*, 2 vols (Paris, 1769).

[50]   Delacoux, *Biographie des sages-femmes célèbres*, pp. 42–3. Ann Carol, 'Sage-femme ou gynécologue? M.-A. Boivin (1773–1841)', *Clio: Histoire, femmes et sociétés*, 33 (2011), p. 254, n. 36 on Wyttenbach; p. 243 on Boivin's combination of the practical and theoretical; p. 247 on women's hands.

and success in medicine' that led to 'the legal opening of the medical profession to all the free-born women of the state'.[51]

Jex-Blake was writing at a time when women were thought to be in danger of damaging their health if they studied. In 1874, Henry Maudsley claimed that 'women whose reproductive organs remain from some cause in a state of arrested development, approach the mental and bodily habits of men'.[52] In the 1880s, Thomas Smith Clouston warned of the dangers to 'body and mind' for 'The girl student who has concentrated all her force on cramming book knowledge, neglecting her bodily requirements.'[53] He stated that 'The unceasing grind at book-knowledge, from thirteen to twenty, has actually warped the woman's nature, and stunted some of her most characteristic qualities. She is, no doubt, cultured, but then she is unsympathetic; learned, but not self-denying. The nameless graces and charms of manner have not been evoked as much as they might have been. Softness is deficient.'[54] Because by this period it was believed that a woman who studied would become masculine, one possibility here was that Agnodice was able to pass as a man simply because her efforts to learn medicine had altered her body.

Being Too Smooth

In Hyginus' version of her story, Agnodice is not 'soft' so much as 'smooth'; she is, in the Latin, *glaber*, 'smooth/hairless'. While this refers in particular to her lack of a beard, the word also implies that in some way this makes her attractive to the women patients, a point addressed in different ways by Hyginus' modern translators. Grant has the doctors saying that 'he' was 'a seducer and corruptor of women'; Smith and Trzaskoma instead give 'asserting that she was an effeminate gigolo and seducing them'.[55] A better translation, separating out the two concepts a little more, is found in Green: 'they said she was a "smooth-faced boy" and a corrupter of women'.[56] Early modern translations have some sense of this too; for example, in Heywood she is thought to be 'a loose and intemperate yong man'.[57]

---

[51]   Jex-Blake, 'Medicine as a Profession for Women', p. 85 and *Medical Women. A Thesis and a History*, 2nd edition (Edinburgh and London, 1886), pp. 10–11.

[52]   Henry Maudsley, 'Sex in Mind and in Education', *Popular Science Monthly* (June 1874), p. 202.

[53]   Thomas Smith Clouston, 'Female Education from a Medical Point of View (I)', *Popular Science Monthly*, 24 (1883), p. 214, discussed by Farkas, *Aesculapia Victrix*, pp. 57–8.

[54]   Thomas Smith Clouston, 'Female Education from a Medical Point of View (II)', *Popular Science Monthly*, 24 (1884), p. 332.

[55]   The Latin is *quod dicerunt eum glabrum esse et corruptorem earum*.

[56]   M.H. Green, *Making Women's Medicine Masculine*, p. 31.

[57]   Heywood, *Gynaeikeion*, p. 203.

Agnodice's smoothness of course contrasts strongly with Phaethousa, who is not only bearded but has hair all over her body.

Body hair, in antiquity and beyond, could distinguish between child and adult, male and female, human and animal.[58] Hairiness, in both quantity and location, was a relative concept. For example, Aristotle used hair to distinguish between men and beasts. In comparison with women, men were characterised as 'hairy', but in comparison with animals men are relatively hair*less*, making them the exception among the viviparous animals; men also have more hair on the head than any animal, and more hair on the front of the body than on the back.[59] In his discussion of apes, Aristotle noted that to have hair on the front is to be anthropoid, 'man-like'.[60] He noted that, among animals, man is also distinctive in being the only animal to have some hair that only comes later in life, and that in both men and women, to have no pubic hair is a sign of sterility.[61] He stated that the hair on the chin grows only after that of the pubic area and the armpits, making it the last hair to appear.[62] In humans, he stated that the hair is hard in warm parts of the body, and soft in cold parts; again, the production of very strong hair is associated with heat, gendered masculine.[63] The meaning of body and facial hair thus differs according to whether men are being compared to women (in which case, men are very hairy) or to beasts (in which case, men are not very hairy at all, and have most of theirs on the front, and develop it in different parts during the life cycle).[64]

Even the body hair which is the result of the greater heat of the man and thus a marker of masculinity should be neither too skimpy nor too excessive. Dominic Montserrat showed how ordinary people in Roman Egypt used 'wispy-bearded' as one of the characteristics employed to identify men.[65] The adjective is *spanopôgôn* or *kakopôgôn*: a wispy beard is *kakos*, 'bad of its kind', because a beard should be a substantial thing, not a mere wisp. But it should not be excessively big; it needs to be trimmed, rather than shaggy. On late fifth-century

---

[58]   Mireille M. Lee, 'Body-Modification in Classical Greece', in Thorsten Fögen and Mireille M. Lee (eds), *Bodies and Boundaries in Graeco-Roman Antiquity* (Berlin, 2009), pp. 168–9. This section draws on King, 'Barbes, sang et genre'.

[59]   Aristotle, *Generation of Animals*, 782b10–11; *History of Animals*, 498b16–22.

[60]   Aristotle, *History of Animals*, 502a24.

[61]   Aristotle, *History of Animals*, 518a19–20; Gk *agonos*, Aristotle, *History of Animals*, 518a33–b3.

[62]   Aristotle, *History of Animals*, 518a22.

[63]   Aristotle, *History of Animals*, 517b19–20.

[64]   Dean-Jones, *Women's Bodies in Classical Greek Science*, p. 85 further notes that 'Aristotle has difficulty in attaining consistency in his theory of hair growth because while adult men produce more they also lose more, and he wants both to be indications of male superiority.'

[65]   Dominic Montserrat, 'Experiencing the Male Body in Roman Egypt', in Lin Foxhall and John Salmon, *When Men Were Men: Masculinity, Power and Identity in Classical Antiquity* (London and New York, 1998), p. 162.

BC Greek vases, painters showed Sleep as a beardless youth, Death as an older, bearded and 'often unkempt' figure.[66] This brought Death into the dangerously hairy world of the ancient bandit, a figure also associated with long shaggy beards.[67] For Clement of Alexandria, a contemporary of Galen, man, like the lion, is adorned with a beard, but this beard must still be trimmed.[68] As in all other areas of ancient body-maintenance, there was a thin line between control, and too much control. Excessive care for the physical appearance – grooming – was believed not only to alter the externals, but also to affect the core masculinity: Clement added that such men 'cease to enjoy good health, and decline in the direction of greater softness until they play the woman's part'.[69]

As for hair removal, both the Greeks and the Romans regarded depilation by men – particularly on the legs and chest – as a sign of effeminacy.[70] In Aristophanes' play *The Acharnians*, the politician Cleisthenes was ridiculed for his effeminacy; his lack of a beard and of pubic hair due to shaving was associated with his willingness to take the 'female' (subordinate) role in sex.[71] In a mature man, excessive care for one's appearance was always gendered 'feminine'. This is common to both Greek and Latin sources, over a long period of time. According to a fragment of the Roman Republican writer Scipio Aemilianus preserved by Aulus Gellius, P. Sulpicius Gallus shaved his eyebrows and plucked his beard and thighs; such hairlessness was seen as a sign of effeminacy and of taking the 'female role', but it was also thought to appeal to women.[72] There were variations in fashion; in the first century AD, Seneca poured scorn on men who shave around the lips while leaving the rest of the beard (*Epistula* 114.21), while in the second century AD the

[66]   Emma Stafford, 'Masculine Values, Feminine Forms: On the Gender of Personified Abstractions', in Lin Foxhall and John Salmon, *Thinking Men: Masculinity and its Self-Representation in the Classical Tradition* (London and New York, 1988), p. 50.

[67]   Keith Hopwood, '"All that May Become a Man": The Bandit in the Ancient Novel', in Foxhall and Salmon, *When Men Were Men*, pp. 201–2.

[68]   Clement of Alexandria, *Paidagôgas* 3.3; cf. Lucian, *The Cynic* 14; Gillian Clark, 'The Old Adam: The Fathers and the Unmaking of Masculinity', in Foxhall and Salmon, *Thinking Men*, pp. 172–3.

[69]   Clement, *Paidagôgas* 3.15.1, cited in Gleason, 'The Semiotics of Gender', p. 400; Gleason, *Making Men: Sophists and Self-Presentation in Ancient Rome* (Princeton, NJ, 1995), p. 68. Clement also believed that Eve was made out of the sole hairless part of the body of Adam, her removal leaving him entirely 'male': what is covered with hair is dry/hot (Clement, *Paidagôgas* 3.19.2, cited in Gleason, 'The Semiotics of Gender', p. 401; *Making Men*, p. 69).

[70]   Gleason, *Making Men*, pp. 67–70; Craig A. Williams, *Roman Homosexuality: Ideologies of Masculinity in Classical Antiquity* (New York and Oxford, 1999), p. 129.

[71]   *Acharnians* 118–21; further references in Adriaan Rademaker, '"Most Citizens Are *Euruprôktoi* Now": (Un)manliness in Aristophanes', in Ralph Rosen and Ineke Sluiter (eds), *Andreia: Studies in Manliness and Courage in Classical Antiquity* (Leiden, 2003), p. 122 n. 21.

[72]   Aulus Gellius, *Attic Nights*, 6.12.5; Williams, *Roman Homosexuality*, p. 129–30.

Roman emperor Hadrian's beard may have been a deliberate way of setting his reign apart from that of his predecessor, and quickly started a trend.[73]

Boys were a different matter, and the Romans and Greeks shared 'a taste for smooth young bodies'.[74] To be hairless – boy or woman – is to be submissive. It is here that we meet the adjective *glaber*, applied to Agnodice; for example, the poet Catullus describes Manlius Torquatus having 'a hard time keeping his hands off his hairless boy (*glaber*)'.[75] In Roman society, as in classical Athenian sources, a full beard was a signifier of sexual maturity and, in particular, of the end of the period when the boy was a desirable sexual partner.[76] Roman epitaphs to boys who died before the ceremony of the *depositio barbae*, in which beard clippings were dedicated to the gods, and which usually occurred in the twentieth year,[77] use what Williams has called 'the language of flowering youth'; *flos aetatis*.[78] Indeed, the beard itself could be described as 'the new flower' on the face of a young man.[79] This is an example of the use of the head and its hair as a metonym for the genitalia and the pubic hair; the head and facial hair are used to display meanings that are otherwise hidden under clothing.[80]

What, then, does Agnodice's apparent 'smoothness' indicate? In Guillemeau we read that the jealous physicians 'accused the said Agnodicea, that she had shaved off her beard, that thereby she might abuse women, faining themselves to be sicke'.[81] This was copied by Cellier: 'This so incensed the Physicians that they conspired her Ruin, saying she shaved off her Beard to abuse the Women, who feigned themselves sick to enjoy her Company.'[82] In the version told by Jean Astruc in the 1760s, in contrast, her rivals 'accused Agnodice of being a

---

[73]   Paul Zanker, *The Mask of Socrates: The Image of the Intellectual in Antiquity* (Berkeley, CA, 1995), pp. 217–32.

[74]   Williams, *Roman Homosexuality*, p. 73.

[75]   Catullus, 61.134–6.

[76]   Williams, *Roman Homosexuality*, pp. 26, 73.

[77]   Aristotle, *History of Animals*, 582a32–33 puts the development of the beard at between 14 and 21. On the Roman rituals surrounding the first beard, see Mary Harlow and Ray Laurence, *Growing Up and Growing Old in Ancient Rome: A Life Course Approach* (London and New York, 2002), pp. 72–4.

[78]   Williams, *Roman Homosexuality*, p. 74 and p. 296 n. 60.

[79]   *CLE* 1170.3–4, cited by Williams, *Roman Homosexuality*, p. 297 n. 62.

[80]   Judith Lynn Sebesta, 'Women's Costume and Feminine Civic Morality in Augustan Rome', in Maria Wyke (ed.), *Gender and the Body in the Ancient Mediterranean* (Oxford, 1998), p. 109.

[81]   Guillemeau, *Child-Birth*, p. 80; *De l'heureux accouchement*, 1620 edition, p. 155: 'accuserent ladite Agnodicee de s'estre fait raser la barbe, afin d'abuser les femmes, seignant qu'elles estoient malades'.

[82]   Cellier, *To Dr ...* p. 4.

eunuch, as it appeared she had no beard; and of debauching women'.[83] So in one version she is assumed to be bearded, but shaving in order to make 'himself' seem more attractive to women: in the other, she is a eunuch. In the first version, she is deliberately changing her external signs of sex: in the second, her identity is neither that of a man nor that of a woman. To have a eunuch 'debauching women' may seem odd, but eunuchs created after puberty could still achieve erection; however, it was those created prior to puberty who had the characteristic lack of facial and body hair which *glaber* suggests.[84]

According to 'Philalethes' in his 1649 attack on men's attempts to take over midwifery, the London midwives were not prepared to listen to Peter Chamberlen III because they 'scorn'd to learn from a man, that had no more beard than themselves'; as in the Agnodice story, the beard is used here as a marker of gender identity.[85] In 1670, the elder Hugh Chamberlen travelled to Paris and met François Mauriceau, whose treatise *Traité des maladies des femmes grosses et accouchées* had first appeared in 1668.[86] Mauriceau does not tell the story of Agnodice, but I would suggest that he knew it. He considered whether the male surgeon who wants to practise midwifery should 'be slovenly, or at least very careless, growing a long dirty beard, so as not to afford any occasion for jealousy to the husbands of the women who send for him to help them'.[87] He concluded, however, that an attractive appearance was better; as Lianne McTavish puts it, 'appealing to women [rather] than reassuring their husbands'.[88] Discussing this passage, McTavish notes that Mauriceau finally comes down in favour of what she summarises as 'a clean-shaven, gentle male midwife able to comfort his female clients'.[89] Or, as we could argue from the discussions throughout this book, a man-midwife like Agnodice,

---

[83]   Astruc, *Elements of Midwifery*, p. xxiv; the French original, *L'Art d'accoucher*, p. xli, includes the Latin here, *glabrum esse*. *Glaber* is translated 'a man without a beard' in Bayle's *Dictionary*, p. 172, s.v. Hierophilus.

[84]   Shaun Tougher, 'Byzantine Eunuchs: An Overview, with Special Reference to their Creation and Origin', in Liz James (ed.), *Women, Men and Eunuchs: Gender in Byzantium* (London and New York, 1997), p. 170 points out that eunuchs did have sex with women, although this could not result in pregnancy. See also Mathew Kuefler, *The Manly Eunuch: Masculinity, Gender Ambiguity and Christian Ideology in Late Antiquity* (Chicago, IL, 2001), pp. 34–6.

[85]   'Philalethes', *An Answer to Doctor Chamberlaines Scandalous and False Papers* (London, 1649), p. 2.

[86]   François Mauriceau, *Traité des maladies des femmes grosses et accouchées* (Paris, 1668). It was reprinted many times, and translated into six other languages; in English, *The Diseases of Women with Child, and in Child-Bed: As Also, the Best Means of Helping Them in Natural and Unnatural Labours*, 4th edition (London, 1710). See McTavish, *Childbirth and the Display of Authority*, p. 26.

[87]   Mauriceau, *Des maladies des femmes*, p. 267; translated by McTavish, *Childbirth and the Display of Authority*, p. 113.

[88]   Ibid., p. 113.

[89]   Ibid., pp. 113–4. Clean-shaven recalls Agnodice as *glaber*.

attractively beardless even though this puts him at risk of accusations of seducing the women he attends, or of being seen by female midwives as lacking authority.

'A man's mind in a woman's form': The Transgender Agnodice

Considering Agnodice as a eunuch brings us to one further version of the story. As we have seen, she has been a historical precedent and a role model for women since the sixteenth century, used by Catherine Des Roches and Elizabeth Cellier, among others. At the end of Chapter 5, discussing Agnodice as a role model today, I mentioned the Swiss Fondation Agnodice, which includes on its website a page on 'Who was Agnodice?' The group promotes understanding of people with 'atypical gender', including transgender, transsexual and intersex; members are involved either professionally or personally with this work.[90] In correspondence with the president, Dr Erika Volkmar, I asked her why Agnodice had been chosen. She replied 'We can assume that if Agnodice was successful in practising OBG as a man, she must have been at least very androgyne and gender variant ... Agnodice is perfect as she was both gender variant AND an outstanding professional. Equally, our foundation council is composed of a majority of great professionals with atypical gender identity. She is a model because as a gender variant person she obtained a major victory against the prejudice and sexism of our society, i.e. making medical studies accessible to women.' In response to a further question as to why Agnodice had been chosen rather than Phaethousa, she added 'she is much more appropriate (and credible) than some kind of phantasy that would just reinforce the mythical prejudice trans people already suffer from, i.e. the fascination of people for something weird and bizarre'.[91]

I find this an interesting response. Here, the questions about how Agnodice was so easily able to disguise herself are answered by making her gender variant. In terms of the questions raised in Chapter 7, she is not a midwife, but the pioneer who made it possible for women to study medicine as a whole. In this book, I have argued that – despite attempts to locate her historically – Agnodice is more of a fantasy than Phaethousa. But Phaethousa is a patient, a victim, whereas Agnodice is an active agent, and hence more attractive as an ally. Phaethousa, the bearded woman, is passive, the object of male discussion, and she dies: Agnodice, the smooth 'man', is active, an agent controlling her own image, and she lives. As we have seen in this book, both stories were popular in previous

---

[90]   <http://www.agnodice.ch/> accessed 20 March 2010: 'de promouvoir en Suisse une société bienveillante et juste envers toute personne manifestant une identité de genre atypique'.

[91]   Erika Volkmar, pers. comm., 22 March 2010.

ages because of the 'weird and bizarre' elements in them. Agnodice has another life on websites hailing her as transgender.[92]

The transgender Agnodice is not, in fact, a new reading. Her emergence can be traced back to an elaborate version published in 1912, where – rather than giving a three-word statement of her true sex – she told the court,

> As a child I saw my brothers at their games and books, wherein they told me I could have no part, because forsooth, I was a woman-child! That to my sex forever was denied the boon of knowledge, for the gods ordained that woman by her nature was but fit for household tasks and bearing of the young. I answered naught, but in my heart was born faint stirring of rebellion 'gainst my fate. I mused – 'How strange that these same mighty gods have placed such aspirations in my breast that do of right belong to men alone!'

Later she says 'And so I reasoned, 'twas a blunder made, for which the gods were not responsible. Dame Nature 'twas who in erratic mood had linked a man's mind to a woman's form.'[93]

Conclusion

What, then, does the classical and early modern evidence say to Laqueur's thesis, in *Making Sex*? Most fundamentally, that the 'two-sex' body is not a modern development, tied to specific changes in the eighteenth century. Throughout this book I have demonstrated the coexistence of 'one-sex' and 'two-sex' models over the period from Hippocratic Greece to the nineteenth century, and their presence alongside other ways of understanding the body. 'One-sex' bodies can be fluid, with each sex able to become the other, or hierarchical, with movement only in one direction, and women regarded as perpetually failed males. I have shown that Galen's 'inside-out' body is not as simple as it may appear; it was phrased as a thought experiment, with conflicting models appearing elsewhere in his work. I have identified the second half of the sixteenth century – when not only Hippocratic 'two-sex' models, but also the story of Agnodice, were becoming more widely known – as the nearest thing to a Laqueur-style watershed in how the body was seen, as it was then that ideas that men were women, but 'inside-out', were rejected as ridiculous.

Like Laqueur, I agree that denials of the 'one-sex' body were not due to an increased focus on what could actually be seen, in anatomy; what was seen depended on what the viewer expected to see. In contrast to him, I would stress that expectations were affected by such factors as the return of Hippocratic

---

[92] For example, *A Gender Variance Who's Who*, <http://zagria.blogspot.co.uk/2012/06/hagnodike-3rd-century-bce-physician.html> accessed 15 November 2012.

[93] Sprague, 'Agnodice', p. 13.

gynaecology to Western European medicine following the publication of the complete Hippocratic corpus in 1525. However, I have emphasised throughout that this viewer – ancient, early modern, male, female – must be properly read in his or her own time. The Vesalius Figure 27 would, I have argued, have been seen not as a womb-as-penis, but as an empty womb with its extendable neck. The same cautions apply to reading texts; we must read closely, so that we do not depend on our conflicting assumptions about apparent similarity (leading us to take Phaethousa at face value as a case history, trusting in her connection with the 'Father of Medicine') and about apparent difference (encouraging us to construct the past as alien territory and to marvel at the possibility of a time when people did not feel secure in their sex). Every source should be interrogated closely; a book such as the *Masterpiece* is complex, drawing on previous texts in both Latin and English, and also went into many versions. Sixteenth-century discussions of Phaethousa could engage closely with the Hippocratic story, or could range widely, selecting features from it, and finding connections between it and other ancient medical or non-medical writing. We have seen stories echoing each other; Agnodice recalls the Hippocratic statement of women's reluctance to speak to men about their diseases, and Caelius Aurelianus' story of how women physicians came into being, while there are striking parallels between Diodorus' Heraïs and Phaethousa in the absence of their husbands which precipitates their physical changes, and in their status as *oikouros*. In Phaethousa's case this status seems to demonstrate her underlying femininity, while for Heraïs it is an assumed behaviour that allows her to disguise the penis beneath her female clothing. It is rarely possible to lay out a neat pattern of direct connection, an intellectual family tree in which the writers of these stories read the previous versions, but maybe that is the point.

Another point follows from this: our source base should be widened beyond the major medical texts, and even within medicine the sources should be read according to their genre. The stories I have chosen here, however, are interesting precisely because neither fits neatly into a single genre. Agnodice is a novel, a historical account, a myth, and/or a role model: Phaethousa is a case history, a thought experiment, a cautionary tale, a precedent. And these categories are not exclusive – a story can be more than one, over time, or at the same time. Phaethousa shows how a story can escape from the clutches of medical writers and become something else; how a medical text can merge with myths. Furthermore, our sources should be read where possible 'against the grain'; for example, Diodorus Siculus' story of the sex change of Heraïs is surrounded by distancing devices that work to undercut a straightforward interpretation. Claims to have seen something for oneself are rarely straightforward, and could be copied from one writer to another. Throughout this book I have also used the variations on these stories in later historical periods as a way of returning to the original texts and thinking about what they meant when they were composed. In neither case is it possible to tie them very precisely to social or cultural changes; the Hippocratic *Epidemics* 6 can only be located approximately, while Hyginus' *Fabulae* is impossible even to date firmly to any one century. We can say more about these stories' readers and users, and how Agnodice and Phaethousa met their specific needs.

In the stories of both Phaethousa and Agnodice, there is a true sex that does not depend on the externals: voice, facial and body hair, clothing. In each case, judging from what one sees leads to error. For Phaethousa, her true sex is shown not by externals but by what is inside: the womb, invisible, but known through her status as a previously prolific mother, *epitokos*. She was not a woman trying to play a male role – she was not an Amazon – but a woman influenced by what was then believed about her biology; her blood simply could not stop becoming a beard when its normal flow was blocked. Her very femininity is her downfall; an entirely successful woman in that she had previously been highly fertile, the fact that she could not divorce her husband – or, in other versions, her faithfulness to him and her continued desire for him – meant that she could not find the proper outlet for her blood. The womb was always a problem for a 'one-sex' model, as it had no obvious analogue with the body, and attempts to match it to the scrotum were not persuasive. Performing the comparison the other way around, and starting with the man, the penis was hard to match to the female body: was it the womb, the vagina, or the clitoris?

Phaethousa's body needs to be read with specialist knowledge: Agnodice chooses who reads her body, and how. Over time, Phaethousa – originally, I have argued, a 'two-sex' story about difference – was brought into lists of sex change stories that emphasised change over time, even being said to have 'turned into a man', but alongside this reading other early modern users insisted that she was the best evidence of the impossibility of such a change. For her, much hinged on whether a key element of the original story – her death – was included, or was conveniently forgotten by 'one-sex' readers who wanted to keep her as the Hippocratic icing at the top of their list of cases of sex change. As for Agnodice's story, its value for readers could depend on whether it was presented as a story about midwifery – 'The ancients had no midwives' – or was seen as evidence that women could be physicians; I have suggested that it could originally have been a story about women physicians, shaped to fit a list of 'Who invented what', but in any case it is clear that its sixteenth-century readers understood her to be a physician, while in the eighteenth century some took her instead as a midwife. Like the womb in the body, birth became the sticking point, the situation in which women's difference is most obvious, and where a 'two-sex' reading may suggest that they should insist on medical help from someone of their own sex. But if women are radically different, should only a woman care for a woman, or is this something that can be done by a specialised male physician?

Applying 'one-sex'/'two-sex' labels here obscures the complexity of the different interest groups, readers and tellers of my chosen stories. Like retrospective diagnosis, it hides the historically specific detail, the mindset of the historical subjects. These stories and themes are fluid, prefiguring and echoing each other, in a dance that never ends.

Appendix: Agnodice in Latin and in Selected English Translations

(A) Hyginus, *Fabula* 274:

Antiqui obstetrices non habuerunt, unde mulieres verecundia ductae interierant (nam Athenienses caverant, ne quis servus aut f[o]emina artem medicinam disceret) Agnodice quaedam puella virgo concupivit medicinam discere. quae cum concupisset, demptis capillis habitu virili se H[i]erophilo cuidam tradidit in disciplinam. quae cum artem didicisset et f[o]eminam laborantem audisset ab inferiore parte, veniebat ad eam. quae cum credere se noluisset existimans virum esse illa tunica sublata ostendebat se f[o]eminam esse: et ita eas curabat. quod cum vidissent medici se ad f[o]eminas non admitti Agnodicen accusare coeperunt, quod dicerunt eum glabrum esse et corruptorem earum et illas simulare imbecillitatem. quod cum Areopagitae consedissent Agnodicen damnare coeperunt. quibus Agnodice tunicam allevavit et se ostendit f[o]eminam esse. et validius medici accusare coeperunt, quare tum feminae principes ad iudicium venerunt et dixerunt, Vos coniuges non estis sed hostes, quia quae salutem nobis invenit eam damnatis. tunc Athenienses legem emendarunt, ut ingenuae arte medicinam discerent (ed. Rose, emended).

(B) Jacques Guillemeau, *Child-Birth or, the Happy Deliverie of Women* (London: A. Hatfield, 1612), pp. 80–81:

Beside this curiositie; necessitie, (the mistress of Arts) hath constrained women, to learne and practise Physicke, one with an other. For finding themselves afflicted, and troubled with divers diseases in their naturall parts, and being destitute of all remedies, (for want whereof many perished, and died miserably) they durst not discover, and lay open their infirmities, to any but themselves, accounting it to be dishonest: As Higinus testifies, who relateth, how the Athenians had forbidden women, by their Lawes, to studie in Physicke; and that at the same time there was a certain maide named Agnodicea, verie desirous to studie therein, who the better to attaine unto her purpose, did cut off her haire, and apparell herself like a man: and being so disguised, she became the scholler of Herophylus the Physition: And when she had learned Physicke, having notice of a certaine woman that was troubled in her naturall parts; she went unto her, and made proffer of her service; which the sicke party refused, thinking she had been a man: But when Agnodicea had assured her (by discovering of her selfe) that she was a maide, the woman committed her selfe, into her hands, who drest, and cured her perfectly: and with the like care and industrie she looked to many others, and cured them. Which being knowen by the Physitions, because they were not called any more to the cure of women, they accused the said Agnodicea, that she had shaved off her beard, that thereby she might abuse women, faining themselves to be sicke. Then she putting aside her garments, made it evident that she was a maide: which caused the Physitions then to accuse her of a greater fault, for transgressing the Law, which forbad women either to studie or to practize Physicke. This being come to the eares of the chiefest women, they presently went to the chiefe Magistrates, and Judges of the Citie, called the Areopagites, and told them, that they did not account them, for their husbands, and friends, but for enemies; that they would condemne her, which restor'd them to their health: which made the Athenians to revoke and disanull that Law, giving Gentle-women leave to studie and practise Physicke.

(C) Thomas Heywood, *Gynaikeion: or, Nine bookes of various history concerning women* (London: Adam Islip, 1624), 'Of such as have died in child-birth', pp. 203–4:

Higinus in his two hundred threescore and fourth Fable tells this tale: In the old time sayth he, there were no midwives at all, and for that cause many women in their modestie, rather suffered themselves to perish for want of helpe, than that any man should bee seene or knowne to come about them. Above all, the Athenians were most curious that no servant or woman should learn the art of Chyrurgerie. There was a damosell of that City, that was verie industrious in the search of such mysteries, whose name was *Agnodice*, but wanting meanes to attaine unto that necessarie skill, she caused her haire to be shorne, and putting on the habit of a yong man, got her selfe into the service of one *Heirophilus* a Phisitian, and by her industrie and studie having attained to the deapth of his skill, and the height of her own desires, upon a time hearing where a noble ladie was in child-birth, in the middest of her painfull throwes, she offered her selfe to her helpe, whom the modest Ladie (mistaking her Sex) would by no persuasion suffer to come neere her, till she was forced to strip her selfe before the women, and to give evident signes of her woman-hood. After which shee had accesse to many, prooving so fortunate, that she grew verie famous. Insomuch that being envied by the colledge of the Phisitians, she was complained on to the Areopagitae, or the nobilitie of the Senat: such in whose power it was to censure and determine of all causes and controversies. *Agnodice* thus convented, they pleaded against her youth and boldnesse, accusing her rather a corrupter of their chastities, than any way a curer of their infirmities: blaming the matrons, as counterfeiting weaknesse, onely of purpose to have the companie and familiaritie of a loose and intemperate yong man. They prest their accusations so farre, that the Judges were readie to proceede to sentence against her; when shee opening her brest before the Senat, gave manifest testimonie that she was no other then a woman: at this the Phisitians the more incenst, made the fact the more henious, in regard that being a woman, she durst enter into the search of that knowledge, of which their Sex by the law was not capable. The cause being once more readie to goe against her, the noblest matrons of the cittie assembled themselves before the Senat, and plainely told them, they were rather enemies than husbands, who went about to punish her, that of all their Sex had beene the most studious for their generall health and safetie. Their importancie so farre prevailed, after the circumstances were truely considered, that the first decree was quite abrogated, and free libertie granted to women to imploy themselves in those necessarie offices, without the presence of men. So that Athens was the first cittie of Greece, that freely admitted of Mid-wives by the meanes of this damosell *Agnodice*.

(D) Elizabeth Nihell, *A Treatise on the Art of Midwifery setting forth Various Abuses Therein, especially as to the Practice with Instruments* **(London: A. Morley, 1760), pp. 219–21, note on p. 219:**

As the story is told in Hyginus, it should seem that the practice of midwifery at Athens, was, on a reason interdicted to the women, who, by a fixt resolution to die rather than submit to be delivered by the men, procured from the Areopagus the repeal of that statute, and the saving from imminent condemnation one Agnodice, who had dressed herself in mens cloaths, to elude the cognizance of the law. The great practice she had obtained by this means had alarmed the physicians, who thereon accused her as a seducer of the women: against which she easily defended herself by a declaration of her sex. But this brought her under the penalty of the law against women exercising the midwife's profession. The story imperfectly related in Hyginus, at the same time that it does honor to the modesty of the Athenian women, that is to say, if modesty is not, according to the men-midwives, a false honor, gives room to suspect, that the midwives themselves had perhaps occasioned the promulgation of so absurd a law. It is well known, than in those antient times, there were for female disorders women-physicians in form. Perhaps their encroachments on the province of the men, by exercising the art of physic in general, might make a restraint necessary, which was only so far faulty as that the remedy was in this, as it often is in other cases, carried into extremes. I would no more justify the women overstepping their proper sphere of employment into that of the men, than I would the men sinking into that of women. They are both reprehensible, both dangerous, but assuredly, the last must be the most ridiculous.

(E) Mary Grant (ed. and tr.), *The Myths of Hyginus*, **University of Kansas Publications in Humanistic Studies, no. 34 (Lawrence, KS: University**

of Kansas Press, 1960); <http://www.theoi.com/Text/HyginusFabulae5.
html#274> accessed 4 July 2011:

The ancients didn't have obstetricians, and as a result, women because of modesty
perished. For the Athenians forbade slaves and women to learn the art of medicine.
A certain girl, Hagnodice, a virgin desired to learn medicine, and since she desired
it, she cut her hair, and in male attire came to a certain Herophilus for training.
When she had learned the art, and had heard that a woman was in labor, she came
to her. And when the woman refused to trust herself to her, thinking that she was
a man, she removed her garment to show that she was a woman, and in this way
she treated women. When the doctors saw that they were not admitted to women,
they began to accuse Hagnodice, saying that 'he' was a seducer and corruptor of
women, and that the women were pretending to be ill. The Areopagites, in session,
started to condemn Hagnodice, but Hagnodice removed her garment for them
and showed that she was a woman. Then the doctors began to accuse her more
vigorously, and as a result the leading women came to the Court and said: 'You
are not husbands, but enemies, because you condemn her who discovered safety
for us.' Then the Athenians amended the law, so that free-born women could learn
the art of medicine.

(F) R. Scott Smith and Stephen Trzaskoma, *Apollodorus' Library and Hyginus'
Fabulae (Indianapolis, IN: Hackett Publishing, 2007), p. 180:

The ancients did not have midwives, and because of this many women died
from a sense of shame because the Athenians made sure that no slave or woman
learned medicine. A certain young girl named Agnodice desired to learn medicine;
because of this desire she cut off her hair, put on men's clothing, and became
the student of a certain Herophilus for formal instruction. After she was trained,
whenever she heard a woman was having trouble below her waist, she went to her.
Women did not trust her, thinking that she was a man, so Agnodice would lift up
her tunic and prove that she was a woman. In this guise Agnodice would take care
of these women. But when doctors saw that their services were not being called
upon by women, they accused Agnodice, asserting that she was an effeminate
gigolo and seducing them and that the women were only pretending to be sick.
The Areopagites assembled and found Agnodice guilty. She lifted her tunic and
showed them that she was a woman. The doctors then raised stronger accusations
against her. Because of this the women leaders converged on the court and said,
'You are not our husbands but our enemies, for you have condemned the woman
who discovered a means to provide for our well-being.' The Athenians then
changed the law to allow free-born women to learn medicine.

Bibliography

Manuscript Sources

British Library
    Cup.366.e.20, *Certificates of a Very Rare Specimen of Hermaphroditism, Dublin 5 July 1835.*

London Metropolitan Archives
    WJ/SR II/146

Royal College of Surgeons, Edinburgh
    Ms lectures of Thomas Young, 1771

Printed Sources

Adams, James N., *The Latin Sexual Vocabulary* (London: Duckworth, 1982).

Adelman, Janet, 'Making Defect Perfection: Shakespeare and the One-Sex Model', in Viviana Comensoli and Anne Russell (eds), *Enacting Gender on the English Renaissance Stage* (Urbana/Chicago, IL: University of Illinois Press, 1999), 23–52.

Aetius of Amida, *Aetii Amideni medici ... Libri sexdecim nunc primum Latinitate* (Venice: in aedibus haeredum Aldi Manutii, & Andreae Asulani, 1534).

Albucasis: Martin S. Spink and G.L. Lewis, *Albucasis, On Surgery and Instruments. A Definitive Edition of the Arabic Text with English Translation and Commentary* (London: Wellcome Institute of the History of Medicine, 1973).

Alic, Margaret, *Hypatia's Heritage: A History of Women in Science from Antiquity through the Nineteenth Century* (Boston, MA: Beacon Press, 1986).

Allen, Don Cameron (ed.), *Palladis Tamia (1598)* (New York: Scholars' Facsimiles and Reprints, 1938).

Allott, Robert, *Wits Theatre of the Little World* (London: J[ames] R[oberts] for N[icholas] L[ing], 1599).

Alsop, Gulielma Fell, *History of the Woman's Medical College, Philadelphia, Pennsylvania, 1850–1950* (Philadelphia, PA: J.B. Lippincott, 1950).

Amatus Lusitanus, *Centuria secunda* (Venice: Vincentus Valgrisus, 1552).

Amussen, Susan Dwyer, 'Review of Thomas Laqueur, *Making Sex*', *Journal of Interdisciplinary History*, 24 (1994): 521–3.

The Anatomie of the Inward parts of Woman, very necessary to be knowne to physitians, surgians, and all other that desire to know themselues (London: Blackfriars, 1599).

Aristotle's Compleat Master-piece, in Three Parts: Displaying the Secrets of Nature in the Generation of Man (London, 1771).

Aristotle's Master-piece (London: J. How, 1690).

Aristotle's Master-piece (London: B. Harris, 1697).

Aristotle's Master-piece, or, The Secrets of Generation ... very necessary for all midwives, nurses, and young-married women (London: printed for W.B, 1694).

Aristotle's Masterpiece (New York: Arno Press, 1974).

Artemidorus: Rudolph Hercher, *Artemidori Daldiani, Onirocriticon Libri V* (Leipzig: Teubner, 1864).

— White, Robert J. (tr.), *Interpretation of Dreams. Oneirocritica by Artemidorus* (New Jersey: Noyes Press, 1975).

'Artium Magister', *An Apology for the Beard* (London: Rivingtons, 1862).

Astruc, Jean, *L'Art d'accoucher réduit a ses principes* (Paris: P. Guillaume Cavelier, 1766).

— *Elements of Midwifery. Containing the Most Modern and Successful Method of Practice* (London: S. Crowder, 1767).

Atkinson, Catherine, *Inventing Inventors in Renaissance Europe: Polydore Vergil's De inventoribus rerum*, Spätmittelalter und Reformation Neue Reihe 33 (Tübingen: Mohr Siebeck, 2007).

Avicenna, *Canon* (Venice: n.p., 1507).

Azzolini, Monica, 'Exploring Generation: A Context to Leonardo's Anatomies of the Female and Male Body', in Alessandro Nova and Domenico Laurenza (eds), *Leonardo da Vinci's Anatomical World: Language, Context and 'Disegno'* (Florence: Marsilio, 2011), 79–97.

B., J. [Bulwer], *Anthropometamorphosis: Man Transformed; or, the Artificial Changeling* (London: J. Hardesty, 1650).

Bambach, Carmen C., 'Leonardo's Drawing of Female Anatomy and his "Fassciculu Medjcine Latino"', in Alessandro Nova and Domenico Laurenza (eds), *Leonardo da Vinci's Anatomical World: Language, Context and 'Disegno'* (Florence: Marsilio, 2011), 109–30.

Banister, John, *The Historie of Man, Sucked from the Sappe of the most Approved Anathomistes* (London: John Day, 1578).

Barnard, L.W., *John Potter. An Eighteenth Century Archbishop* (Ilfracombe: Arthur J. Stockwell, 1989).

Barret, Robert, *A Companion for Midwives, Child-bearing women, and Nurses Directing them how to Perform their Respective Offices* (London: Thomas Ax, 1699).

Bartholin, Caspar, *Anatomicae institutiones corporis humanis* ([Wittenberg]: A. Rüdinger apud Bechtoldum Raaben, 1611).

Bartholinus Anatomy, tr. Nicholas Culpeper and Abdiah Cole (London: Peter Cole, 1663).

Barton, Carlin A., *The Sorrows of the Ancient Romans: The Gladiator and the Monster* (Princeton, NJ: Princeton University Press, 1995).

Bartsch, Shadi, *The Mirror of the Self: Sexuality, Self-Knowledge and the Gaze in the Early Roman Empire* (Chicago, IL: University of Chicago Press, 2006).

Baruch, Elaine Hoffman, *Women, Love, and Power: Literary and Psychoanalytic Perspectives* (New York: New York University Press, 1991).

Bate, Walter J., *Keats: A Collection of Critical Essays* (Englewood Cliffs, NJ: Prentice-Hall, 1964).

Bauhin, Caspar, *Institutiones Anatomicae Corporis Virilis et Muliebris Historiam Exhibentes* (Berne: apud Ioannem le Preux, 1604).

— *Theatrum Anatomicum* (Frankfurt am Main: Matthaeus Becker, 1605).

Bayle, Pierre, *Dictionnaire Historique et Critique*, vol. 2, H–O (Rotterdam: chez Reinier Lees, 1697), translated into English as *A General Dictionary, Historical and Critical* (London: C. Harper, D. Brown, J. Tonson, et al., 1710).

— *The Dictionary Historical and Critical of Mr Peter Bayle*, vol. 3, F–L, 2nd edition (London: J.J. and P. Knapton, 1736).

Beagon, Mary, *The Elder Pliny on the Human Animal. Natural History Book 7. Translation with Introduction and Historical Commentary* (Oxford: Clarendon Press, 2005).

Beard, Mary, 'Did the Romans Have Elbows? or Arms and the Romans', in Pierre Borgeaud (ed.), *Corps Romains* (Grenoble: Editions Jérôme Millon, 2002), 47–59.

Beecher, Donald, 'Concerning Sex Changes: The Cultural Significance of a Renaissance Medical Polemic', *The Sixteenth Century Journal*, 36 (2005): 991–1016.

Benedetti, Alessandro, *Anatomice: sive, de historia corporis humani libri quinque* (Venice: a Bernardino Guerraldo, 1502).

Berengario da Carpi, Jacopo, *Isagogae breves* (Bologna: Benedictus Hectoris, 1522).

— (L.R. Lind, ed. and tr.), *A Short Introduction to Anatomy* (Chicago, IL: University of Chicago Press, 1959).

Beusterien, John L., 'Jewish Male Menstruation in Seventeenth-Century Spain', *Bulletin of the History of Medicine*, 73 (1999): 447–56.

Bicks, Caroline, *Midwiving Subjects in Shakespeare's England* (Aldershot: Ashgate, 2003).

Billing, Christian, *Masculinity, Corporality and the English Stage 1580–1635* (Aldershot: Ashgate, 2008).

Blackman, Janet, 'Popular Theories of Generation: The Evolution of *Aristotle's Works*; The Study of an Anachronism', in John Woodward and David Richards (eds), *Health Care and Popular Medicine in Nineteenth-Century England* (London: Croom Helm, 1977), 56–88.

Blair, Ann, 'The Rise of Note-Taking in Early Modern Europe', *Intellectual History Review*, 20 (2010): 303–16.

— *Too Much to Know: Managing Scholarly Information before the Modern Age* (New Haven, CT: Yale University Press, 2010).

Blake, Catriona, *The Charge of the Parasols: Women's Entry to the Medical Profession* (London: Women's Press, 1994).

Blundell, Sue, *Women in Ancient Greece* (London: British Museum Press, 1995).

Bogdan, Robert, 'The Social Construction of Freaks', in Rosemarie Garland Thomson (ed.) *Freakery. Cultural Spectacles of the Extraordinary Body* (New York: New York University Press, 2006), 23–37.

— *Freak Show: Presenting Human Oddities for Amusement and Profit* (Chicago, IL: University of Chicago Press, 1988).

Bolton, Henry Carrington, 'The Early Practice of Medicine by Women', *Popular Science Monthly*, 18 Dec. 1880: 191–202.

Bonner, Campbell, 'The Trial of St Eugenia', *American Journal of Philology* 41 (1920): 253–64.

Booth, George, *The Historical Library of Diodorus the Sicilian, in Fifteen Books*, vol. II (London: J. Davis, 1814).

Boriaud, Jean-Yves, ed., *Hygine, Fables* (Collection Budé; Paris: Les Belles Lettres, 1997).

Bost, Hubert, *Pierre Bayle historien, critique et moraliste* (Turnhout: Brepols, 2006).

Boter, Gerard, *The Textual Tradition of Plato's Republic* (Leiden: Brill, 1989).

Botteri, Paula, *Les Fragments de l'histoire des Gracques dans la Bibliothèque de Diodore de Sicile* (Geneva: Droz, 1992).

Bourgeois (Boursier), Louise, *Introduction à ma fille* in *Observations diverses, sur la sterilité, perte de fruict, foecondité, accouchements, et maladies des femmes, et enfants nouveaux naiz*, vol. 2 (Paris: A. Saugrain, 1617), 199–251.

— *Fidelle Relation de l'accouchement, maladie et ouverture du corps de feu Madame* (Paris, n.p., 1627).

— Boursier, Louise, *Récit véritable de la naissance des messeigneurs et dames les enfans de France, Instruction à ma fille, et autres textes*. Critical edition by François Rouget and Colette H. Winn (Geneva: Librairie Droz, 2000).

Boyd, M.J., Review of Mary Grant (ed. and tr.), *The Myths of Hyginus*, *Classical Review*, 13 (1963): 350.

Bréjon, Jacques, *André Tiraqueau (1488–1558): un jurisconsulte de la Renaissance* (Paris: Librairie du Recueil Sirey, 1937).

Brisson, Luc, *Le Sexe incertain. Androgynie et hermaphrodisme dans l'Antiquité gréco-romaine* (Paris, Les Belles Lettres, 1997, tr. as *Sexual Ambivalence: Androgyny and Hermaphroditism in Graeco-Roman Antiquity*, Berkeley, CA and London: University of California Press, 2002).

Broc-Lapeyre, Monique, 'Pourquoi Baubo a-t-elle fait rire Demeter?', in *Recherches sur la philosophie et le langage*, 5 (1985): *Pratiques de langage dans l'Antiquité*, 59–76.

Brooten, Bernadette J., *Love between Women: Early Christian Responses to Female Homoeroticism* (Chicago, IL: Chicago University Press, 1996).

Browder, Clifford, *The Wickedest Woman in New York: Madame Restell, the Abortionist* (Hamden, CT: Archon Books, 1988).

Brown, Kathleen, "'Changed … into the Fashion of Man": The Politics of Sexual Difference in a Seventeenth-Century Anglo-American Settlement', *Journal of the History of Sexuality*, 6 (1995): 171–93.

Browner, Stephanie, 'Review of Thomas Laqueur, *Making Sex*', *Victorian Studies*, 35 (1992): 221–2.

Bullough, Vern L. 'An Early American Sex Manual, or, Aristotle Who?', *Early American Literature*, 7 (1972–73): 236–46.

Burrows, Erin N., 'By the Hair of her Chin: A Critical Biography of Bearded Lady Jane Barnell' (MA thesis, Sarah Lawrence College, 2009).

Burton, Thomas, *The Anatomy of Melancholy* (Oxford: John Lichfield and James Short, for Henry Cripps, 1621).

C., R., I. D., M. S. and T. B., *The Compleat Midwife's Practice Enlarged … The second edition corrected* (London: Nathaniel Brook, 1663).

Cabré, Montserrat, 'Kate Campbell Hurd-Mead (1867–1941) and the Medical Women's Struggle for History', *Collections. The Newsletter of the Archives and Special Collections on Women in Medicine. The Medical College of Pennsylvania*, 26 (1993): 1–4, 8.

Cadden, Joan, *Meanings of Sex Difference in the Middle Ages: Medicine, Science, and Culture* (Cambridge: Cambridge University Press, 1993).

Cairns, Douglas, *Aidos. The Psychology and Ethics of Honour and Shame in Ancient Greek Literature* (Oxford: Clarendon Press, 1993).

Canton, Dan W., *The Good, the Bold, and the Beautiful: The Story of Susanna and its Renaissance Interpretations* (New York and London: T. & T. Clark, 2006).

Carey, Sorcha, *Pliny's Catalogue of Nature: Art and Empire in the Natural History* (Oxford: Oxford University Press, 2003).

Carlino, Andrea, *Books of the Body: Anatomical Ritual and Renaissance Learning* (Chicago, IL: University of Chicago Press, 1999).

Carol, Ann, 'Sage-femme ou gynécologue? M.-A. Boivin (1773–1841)', *Clio: Histoire, femmes et sociétés*, 33 (2011): 237–60.

Cartari, Vincenzo, *Imagines Deorum* (Lyon: G. Jullieron for B. Honorat, 1581).

Castro, Roderigo de, *De universa mulierum medicina* (Hamburg: ex officina Frobenianus, 1603).

A Catalogue and Particular Description of the Human Anatomy in Wax-Work, and several other preparations to be seen at the Royal-Exchange (London: T. White, 1736).

Cellier, Elizabeth, *Malice Defeated, Or, a brief Relation of the Accusation and Deliverance of Elizabeth Cellier* (London, 1680).

— *A Scheme for the Foundation of a Royal Hospital, and Raising a Revenue of Five or Six-thousand Pounds a Year, by, and for the Maintenance of a Corporation of skilful Midwives …* (London, 1687).

— *To Dr … an Answer to his Queries, concerning the Colledg of Midwives* (London, 1688).

Chamberlen, Peter, *A Voice in Rhama: Or, The Crie of Women and Children* (London: printed by William Bentley, 1647).

Chantraine, Pierre, *Dictionnaire étymologique de la langue grecque* (Paris: Klincksieck, 1999; first published 1968).

Chiang, Howard Hsueh-Hao, 'Epistemic Gender, Sex Beyond the Flesh: Science, Medicine, and the Two-Sex Model in Modern America', *eSharp*, 9 (2007), *Gender: Power and Authority*, <http://www.gla.ac.uk/media/media_41212_en.pdf> accessed 1 July 2011.

Churchill, Wendy, 'The Medical Practice of the Sexed Body: Women, Men and Disease in Britain, *c*.1600–1740', *Social History of Medicine*, 18 (2005): 3–22.

Clark, G.N., 'Edward Grimeston, the Translator', *English Historical Review*, 43 (1928): 585–98.

Clark, Gillian, 'The Old Adam: The Fathers and the Unmaking of Masculinity', in Lin Foxhall and John Salmon (eds), *Thinking Men: Masculinity and its Self-Representation in the Classical Tradition* (London and New York: Routledge, 1988), 170–82.

— *Women in Late Antiquity: Pagan and Christian Lifestyles* (Oxford: Oxford University Press, 1993).

Clark, Stuart, *Thinking with Demons: The Idea of Witchcraft in Early Modern Culture* (Oxford: Oxford University Press, 1997).

Clark, William, *The Province of Midwives in the Practice of their Art* (London: M. Cooper, 1751).

Clay, Charles, *A Cyclopaedia of Obstetrics, Theoretical, Practical, Historical, Biographical, and Critical, Including the Diseases of Women and Children* (Manchester: W.M. Irwin and London: H. Renshaw, 1848).

Cleminson, Richard and Francisco Vázquez García, 'Breasts, Hair and Hormones: The Anatomy of Gender Difference in Spain, 1880–1940', *Bulletin of Spanish Studies*, 86:5 (2009): 627–52.

Clouston, Thomas Smith, 'Female Education from a Medical Point of View (I)', *Popular Science Monthly*, 24 (1883): 214–29.

— 'Female Education from a Medical Point of View (II)', *Popular Science Monthly*, 24 (1884): 319–34.

Cody, Lisa Forman, 'The Politics of Reproduction: From Midwives' Alternative Public Sphere to the Public Spectacle of Man-Midwifery', *Eighteenth-Century Studies*, 32 (1999): 477–95.

— *Birthing the Nation. Sex, Science, and the Conception of Eighteenth-Century Britons* (Oxford: Oxford University Press, 2005).

Coles, Elisha, *A Dictionary, Latin and English* (London: John Richardson, for Peter Parker, 1679).

Commelinus, Hieronymus, *Mythologici Latini* ([Heidelberg]: Ex Bibliopolio Commeliniano, 1599).

Condrau, Flurin, 'The Patient's View Meets the Clinical Gaze', *Social History of Medicine*, 20 (2007): 525–40.

Considine, John and Sylvia Brown (eds), *N.H., The Ladies Dictionary* (Aldershot and Burlington, VT: Ashgate, 2010).

Conti, Natali, *Mythologiae, sive Explicationum fabularum libri decem* (Venice: Comin da Trino, 1568).

Le Contre-Poison, ou la nation vengée (Amsterdam, 1761).

Cook, Harold J., *The Decline of the Old Medical Regime in Stuart London* (Ithaca, NY and London: Cornell University Press, 1986).

Copenhaver, Brian P., 'The Historiography of Discovery in the Renaissance: The Sources and Composition of Polydore Vergil's *De inventoribus rerum*, I–III', *Journal of the Warburg and Courtauld Institutes*, 41 (1978): 192–214.

— *Polydore Vergil On Discovery* (Cambridge, MA: Harvard University Press, 2002).

Corde, Maurice de la, *Hippocratis Coi, Medicorum principis, liber prior de morbis mulierum* (Paris: apud Dionysium Duvallium, 1585).

Cornarius, Janus, *Hippocratis Coi medicorum omnium longe principis, opera quae apud nos extant* (Paris: apud Carolam Guillard, 1546).

— *Opera quae nos extant omnia* (Basle: Froben, 1558).

Craik, Elizabeth, (ed.) *Hippocrates, Places in Man* (Oxford: Oxford University Press, 1988).

— *Two Hippocratic Treatises: On Sight and On Anatomy*, Studies in Ancient Medicine, vol. 33 (Leiden: Brill, 2006).

Crawford, Katherine, *European Sexualities, 1400–1800* (Cambridge: Cambridge University Press, 2007).

Crooke, Helkiah, *Microcosmographia: A Description of the Body of Man* (London: William Jaggard, 1615).

— *Somatographia Anthropine. Or, A description of the body of man. By artificiall figures representing the members, and fit termes expressing the same. Set forth either to pleasure or to profite those who are addicted to this study* (London: William Jaggard, 1616).

Crowther, Margaret A. and Marguerite Dupree, *Medical Lives in the Age of Surgical Revolution* (Cambridge: Cambridge University Press, 2007).

Crozier, Ivan, 'Pillow Talk: Credibility, Trust and the Sexological Case History', *History of Science*, 46 (2008): 375–404.

Cuir, Raphael, *The Development of the Study of Anatomy from the Renaissance to Cartesianism: da Carpi, Vesalius, Estienne, Bidloo* (Lewiston, Queenston and Lampeter: Edwin Mellen Press, 2009).

Culpeper, Nicholas, *A Directory for Midwives or, a Guide for Women, in their Conception, Bearing, and Suckling their Children* (London: Peter Cole, 1651).

Cunningham, Andrew, *The Anatomical Renaissance: The Resurrection of the Anatomical Projects of the Ancients* (Aldershot: Scolar Press, 1997).

— *The Anatomist Anatomis'd: An Experimental Discipline in Enlightenment Europe* (Aldershot and Burlington, VT: Ashgate, 2010).

Cuomo, Serafina, *Technology and Culture in Greek and Roman Antiquity* (Cambridge: Cambridge University Press, 2007).

d'Ardène, Jean-Paul Rome, *Lettres interessantes pour les médecins de profession*, vol. 2 (Avignon: chez Louis Chambeau, 1759).

Dasen, Véronique and Sandrine Ducaté-Paarmann, 'Hysteria and Metaphors of the Uterus in Classical Antiquity', in Silvia Schroer (ed.), *Images and Gender. Contributions to the Hermeneutics of Reading Ancient Art, Orbis Biblicus et Orientalis* 220 (Fribourg: Academic Press, 2006), 239–62.

Daston, Lorraine and Katharine Park, 'The Hermaphrodite and the Orders of Nature: Sexual Ambiguity in Early Modern France', in Louise Fradenburg and Carla Freccero (eds), *Premodern Sexualities* (New York: Routledge, 1996), 117–36.

Davis, Natalie Zemon, *The Return of Martin Guerre* (Cambridge, MA: Harvard University Press, 1984).

Dawkes, Thomas, *The Midwife Rightly Instructed* (London: J. Oswald, 1736).

Dean-Jones, Lesley, *Women's Bodies in Classical Greek Science* (Oxford: Clarendon Press, 1994).

— '*Autopsia, Historia* and What Women Know: The Authority of Women in Hippocratic Gynaecology', in Don Bates (ed.), *Knowledge and the Scholarly Medical Traditions* (Cambridge: Cambridge University Press, 1995), 41–59.

Debru, Armelle, 'La Suffocation hystérique chez Galien et Aetius: réécriture et emprunt de "je"', in Antonio Garzya (ed.), *Tradizione e ecdotica dei testi medici tardoantichi e bizantini* (Naples: M. D'Auria, 1992), 79–89.

Delacoux, Alexis, *Biographie des sages-femmes célèbres* (Paris: Trinquart, 1834).

Delacroix, Jean-François, *Dictionnaire historique portatif des femmes célèbres*, 2 vols (Paris: L. Cellot, 1769).

Delcourt, Marie, *Hermaphrodite: mythes et rites de la bisexualité dans l'antiquité classique* (Paris: Presses Univ. de France, 1958), tr. as *Hermaphrodite: Myths and Rites of the Bisexual Figure in Classical Antiquity* (London: Studio Books, 1961).

Demand, Nancy, *Birth, Death, and Motherhood in Classical Greece* (Baltimore, MD and London: Johns Hopkins University Press, 1994).

Desclos, Marie-Laurence and William W. Fortenbaugh (eds), *Strato of Lampsacus: Text, Translation, and Discussion*, Rutgers University Studies in Classical Humanities, XVI (New Brunswick, NJ: Rutgers University Press, 2011).

Des Roches, Catherine, *Les Oeuvres des Mes-dames des Roches de Poetiers mere et fille* (Paris: L'Angelier, 1578).

Devereux, Georges, *Baubo. La Vulve mythique* (Paris: J.-C. Godefroy, 1982).

Dickey, Eleanor, *Ancient Scholarship* (Oxford: Oxford University Press, 2007).

Dickie, Matthew, *Magic and Magicians in the Greco-Roman World* (London: Routledge, 2001).

Diepgen, Paul, *Die Frauenheilkunde der Alten Welt*, Handbuch der Gynäkologie 12, 1, Geschichte der Frauenheilkunde 1 (Munich: J. Bergmann, 1937).

Dillon, Elizabeth Maddock, 'Nursing Fathers and Brides of Christ: The Feminized Body of the Puritan Convert', in Janet Moore Lindman and Michele Lise Tarter (eds), *A Centre of Wonders: The Body in Early America* (Ithaca, NY: Cornell University Press, 2001), 129–44.

Dionis, Pierre, *Traité general des accouchemens* (Paris: chez Charles-Maurice d'Houry, 1718).

— *A General Treatise of Midwifery* (London: A. Bell, J. Darby et al., 1719).

Dodds, E.R., *The Greeks and the Irrational* (Berkeley, CA and London: University of California Press, 1951).

Dolan, Frances, *Whores of Babylon: Catholicism, Gender, and Seventeenth-Century Print Culture* (Ithaca, NY: Cornell University Press, 1999).

Donati, Gemma, *L'Orthographia di Giovanni Tortelli. Percorsi dei classici*, 11 (Messina: Centro Interdipartimentale di Studi Umanistici, 2006).

Dover, Kenneth J., 'The Political Aspects of Aeschylus' *Eumenides*', *Journal of Hellenic Studies*, 77 (1957): 230–37.

Drabkin, Miriam F. and Israel E. Drabkin, *Caelius Aurelianus, Gynaecia: Fragments of a Latin Version of Soranus' Gynaecia from a Thirteenth Century Manuscript* (Baltimore, MD: Johns Hopkins Press, 1951).

Dreger, Alice Domurat, *Hermaphrodites and the Medical Invention of Sex* (Cambridge, MA: Harvard University Press, 1998).

Dreux du Radier, Jean-François, *Bibliothèque historique et critique du Poitou, contenant les vies des Savans de cette Province*, vol. 2 (Paris: chez Ganeau, 1754).

Duckworth, W.L.H. (tr.), *Galen On Anatomical Procedures: The Later Books* (Cambridge: Cambridge University Press, 1962).

Dumont, Martial, 'La délirante "Luciniade" de l'anticésarien Jean-François Sacombe', *Revue Française de Gynécologie et d'Obstétrique* 66 (1971): 199–204.

Durbach, Nadja, *Spectacle of Deformity. Freak Shows and Modern British Culture* (Berkeley, CA and London: University of California Press, 2010).

Duval, Jacques, *Des hermaphrodits, accouchemens des femmes, et traitement qui est requis pour les relever en santé, et bien élever leurs enfants* (Rouen: David Geuffroy, 1612).

Egmond, Florike and Robert Zwijnenberg (eds), *Bodily Extremities: Preoccupations with the Human Body in Early Modern European Culture* (Aldershot: Ashgate, 2003).

Eijk, Philip van der and Robert W. Sharples (eds and tr.), *Nemesius On the Nature of Man* (Liverpool: Liverpool University Press, 2008).

Elsom, Helen, 'Callirhoe: Displaying the Phallic Woman', in Amy Richlin (ed.), *Pornography and Representation in Greece and Rome* (New York and Oxford: Oxford University Press, 1992), 212–30.

Eriksson, Maria, 'Biologically Similar and Anatomically Different? The One-Sex Model and the Modern Sex/Gender Distinction', *NORA: Nordic Journal of Women's Studies*, 6 (1998): 31–8, online version <http://baer.rewi.hu-berlin.de/w/files/lsbpdf/eriksson.pdf> accessed 12 August 2012.

Eriksson, Ruben (tr.), *Andreas Vesalius' First Public Anatomy at Bologna, 1540: An Eyewitness Report* (Uppsala and Stockholm: Almquist and Wiksells, 1959).

Estienne, Charles, *Dictionarium historicum ac poeticum* (Geneva: apud Jacobum Stoer, 1590).

Evenden, Doreen, *The Midwives of Seventeenth-Century London* (Cambridge: Cambridge University Press, 2000).

Fabricius, Johann Albert, *Bibliothecae graecae*, vol. 13 (Hamburg: sumptu Theodori Christophori Felgineri, 1726).

Faderman, Lillian, 'Review: Thomas Laqueur, *Making Sex: Body and Gender from the Greeks to Freud*', *Signs*, 17 (1992): 820–24.

Falloppio, Gabriele, *Observationes anatomicae* (Venice: Marcus Antonius Ulmus, 1561).

Faraone, Christopher A. and Laura McClure (eds), *Prostitutes and Courtesans in the Ancient World* (Madison, WI: University of Wisconsin Press, 2006).

Farkas, Carol-Ann, 'Aesculapius Victrix: Fiction about Women Doctors, 1870–1900' (PhD thesis, University of Alberta, Edmonton, Alberta, 2000).

Fausto-Sterling, Anne, 'The Five Sexes: Why Male and Female Are Not Enough', *The Sciences* (March/April 1993): 20–24.

— *Sexing the Body: Gender Politics and the Construction of Sexuality* (New York: Basic Books, 2000).

— 'The Five Sexes, Revisited', *The Sciences* (July/August 2000): 19–23.

Ferguson, John K., *Bibliographical Notes on Histories of Inventions and Books of Secrets*, 2 vols (Glasgow: R. Maclehose, 1895; reprinted London: Holland Press, 1959).

Ferrand, Jacques, *De la maladie d'amour ou melancholie erotique* (Paris: Chez Denis Moreau, 1623); translated as Donald A. Beecher and Massimo Ciavolella (tr. and ed.), *Jacques Ferrand, A Treatise on Lovesickness* (Syracuse, NY: Syracuse University Press, 1990).

— *Erotomania or a Treatise Discoursing of the Essence, Causes, Symptomes, Prognosticks, and Cure of Love or Erotique Melancholy* (Oxford: L. Lichfield, 1640).

Ferrari, Gian A. and Mario Vegetti, 'Science, Technology and Medicine in the Classical Tradition', in Pietro Corsi and Paul Weindling (eds), *Information Sources in the History of Science and Medicine* (London and Boston, MA: Butterworth Scientific, 1983), 197–220.

Ferrari, Giovanna, 'Public Anatomy Lessons and the Carnival: The Anatomy Theatre of Bologna', *Past and Present*, 117 (1987): 50–106.

— *L'Esperienza del Passato. Alessandro Benedetti Filologo e Medico Umanistica* (Florence: Leo S. Olshki, 1996).

Finucci, Valeria, 'Maternal Imagination and Monstrous Birth: Tasso's *Gerusalemme liberata*', in Valeria Finucci and Kevin Brownlee (eds), *Generation and Degeneration: Tropes of Reproduction in Literature and History from Antiquity to Early Modern Europe* (Durham, NC and London: Duke University Press, 2001), 41–80.

Fisher, Will, 'The Renaissance Beard: Masculinity in Early Modern England', *Renaissance Quarterly*, 54 (2001): 155–87.

Fissell, Mary, 'Hairy Women and Naked Truths: Gender and the Politics of Knowledge in *Aristotle's Masterpiece*', *William and Mary Quarterly*, 3rd ser., 60 (2003): 43–74.

— 'Making a Masterpiece: The Aristotle Texts in Vernacular Medical Culture', in Charles E. Rosenberg (ed.), *Right Living: An Anglo-American Tradition of Self-Help Medicine* (Baltimore, MD: Johns Hopkins University Press, 2003), 59–87.

Flemming, Rebecca, *Medicine and the Making of Roman Women. Gender, Nature, and Authority from Celsus to Galen* (Oxford: Oxford University Press, 2000).

— 'Women, Writing and Medicine in the Classical World', *Classical Quarterly*, 57 (2007): 257–79.

Fletcher, Anthony, *Gender, Sex, and Subordination in England, 1500–1800* (New Haven, CT: Yale University Press, 1995).

Foës, Anuce, *Hippocrates: Opera omnia, quae extant* (Frankfurt: Heirs of Andreas Wechel, Claude Marne & Jean Aubry, 1596).

Foucault, Michel, *Herculine Barbin, dite Alexina B.* (Paris: Gallimard, 1978); tr. as *Herculine Barbin: Being the Recently Discovered Memoirs of a Nineteenth-Century French Hermaphrodite*, tr. Richard McDougall (New York: Pantheon, 1980).

— 'Le vrai sexe', *Arcadie*, 323 (1980): 617–25.

Fraser, Peter M., *Ptolemaic Alexandria* (Oxford: Oxford University Press, 1972).

Freeman, Stephen, *The Ladies Friend* (London: printed for the author, 1787).

French, Roger, *Ancient Natural History* (London: Routledge, 1994).

— *Dissection and Vivisection in the European Renaissance* (Aldershot: Ashgate, 1999).

Freud, Sigmund, 'On the Universal Tendency to Debasement in the Sphere of Love' (1912), James Strachey (ed. and tr.), *The Standard Edition of the Complete Psychological Works* (London, 1957), vol. 11, 177–90.

Freund, Julien, *The Sociology of Max Weber* (New York: Random House, 1969).

Friedman, David M., *A Mind of its Own: A Cultural History of the Penis* (New York: The Free Press, 2001).

Galen, *De uteri dissectione*, ed. Diethard Nickel, *Corpus Medicorum Graecorum* V 2, 1 (Berlin: Akademie-Verlag, 1971).

— *On Seed*, ed. Philip de Lacy, *Corpus Medicorum Graecorum* V 3, 1 (Berlin: Akademie-Verlag, 1992).

— *Doctrines of Hippocrates and Plato*, ed. Philip de Lacy, *Corpus Medicorum Graecorum* V. 4.1, 2 (Berlin: Akademie-Verlag, 2005).

Gardiner, Anne Barbeau, 'Elizabeth Cellier in 1688 on Envious Doctors and Heroic Midwives Ancient and Modern', *Eighteenth Century Life*, 14 (1990): 24–34.

Gardner, Augustus, *A History of the Art of Midwifery: A Lecture Delivered at the College of Physicians and Surgeons, November 11th, 1851, Introductory to a Course of Private Instruction on Operative Midwifery; Showing the Past Inefficiency and Present Natural Incapacity of Females in the Practice of Obstetrics by Augustus K. Gardner* (New York: Stringer and Townsend, 1852); reprinted in *The Modern Practice of Midwifery: A Course of Lectures on Obstetrics: Delivered at St Mary's Hospital, London, by Wm Tyler Smith MD* (New York: Robert M. De Witt, 1858).

Garland, Robert, *The Eye of the Beholder: Deformity and Disability in the Graeco-Roman World* (London: Duckworth, 1995).

Gazzaniga, Valentina, 'Phanostrate, Metrodora, Lais and the Others. Women in the Medical Profession', *Medicina nei Secoli, Arte e Scienza*, 9 (1997): 277–90.

Geminus, Thomas, *Compendiosa totius Anatomie delineatio* (London: Nicholas Hill, 1553).

Gerber, David A., 'The "Careers" of People Exhibited in Freak Shows: The Problem of Volition and Valorization', in Rosemarie Garland Thomson (ed.) *Freakery. Cultural Spectacles of the Extraordinary Body* (New York: New York University Press, 2006), 38–54.

Gibson, Thomas, *The Anatomy of Humane Bodies Epitomized* (London: M. Fisher for T. Fisher, 1682).

— (1703) *The Anatomy of Humane Bodies Epitomized*, 6th edition (London: T.W.).

Gilbert, Ruth, *Early Modern Hermaphrodites: Sex and Other Stories* (Basingstoke: Palgrave, 2002).

Glazebrook, Alison and Madeleine M. Henry (eds), *Greek Prostitutes in the Ancient Mediterranean, 800 BCE–200 CE* (Madison, WI: University of Wisconsin Press, 2011).

Gleason, Maud, 'The Semiotics of Gender', in David Halperin, John J. Winkler and Froma Zeitlin (eds), *Before Sexuality: The Construction of Erotic Experience in the Ancient Greek World* (Princeton, NJ: Princeton University Press, 1990), 389–415.

— *Making Men: Sophists and Self-Presentation in Ancient Rome* (Princeton, NJ: Princeton University Press, 1995).

Goldberg, Marilyn Y., 'Spatial and Behavioural Negotiation in Classical Athenian City Houses', in Penelope M. Allison (ed.), *The Archaeology of Household Activities* (London and New York: Routledge, 1999), 142–61.

Golding, William, *Fire Down Below* (London: Faber & Faber, 1989).

Goulart, Simon, *Thresor d'histoires admirables et memorables de nostre temps* (Paris, Jean Houzé, 1600).

— *Admirable and memorable histories containing the wonders of our time. Collected into French out of the best authors. By I. [sic] Goulart. And out of French into English. By Ed. Grimeston* (London: George Eld, 1607).

Gould, George M. and Walter L. Pyle, *Anomalies and Curiosities of Medicine* (Philadelphia, PA: W.B. Saunders, 1896).

Gourevitch, Danielle, 'Pudeur et pratique médicale dans l'Antiquité classique', *La Presse médicale*, 3 (1968): 544–6.

Gowing, Laura, *Common Bodies. Women, Touch and Power in Seventeenth-Century England* (New Haven, CT: Yale University Press, 2003).

Grant, Mary (ed. and tr.), *The Myths of Hyginus*, University of Kansas Publications in Humanistic Studies, no. 34 (Lawrence: University of Kansas Press, 1960).

Green, Monica H., 'Women's Medical Practice and Health Care in Medieval Europe', in Judith Bennett et al. (eds), *Sisters and Workers in the Middle Ages* (Chicago, IL: University of Chicago Press, 1989), 39–78.

— *The Trotula. A Medieval Compendium of Women's Medicine* (Philadelphia, PA: University of Pennsylvania Press, 2001).

— *Making Women's Medicine Masculine: The Rise of Male Authority in Pre-Modern Gynaecology* (Oxford: Oxford University Press, 2008).

— 'The Sources of Eucharius Rösslin's *Rosegarden for Pregnant Women and Midwives*', *Medical History*, 53 (2009): 167–92.

— 'Bodily Essences: Bodies as Categories of Difference', in Linda Kalof (ed.), *A Cultural History of the Human Body: The Medieval Age* (New York: Berg, 2010), 141–62.

Green, Peter (tr.), *Diodorus Siculus: Books 11–12.37.1. Greek History, 480–431 BC, the Alternative Version* (Austin, TX: University of Texas Press, 2006).

Grell, Ole P., 'Caspar Bartholin and the Education of the Pious Physician', in Ole P. Grell and Andrew Cunningham (eds), *Medicine and the Reformation* (London, 1993), 78–100.

Guillemeau, Jacques, *De l'heureux accouchement des femmes* (Paris: Nicolas Buon, 1609).

— *Child-Birth or, the Happy Deliverie of Women* (London: A. Hatfield, 1612).

Hägg, Tomas, *The Novel in Antiquity* (Berkeley and Los Angeles, CA: University of California Press, 1983).

Hammond, William A. (ed.), *Polydori Virgilii de rerum inventoribus; translated into English by John Langley* (New York: Agathynian Club, 1868).

Handyside, Peter D., 'Account of a Case of Hermaphroditism', *Edinburgh Medical and Surgical Journal*, 43 (1835): 313–18.

Hansen, William, *Phlegon of Tralles' Book of Marvels* (Exeter: University of Exeter Press, 1996).

Hanson, Ann Ellis, 'Hippocrates: *Diseases of Women 1*', *Signs: Journal of Women in Culture and Society*, 1 (1975): 567–84.

— 'Diseases of Women in the *Epidemics*', in Gerhaad Baader and Rolf Winau (eds), *Die Hippokratischen Epidemien: Theorie–Praxis–Tradition*, *Sudhoffs Archiv*, Beiheft 27 (Stuttgart: Franz Steiner, 1989), 38–51.

— 'A Division of Labor: Roles for Men in Greek and Roman Births', *Thamyris: Mythmaking from Past to Present*, 1 (1994): 157–202.

— 'Doctors' Literacy and Papyri of Medical Content', *Studies in Ancient Medicine*, 35 (2010): 187–204.

— and David Armstrong, 'The Virgin's Voice and Neck: Aeschylus, *Agamemnon* 245 and Other Texts', *Bulletin of the Institute of Classical Studies*, 33 (1986): 97–100.

Harley, David, 'Ignorant Midwives – A Persistent Stereotype', *Society for the Social History of Medicine Bulletin*, 28 (1981): 6–9.

Harlow, Mary and Ray Laurence, *Growing Up and Growing Old in Ancient Rome: A Life Course Approach* (London and New York: Routledge, 2002).

Harris, Joseph, '"La force du tact": Representing the Taboo Body in Jacques Duval's *Traité des hermaphrodits* (1612)', *French Studies*, 57 (2003): 311–22.

Harrison, Wendy Sealey, 'The Shadow and the Substance: The Sex/Gender Debate', in Kathy Davis, Mary Evans and Judith Lorber (eds), *Handbook of Gender and Women's Studies* (London: Sage, 2006), 35–52.

Harvey, Karen, 'The Century of Sex? Gender, Bodies, and Sexuality in the Long Eighteenth Century', *Historical Journal*, 45 (2002): 899–916.

— *Reading Sex in the Eighteenth Century: Bodies and Gender in English Erotic Culture* (Cambridge: Cambridge University Press, 2004).

Hasson, Or, 'On Sex-Differences and Science in Huarte de San Juan's *Examination of Men's Wits*', *Iberoamerica Global*, 2 (2009): 194–212; <http://iberoamericaglobal.huji.ac.il/Num5/Art_15.pdf> accessed 28 August 2012.

Haynes, Katharine, *Fashioning the Feminine in the Greek Novel* (London: Routledge, 2003).

Hecquet, Philippe, *De l'indecence aux hommes d'accoucher les femmes* (Paris: Jacques Estienne, 1708).

— *De l'indecence aux hommes d'accoucher les femmes* (Trevoux: l'Imprimerie de S.A.S. and Paris: chez la Veuve Ganeau, 1744).

Herodotus: *The famous hystory of Herodotus* (London: Thomas Marshe, 1584).

Herrlinger, Robert and Edith Feiner, 'Why Did Vesalius Not Discover the Fallopian Tubes?', *Medical History*, 8 (1964): 335–41.

Heywood, Thomas, *Gynaikeion: or, Nine bookes of various history concerning women* (London: Adam Islip, 1624).

Hillman, David and Carla Mazzi (eds), *The Body in Parts: Fantasies of Corporeality in Early Modern Europe* (London and New York: Routledge, 1997).

[Hippocrates] *Epidemics, Traduction des Oeuvres Médicales d'Hippocrate*, vol. 4 (Toulouse: Faces, Meilhac et Comanie, 1801).

Hirsch, Brett D., '"What are these Faces?" Interpreting Bearded Women in *Macbeth*', in Andrew Lynch and Anne M. Scott (eds), *Renaissance Poetry and Drama in Context, Essays for Christopher Wortham* (Newcastle-upon-Tyne: Cambridge Scholars Press, 2008), 91–114.

Hitchcock, Tim, *English Sexualities, 1700–1800* (New York: St Martin's Press and Basingstoke: Palgrave Macmillan, 1997).

Hobby, Elaine, *Virtue of Necessity. English Women's Writing 1649–88* (Ann Arbor, MI: University of Michigan Press, 1989).

— '"Secrets of the Female Sex": Jane Sharp, the Reproductive Female Body, and Early Modern Midwifery Manuals', *Women's Writing*, 8 (2001): 201–12.

— '"The Head of this Counterfeit Yard is called Tertigo" or, "It is not Hard Words that Perform the Work": Recovering Early Modern Women's Writing', in Jo

Wallwork and Paul Salzman (eds), *Women Writing 1550–1750*, special issue of *Meridian*, 18:1 (2001): 13–23.

— 'Gender, Science and Midwifery: Jane Sharp, The Midwives Book (1671)', in Claire Jowitt and Diane Watt (eds), *The Arts of Seventeenth-Century Science: Representations of the Natural World in European and North American Culture* (Aldershot: Ashgate, 2002), 146–59.

— 'Yarhound, Horrion, and the Horse-Headed Tartar: Editing Jane Sharp, *The Midwives Book* (1671)', in Katherine Binhammer and Jeanne Wood (eds), *Women and Literary History: 'For There She Was'* (Newark, DE and London: Associated University Presses, 2003), 27–42.

— '"Dreams and Plain Dotage": The Value of *The Birth of Mankind*', in Sharon Ruston (ed.), *Literature and Science*: Essays and Studies 2008, The English Association (Cambridge: D.S. Brewer, 2008), 35–52.

— (ed.), *The Birth of Mankind, Otherwise Named, The Woman's Book* (Aldershot and Burlington, VT: Ashgate, 2009).

Holford-Strevens, Leofranc, *Aulus Gellius. An Antonine Scholar and his Achievement*, revised edition (Oxford: Oxford University Press, 2003).

Holmes, Brooke, *Gender: Antiquity and its Legacy* (London: I.B. Tauris, 2012).

Home, Everard, *Lectures on Comparative Anatomy*, vol. 3 (London: Longman, Hurst, Rees, Orme and Brown, 1823).

Hopwood, Keith, '"All that May Become a Man": The Bandit in the Ancient Novel', in Lin Foxhall and John Salmon (eds), *When Men Were Men: Masculinity, Power and Identity in Classical Antiquity* (London and New York: Routledge, 1998), 195–204.

Horstmanshoff, H.F.J., 'The Ancient Physician: Craftsman or Scientist?', *Journal of the History of Medicine and Allied Sciences*, 45 (1990): 176–97.

— and Helen King, Claus Zittel (eds), *Blood, Sweat and Tears: The Changing Concepts of Physiology from Antiquity into Early Modern Europe*, *Intersections*, 25 (Leiden: Brill, 2012).

Huarte, Juan, *Examen de ingenios, para les sciencias* (Baeça, 1575).

— *The Examination of Mens Wits in whicch [sic], by Discouering the Varietie of Natures, is Shewed for what Profession Each One is Apt, and How Far he shall Profit Therein. By Iohn Huarte. Translated out of the Spanish tongue by M. Camillo Camili. Englished out of his Italian, by R[ichard] C[arew] Esquire* (London, 1594) (Gainesville, FL: Scholar's Facsimiles and Reprints, 1959).

Huet, Marie-Hélène, *Monstrous Imagination* (Cambridge, MA: Harvard University Press, 1993).

Huisman, Frank and John Harley Warner (eds), *Locating Medical History: The Stories and their Meanings* (Baltimore, MD: Johns Hopkins University Press, 2006).

Huisman, Tim, *The Finger of God: Anatomical Practice in Seventeenth-Century Leiden* (Leiden: Primavera Press, 2009).

Hurd-Mead, Kate, 'An Introduction to the History of Women in Medicine 1. Medical Women before Christianity (continued)', *Annals of Medical History*, 5 (1933): 171–96.

Hyginus: C. Iulii Hygini Augusti Liberti, *Fabularum Liber* (Lyon: apud Ioannem Degabiano, 1608).

— *Hygini. Quae hodie extant, adcurante Joanne Scheffero ... Accedunt et Thomae Munceri In Fabulas Hygini Annotationes* (Hamburg: Ex officina Gothofredi Schultzen, 1674).

Index Hippocraticus, Fasc. II, E–K (Gottingen: Vandenhoeck & Ruprecht, 1987).

Insigne Artificium Aristotelis: or, Aristotle's Compleat Master-Piece. In two parts. Displaying the secrets of nature in the generation of man (London: n.p., 1702).

Jansson ab Almeloveen, Theodoor, *Opuscula: sive Antiquitatum e sacris profanarum specimen* (Amsterdam: Jansson-Waesberg, 1686).

Jaulin, Annick, 'La Fabrique du sexe, Thomas Laqueur et Aristote', *Clio: Histoire, femmes et sociétés*, 14 (2001): 195–205.

Jenkinson, Sally L., *Bayle: Political Writings* (Cambridge: Cambridge University Press, 2000).

Jenner, Mark and Bernard Taithe, 'The Historiographical Body', in John Pickstone and Roger Cooter (eds), *History of Medicine in the Twentieth Century*: Volume 2, *The Body* (New York: Harwood Publishing, 1999), 187–200.

Jex-Blake, Sophia, 'Medicine as a Profession for Women', in Josephine Butler (ed.), *Woman's Work and Woman's Culture. A Series of Essays* (London: Macmillan and Co., 1869), 78–120.

— *Medical Women: A Thesis and a History* (Edinburgh: Oliphant, Anderson and Ferrier, 1886).

Johnson, Monte Ransome, *Aristotle on Teleology* (Oxford: Clarendon Press, 2005).

Johnston, Mark, *Beard Fetish in Early Modern England* (Aldershot: Ashgate, 2011).

Jordan, Jennifer, '"That ere with Age, his strength is utterly decay'd": Understanding the Male Body in Early Modern Manhood', in Sarah Toulalan and Kate Fisher (eds), *Bodies, Sex and Desire from the Renaissance to the Present* (Basingstoke: Palgrave Macmillan, 2011), 27–48.

Jordanova, Ludmilla, *Sexual Visions: Images of Gender in Science and Medicine between the Eighteenth and Twentieth Centuries* (Hemel Hempstead: Harvester Wheatsheaf, 1989).

Jouanna, Jacques, *Hippocrate* (Paris: Fayard, 1992).

Karaghiorga-Stathacopoulou, Théodora, 'Baubo', *Lexicon Iconographicum Mythologiae Classicae* III.1, 87–90 (Zürich and München: Artemis-Verlag, 1986).

Keller, Eve, 'Mrs Jane Sharp: Midwifery and the Critique of Medical Knowledge in Seventeenth-Century England', *Women's Writing*, 2 (1995): 101–11.

— *Generating Bodies and Gendered Selves: The Rhetoric of Reproduction in Early Modern England* (Seattle and London: University of Washington Press, 2007).

Kelly, Laura, '"Fascinating Scalpel-Wielders and Fair Dissectors": Women's Experience of Irish Medical Education, c.1880s–1920s', *Medical History*, 54 (2010): 495–516.

Ker, Ian Turnbull (ed.), *Letters and Diaries of John Henry Newman*, vol. 18: *New Beginnings in England, April 1857–December 1858* (London and New York: T. Nelson, 1968).

King, Helen, 'Agnodike and the Profession of Medicine', *Proceedings of the Cambridge Philological Society*, 32 (1986): 53–77.

— 'The Politick Midwife: Models of Midwifery in the Work of Elizabeth Cellier', in Hilary Marland (ed.), *The Art of Midwifery* (London: Routledge, 1993), 115–30.

— 'Sowing the Field: Greek and Roman Sexology', in Roy Porter and Mikuláš Teich (eds), *Sexual Knowledge, Sexual Science. The History of Attitudes to Sexuality* (Cambridge: Cambridge University Press, 1994), 29–46.

— *Hippocrates' Woman: Reading the Female Body in Ancient Greece* (London: Routledge, 1998).

— 'The Power of Paternity: The Father of Medicine Meets the Prince of Physicians', in David Cantor (ed.), *Reinventing Hippocrates* (Aldershot: Ashgate, 2001), 21–36.

— *The Disease of Virgins: Green Sickness, Chlorosis and the Problems of Puberty* (London: Routledge, 2003).

— 'The Mathematics of Sex: One to Two, or Two to One?', *Studies in Medieval and Renaissance History*, series 3, vol. II (2005): 47–58.

— *Midwifery, Obstetrics and the Rise of Gynaecology: The Uses of a Sixteenth-Century Compendium* (Aldershot: Ashgate, 2007).

— 'Barbes, sang et genre: afficher la différence dans le monde antique', in Jérôme Wilgaux and Véronique Dasen (eds), *Langages et métaphores du corps* (Rennes: Presses universitaires de Rennes, 2008), 153–68.

— 'Engendrer "la femme": Jacques Dubois et Diane de Poitiers', in Cathy McClive, Jean-François Budin and Nicole Pellegrin (eds), *Femmes en Fleurs: Santé, Sexualité et Génération du Moyen Age aux Lumières* (Université de Saint-Étienne, 2010), 125–38.

— 'Galen and the Widow. Towards a History of Therapeutic Masturbation in Ancient Gynaecology', *EuGeStA: Journal on Gender Studies in Antiquity*, 1 (2011): 205–35.

— 'Inside and Outside, Cavities and Containers: The Organs of Generation in Seventeenth-Century English Medicine', in Patricia A. Baker, Han Nijdam, Karine van 't Land (eds), *Medicine and Space: Body, Surroundings and Borders in Antiquity and the Middle Ages, Visualising the Middle Ages* 4 (Leiden: Brill, 2011), 37–60.

— 'Sex, Medicine and Disease', in Mark Golden and Peter Toohey (eds), *A Cultural History of Sexuality in the Classical World* (Oxford and New York: Berg, 2011), 107–24.

— and Cathy McClive, 'When is a Foetus not a Foetus? Diagnosing False Conceptions in Early Modern France', in Véronique Dasen (ed.), *L'Embryon humain à travers l'histoire: Images, savoirs et rites*, Actes du colloque international de Fribourg, 27–29 octobre 2004 (Gollion: Infolio, 2008), 223–38.

Kivistö, Sari, 'G. F. von Franckenau's *Satyra Sexta* (1674) on Male Menstruation and Female Testicles', in Anu Korhonen and Kate Lowe (eds), *The Trouble with Ribs: Women, Men and Gender in Early Modern Europe*, COLLeGIUM: *Studies Across Disciplines in the Humanities and Social Sciences*, 2 (2007): <http://hdl.handle.net/10138/25752>.

Kleingünther, Adolf, *Prôtos Heuretês: Untersuchungen zur Geschichte einer Fragestellung*, *Philologus* Supplement 26.1 (Leipzig: Akademie Verlag, 1933).

Knibiehler, Yvonne, 'Les Médecins et la "nature féminine" au temps du Code civil', *Annales ESC*, 4 (1976): 824–45.

Knights, Mark, *Politics and Opinion in Crisis, 1678–81* (Cambridge: Cambridge University Press, 1994).

Knox, Vicesimus, *Winter Evenings: or lucubrations on life and letters: In three volumes* (London: printed for Charles Dilly, 1788), vol. 1.

Konstan, David, *The Emotions of the Ancient Greeks: Studies in Aristotle and Classical Literature* (Toronto: University of Toronto Press, 2006).

Kornmann, Heinrich, *De miraculis vivorum* (Frankfurt: Fischer, 1614).

Kudlien, Fridolf, 'Medical Education in Classical Antiquity', in Charles D. O'Malley (ed.), *The History of Medical Education*, UCLA Forum in Medical Sciences, no. 12 (Berkeley and Los Angeles, CA: University of California Press, 1970), 3–37.

Kuefler, Mathew, *The Manly Eunuch: Masculinity, Gender Ambiguity and Christian Ideology in Late Antiquity* (Chicago, IL: Chicago University Press, 2001).

Kukla, Rebecca, *Mass Hysteria: Medicine, Culture, and Mothers' Bodies* (Lanham, MD: Rowman and Littlefield, 2005).

Kusukawa, Sachiko, *Picturing the Book of Nature: Image, Text and Argument in Sixteenth-Century Human Anatomy and Medical Botany* (Chicago, IL: University of Chicago Press, 2012).

Laipson, Peter, 'From Boudoir to Bookstore: Writing the History of Sexuality. A Review Article', *Comparative Studies in Society and History*, 34 (1992): 636–44.

Langholf, Volker, *Medical Theories in Hippocrates: Early Texts and the Epidemics*, Untersuchungen zur antiken Literatur und Geschichte, vol. 34 (Berlin: W. de Gruyter, 1990).

Laqueur, Thomas, 'La Différence: Bodies, Gender, and History', *The Threepenny Review*, 33 (Spring, 1988): 12–14.

— *Making Sex: Body and Gender from the Greeks to Freud* (Cambridge, MA: Harvard University Press, 1990).

— 'One Sex or Two', *London Review of Books*, 12 (6 December 1990).

— 'Sex in the Flesh', *Isis*, 94 (2003): 300–306.

Larsen, Anne R., *From Mother to Daughter: Poems, Dialogues and Letters of Les Dames Des Roches* (Chicago, IL: University of Chicago Press, 2006).

Laurens, André du, *Opera anatomica in quinque libros divisa* (Lyon: John-Baptiste Buisson, 1593).

— *Historia Anatomica Humani Corporis* (Paris: Jamet Mettayer, 1600).

Lawn, Brian, *The Rise and Decline of the Scholastic 'Quaestio Disputata' with Special Emphasis on its Use in the Teaching of Medicine and Science* (Leiden: Brill, 1993).

Le Clerc, Daniel, *Histoire de la médecine ou on voit l'origine et le progress de cet art* (Geneva: J.A. Chouët and D. Ritter, 1696); translated as *The History of Physick, or, an account of the rise and progress of the art* (London: D. Brown, A. Roper, T. Leigh and D. Midwinter, 1699).

— *Histoire de la médecine* (Amsterdam: Compagnie, 1723).

Lee, Mireille M., 'Body-Modification in Classical Greece', in Thorsten Fögen and Mireille M. Lee (eds), *Bodies and Boundaries in Graeco-Roman Antiquity* (Berlin: De Gruyter, 2009), 155–80.

Leitao, David D., *The Pregnant Male as Myth and Metaphor in Classical Greek Literature* (Cambridge: Cambridge University Press, 2012).

Lemnius, Levinus, *De occultis naturae miraculis* (Antwerp: Guilielmus Simonis, 1564).

— *The Secret Miracles of Nature* (London: printed by Jo. Streater, 1658).

— *A Discourse Touching Generation. Collected out of Laevinus Lemnius, a most learned physitian. Fit for the use of physitians, midwives, and all young married people* (London: printed by John Streater, 1664).

Lemos, Maximiano, *Amato Lusitano. A sua vida e a sua obra* (Porto: E. Tavares Martins, 1907).

Lemprière's Biblioteca Classica; Or, A Classical Dictionary, Containing a Full Account of All the Proper Names Mentioned in Antient Authors (London: T. Cadell, 1788).

Lewis, Charlton T. and Charles Short, *A Latin Dictionary* (Oxford: Clarendon Press, 1879).

Lewis, Clive Staple, *Perelandra* (London: John Lane, The Bodley Head, 1943).

Libbon, Stephanie E., 'Pathologizing the Female Body: Phallocentrism in Western Science', *Journal of International Women's Studies*, 8 (2007): 79–92.

Liébault, Jean, *Livres appartenant aux infirmitez et maladies des femmes, pris du Latin de M. Jean Liebaut* (Paris: Jacques de Puys, 1582).

Lindgren, Amy, 'The Wandering Womb and the Peripheral Penis: Gender and the Fertile Body in Late Medieval Infertility Treatises' (PhD thesis, University of California, Davis, 2005).

Ling, Nicholas, *Politeuphuia, Wit's Commonwealth* (London: Printed by I. Roberts for Nicholas Ling, 1597).

Lingo, Alison Klairmont, 'Causes and Cures for Female Infertility, Premature Delivery, and Uterine Disease in the Work of Ambroise Paré and Louise

Bourgeois', in Denis Buican and Denis Thieffry (eds), *Biological and Medical Sciences*, Proceedings of the XXth International Congress of History of Science (Liège, 20–26 July 1997) (Turnhout: Brepols, 2002), 33–8.

— 'Une femme parmi les obstétriciens du XVIIe siècle' (2008), <http://www.societe-histoire-naissance.fr/spip.php?article4> accessed 16 May 2012.

Lipscomb, Harry S. and Hebbel E. Hoff, 'Saint Uncumber or La Vierge Barbue', *Bulletin of the History of Medicine*, 37 (1963): 523–7.

Litoff, Judy Barrett, *The American Midwife Debate: A Sourcebook on its Modern Origin* (Westport, CT and London: Greenwood Press, 1986).

Littré, Emile, *Oeuvres complètes d'Hippocrate*, 10 vols (Paris: Baillière, 1839–1861).

Lloyd, Geoffrey E.R., *Polarity and Analogy: Two Types of Argumentation in Early Greek Thought* (Cambridge: Cambridge University Press, 1966).

Lochrie, Karma, *Margery Kempe and Translations of the Flesh* (Philadelphia, PA: University of Pennsylvania Press, 1991).

Lonie, Iain M., *The Hippocratic Treatises 'On Generation,' 'On the Nature of the Child,' 'Diseases IV'* (Berlin and New York: de Gruyter, 1981).

— 'Literacy and the Development of Hippocratic Medicine', in François Lasserre and Philippe Mudry (eds), *Formes de pensée dans la collection hippocratique: Actes du Colloque hippocratique de Lausanne 1981* (Geneva: Droz, 1983), 145–61.

Loraux, Nicole, 'Sur la race des femmes et quelques-unes de ses tribus', *Arethusa*, 11 (1978): 43–87.

— 'Ponos. Sur quelques difficultés de la peine comme nom du travail', *Annali dell'Instituto Orientale di Napoli*, 4 (1982): 171–92.

McClure, Laura, *Courtesans at Table: Gender and Greek Literary Culture in Athenaeus* (London: Routledge, 2003).

McCrae, Morrice, *Simpson. The Turbulent Life of a Medical Pioneer* (Edinburgh: Birlinn, 2011).

McGrath, Roberta, *Seeing her Sex: Medical Archives and the Female Body* (Manchester: Manchester University Press, 2002).

McLaren, Angus, 'Review: Thomas Laqueur, *Making Sex: Body and Gender from the Greeks to Freud*', *American Historical Review*, 98 (1993): 832–3.

Maclean, Ian, *The Renaissance Notion of Woman: A Study in the Fortunes of Scholasticism and Medical Science in European Intellectual Life* (Cambridge: Cambridge University Press, 1980).

McMaster, Gilbert T., 'The First Woman Practitioner of Midwifery and the Care of Infants in Athens, 300 BC', *American Medicine*, 7 (1912): 202–5.

McTavish, Lianne, *Childbirth and the Display of Authority in Early Modern France* (Aldershot: Ashgate, 2005).

Major, Wilfrid, 'Review of P.K. Marshall, *Hyginus: Fabulae. Editio altera*', *Bryn Mawr Classical Review* (2003), <http://bmcr.brynmawr.edu/2003/2003-06-37.html>.

Mak, Geertje, 'Doubting Sex from Within: A Praxiographic Approach to a Late Nineteenth-Century Case of Hermaphroditism', *Gender & History*, 18 (2006): 332–56.

— 'Hermaphrodites on Show. The Case of Katharina/Karl Hohmann and its Use in Nineteenth-Century Medical Science', *Social History of Medicine*, 25 (2011): 65–83.

— *Doubting Sex. Inscriptions, Bodies and Selves in Nineteenth-Century Hermaphrodite Case Histories* (Manchester and New York: Manchester University Press, 2012).

Manetti, Daniela and Amneris Roselli, *Ippocrate. Epidemie Libro Sesto* (Florence: La Nuova Italia Editrice, 1982).

Mann, Jenny C., 'How to Look at a Hermaphrodite in Early Modern England', *Studies in English Literature*, 46 (2006): 67–91.

Manuli, Paola, 'Donne mascoline, femmine sterili, vergini perpetue. La ginecologia greca tra Ippocrate e Sorano', in Silvia Campese, Paola Manuli and Giulia Sissa, *Madre Materia. Sociologia e biologia della donna greca* (Turin: Boringhieri, 1983).

Marinello, Giovanni, *Le Medicine partenenti alle infirmità delle donne* (Venice: Francesco de' Franceschi, 1563).

Marshall, Peter K., 'The Budé Hyginus', *Classical Review*, 49 (1999): 410–12.

— *Hyginus: Fabulae. Editio altera* (Munich: K.G. Saur, 2002).

Mason, Michael, 'Do Women Like Sex? Review of Thomas Laqueur, *Making Sex*', *London Review of Books*, 8 November 1990, 16–17.

Matthiolus, Petrus Andreas, *Apologia adversus Amathum Lusitanum, cum censura in eiusdem enarrationes* (Venice: ex Officina Erasmiana, V. Valgrisii, 1558).

Maudsley, Henry, 'Sex in Mind and in Education', *Popular Science Monthly* (June 1874): 198–215.

Mauriceau, François, *Traité des maladies des femmes grosses et accouchées* (Paris: J. Henault, 1668).

— *The Diseases of Women with Child, and in Child-Bed: As Also, the Best Means of Helping Them in Natural and Unnatural Labours*, 4th edition (London: Andrew Bell, 1710).

May, Margaret Tallmadge, *Galen, On the Usefulness of the Parts of the Body*, 2 vols (Ithaca, NY: Cornell University Press, 1968).

Mazzini, Innocenzo and Flammini, Guiseppe, *De conceptu: Estratti di un'antica traduzione latina del* Περὶ γυναικείων *pseudoippocratico* (Bologna: Pàtron, 1983).

Mercado, Luis de, *De mulierum affectionibus* Book 2 (Venice: Valgrisi, 1587).

— *De internorum morborum curatione libri IV* in *Opera* (Frankfurt, sumptibus haeredum D. Zachariae Paltheni, 1620).

Mercurialis, Hieronymus, *Variarum lectionum libri* (Basle: Ex officina Petri Pernae, 1576).

— *Variarum lectionum in medicinae scriptoribus et aliis* (Paris: Nicolaus Nivellius, 1585).

— *Variarum lectionum libri* (Venice: apud Iuntas, 1588).

— *Opervm Hippocratis Coi qvae Graece et Latine extant*, 2 vols (Venice: apud Iuntas, 1588).

— *Praelectiones Pisanae* (Venice: apud Iuntas, 1597).

— *Responsorum, et consultationum medicinalium tomus tertius* (Venice: apud Franciscum de Franciscis Senensem, 1597).

Meres, Francis, *Palladis Tamia, Wits Treasury, being the second part of Wits Commonwealth* (London: Printed by P. Short, for Cuthbert Burbie, 1598).

Modesty Triumphing over Impudence. Or, some Notes Upon a late Romance published by Elizabeth Cellier, Midwife and Lady Errant (London: Jonathan Wilkins, 1680).

Montagu, Richard, *The Acts & Monuments of the Church before Christ Incarnate* (London: Miles Flesher and Robert Young, 1642).

Montserrat, Dominic, 'Experiencing the Male Body in Roman Egypt', in Lin Foxhall and John Salmon, *When Men Were Men: Masculinity, Power and Identity in Classical Antiquity* (London and New York: Routledge, 1998), 153–64.

Moreau, Jacques, 'Les Guerriers et les femmes impudiques', *Annuaire de l'Institut de Philologie et d'Histoire orientales et slaves*, 11 (1951): 283–300.

Moreau, Jacques L., *Histoire naturelle de la femme*, 2 vols (Paris: L. Duprat, 1803).

Moréri, Louis, *The Great Historical, Geographical and Poetical Dictionary*, 2 vols (London: printed for Henry Rhodes, 1694).

— *Le grand Dictionnaire historique* (Amsterdam and La Haye: Aux Dépens de la Compagnie, 1702).

Morley, Henry and William Henry Mills, 'Why Shave?', *Household Words*, 13 (August 1853): 560–63.

— H[enry] M[orley], *Why Shave? Or, Beards v. Barbery* (London, 188? [precise date not given]).

Morris, Jan, *Conundrum* (London: Faber and Faber, 1974).

Mr Prance's Answer to Mrs Cellier's Libel ... To which is Added the Adventure of the Bloody Bladder (London: L. Curtis, 1680).

Mulryan, John, 'Translations and Adaptations of Vicenzo Cartari's *Imagini* and Natale Conti's *Mythologiae*: The Mythographic Tradition in the Renaissance', *Canadian Review of Comparative Literature*, 8 (1981): 272–83.

Mundé, Paul F., 'A Case of Presumptive True Lateral Hermaphrodism', *American Journal of Obstetrics and Diseases of Women and Children*, 8 (1876): 615–31.

Murphy, Trevor, *Pliny the Elder's Natural History: The Empire in the Encyclopaedia* (Oxford: Oxford University Press, 2004).

Nance, Brian, 'Wondrous Experience as Text: Valleriola and the *Observationes medicinales*', in Elizabeth Jane Furdell (ed.), *Textual Healing: Essays on Medieval and Early Modern Medicine* (Leiden: Brill, 2005), 101–17.

Nemesius of Emesa, *On the Nature of Man* (William Tefler, ed.) (Philadelphia, PA: Westminster Press, 1955).

Neugebauer, Franz Ludwig von, *Hermaphroditismus beim Menschen* (Leipzig: Verlag von Dr Werner Klinkhardt, 1908).

Newbold, Ronald F., 'Fear of Sex in Nonnus' *Dionysiaca*', *Electronic Antiquity*, 4:2 (1988), <http://scholar.lib.vt.edu/ejournals/ElAnt/V4N2/newbold.html>.

Nickel, Diethard, 'Berufsvorstellungen über weibliche Medizinalpersonen in der Antike', *Klio*, 61 (1979): 515–18.

— 'Medizingeschlichtliches in den "Fabulae" des Hyginus', *International Congress of the History of Medicine*, 16 (1981), vol. II: 170–73.

Nihell, Elizabeth, *A Treatise on the Art of Midwifery setting forth Various Abuses Therein, especially as to the Practice with Instruments* (London: A. Morley, 1760).

— *La Cause de l'humanité, référée au tribunal du bon sens et de la raison: ou traité sur les accouchemens par les femmes: ouvrage tres-utile aux sages-femmes, & tres-interessant pour les familles* (London and Paris: chez Antoine Boudet, 1771).

Nixon, Lucia, 'The Cults of Demeter and Kore', in Richard Hawley and Barbara Levick (eds), *Women in Antiquity: New Assessments* (London: Routledge, 1995), 75–96.

Nutton, Christine, 'Introduction' to *Hieronymus Mercurialis, De arte gymnastica* (Stuttgart: Edition Medicina Rara, 1978).

Nutton, Vivian, '*De placitis Hippocratis et Platonis* in the Renaissance', in Paola Manuli and Mario Vegetti (eds), *Le opere psicologiche di Galeno, Atti del Terzo Colloquio Galenico Internazionale, Pavia 10–12 settembre 1986* (Naples: Bibliopolis, 1988), 281–309.

— 'Representation and Memory in Renaissance Anatomical Illustration', in Fabrizio Meroi and Claudio Pogliano (eds), *Immagini per conoscere: dal Rinascimento alla Rivoluzione scientifica* (Florence, L.S. Olshki, 2001), pp. 61–80.

— 'Vesalius Revised: His Annotations to the 1555 *Fabrica*', *Medical History*, 56 (2012): 415–43.

Oakes, Elizabeth H., *Encyclopedia of World Scientists*, revised edition (New York: Facts on File, 2007).

O'Higgins, Laurie, 'Women's Cultic Joking and Mockery', in André P.M. Lardinois and Laura McClure (eds), *Making Silence Speak: Women's Voices in Greek Literature and Society* (Princeton, NJ: Princeton University Press, 2001), 137–60.

— *Women and Humor in Classical Greece* (Cambridge: Cambridge University Press, 2003).

Olasky, Marvin, *The Press and Abortion, 1838–1988* (Hillsdale, NJ: Lawrence Erlbaum Associates, 1988).

Oldstone-Moore, Christopher, 'The Beard Movement in Victorian Britain', *Victorian Studies*, 48 (2005), 7–34.

Olender, Maurice, 'Aspects de Baubo: textes et contextes antiques', *Revue de l'Histoire des Religions*, 202 (1985): 3–55; abbreviated English translation,

'Aspects of Baubo: Ancient Texts and Contexts', in David Halperin, John J. Winkler and Froma Zeitlin (eds), *Before Sexuality: The Construction of Erotic Experience in the Ancient Greek World* (Princeton, NJ: Princeton University Press, 2001), 83–113.

Panayotakis, Stelios, Maaike Zimmerman and Wytse Hette Keulen, *The Ancient Novel and Beyond, Mnemosyne*, supplement 241 (2003).

Paoletti, Italo, *Gerolamo Mercuriale e il suo tempo* (Lanciano: Cooperativa Editoriale Tipografica, 1963).

Paré, Ambroise, *Les œuvres d'Ambroise Paré, conseiller et premier chirurgien du Roy* (Paris: Gabriel Buon, 1575); English, *On Monsters and Marvels*, tr. Janis L. Pallister (Chicago, IL: University of Chicago Press, 1982).

—— *The Workes of that Famous Chirurgion Ambrose Parey translated out of Latine and compared with the French*, tr. Thomas Johnson (London: Th. Cotes and R. Young, 1634).

Park, Katharine, 'The Rediscovery of the Clitoris', in David Hillman and Carla Mazzio (eds), *The Body in Parts: Fantasies of Corporeality in Early Modern Europe* (London: Routledge, 1997), 171–94.

—— 'Dissecting the Female Body: From Women's Secrets to the Secrets of Nature', in Jane Donawerth and Adele Seeff (eds), *Crossing Boundaries: Attending to Early Modern Women* (Newark, DE: University of Delaware Press and London: Associated University Presses, 2000), 29–47.

—— *Secrets of Women. Gender, Generation and the Origins of Human Dissection* (New York: Zone Books, 2006).

—— 'Cadden, Laqueur, and the "One-sex Body"', *Medieval Feminist Forum*, 46 (2010): 96–100 <http://nrs.harvard.edu/urn-3:HUL.InstRepos:4774909> accessed 10 January 2012.

—— and Robert A. Nye, 'Destiny is Anatomy', *New Republic* (18 February 1991): 53–7.

Parker, Holt, 'Women Doctors in Greece, Rome, and the Byzantine Empire', in Lilian R. Furst (ed.) *Women Healers and Physicians: Climbing a Long Hill* (Lexington, KY: University of Kentucky Press, 1997), 131–50.

—— 'Women and Medicine', in Sharon L. James and Sheila Dillon (eds), *A Companion to Women in the Ancient World* (Oxford: Blackwell, 2012), 107–24.

Parker, Patricia, 'Gender Ideology, Gender Change: The Case of Marie Germain', *Critical Inquiry*, 19 (1993): 337–64.

Parsons, James, *A Mechanical and Critical Enquiry into the Nature of Hermaphrodites* (London: J. Walthoe, 1741).

Peitzman, Steven J., *A New and Untried Course: Woman's Medical College and Medical College of Pennsylvania, 1850–1998* (New Brunswick, NJ: Rutgers University Press, 2000).

Perkins, Wendy, *Midwifery and Medicine in Early Modern France: Louise Bourgeois* (Exeter: University of Exeter Press, 1996).

Peterson, Kaara L., *Popular Medicine, Hysterical Disease, and Social Controversy in Shakespeare* (Aldershot: Ashgate, 2010).

Petit, Samuel, *Leges Atticae* (Leiden: Abraham Kalleweir, 1742).

Petrelli, Richard L., 'The Regulation of French Midwifery during the *Ancien Régime*', *Journal of the History of Medicine and Allied Sciences*, 26 (1971): 276–92.

Petsalis-Diomidis, Alexia, *Truly Beyond Wonders: Aelius Aristides and the Cult of Asklepios* (Oxford and New York: Oxford University Press, 2010).

'Philalethes', *An Answer to Doctor Chamberlaines Scandalous and False Papers* (London, 1649).

Phillips, Mary, 'Midwives Versus Medics. A 17th Century Professional Turf War', *Management and Organizational History*, 2 (2007): 27–44.

Pineau, Severin, *De integritatis et corruptionis virginum notis* (Amsterdam: apud Johannem Ravesteinium, 1663).

Pitaval, François Gayot de, *Bibliotheque des gens de cour, ou mélange curieux* (Paris: Le Gras, 1732).

— *Causes celebres et interessantes avec les jugements qui les ont décidées*, vol. IV (Paris: chez la veuve Delaulne, 1734).

Pitcairn, Archibald, *The Whole Works of Dr. Archibald Pitcairn ...*, tr. George Sewell and J.T. Desaguliers, 2nd edition (London: printed for E. Curll, J. Pemberton, and W. and J. Innys, 1727).

Platner, Johann Zacharias, *Commentatio de arte obstetrica veterum*, in *Facultatis medicae in academia lipsiense* (Leipzig: Literis Langenhemianis, 1735).

— *Opusculorum: Tom. 1: Dissertationes* (Leipzig: Weidmann, 1749).

Pomata, Gianna, 'Menstruating Men: Similarity and Difference of the Sexes in Early Modern Medicine', in Valeria Finucci and Kevin Brownlee (eds), *Generation and Degeneration: Tropes of Reproduction in Literature and History from Antiquity to Early Modern Europe* (Durham, NC and London: Duke University Press, 2001), 109–52.

— (ed. and tr.), *The True Medicine by Olivia Sabuco de Nantes Barrera* (Toronto: Centre for Reformation and Renaissance Studies and ITER: Gateway to the Middle Ages and Renaissance, 2010).

— 'Observation Rising: Birth of an Epistemic Genre, 1500–1600', in Lorraine Daston and Elizabeth Lunbeck (eds), *Histories of Scientific Observation* (Chicago, IL: University of Chicago Press, 2011), 45–80.

Pomeroy, Sarah B., '*Technikai kai mousikai*: The Education of Women in the Fourth Century and in the Hellenistic Period', *American Journal of Ancient History*, 2 (1977): 51–68.

— 'Plato and the Female Physician (*Republic* 454d2)', *American Journal of Philology*, 99 (1978): 496–500.

Pope, Alexander, 'To a Lady in the Name of her Brother', in George Sherburn (ed.), *The Correspondence of Alexander Pope*, 5 vols (Oxford: Clarendon Press, 1956).

Pope, Johnathan H., 'Religion and Anatomy in John Banister's *The Historie of Man* (1578)', *LATCH*, 3 (2010): 1–33.

Pormann, Peter, 'Case Notes and Clinicians: Galen's Commentary on the Hippocratic *Epidemics* in the Arabic Tradition', *Arabic Sciences and Technology*, 18 (2008): 247–84.

— 'New Fragments from Rufus of Ephesus' *On Melancholy*', *Classical Quarterly*, 64 (2014).

Porter, Roy, 'William Hunter: A Surgeon and a Gentleman', in W.F. Bynum and Roy Porter (eds), *William Hunter and the Eighteenth-Century Medical World* (Cambridge: Cambridge University Press, 1985), 7–34.

— '"The Secrets of Generation Display'd": *Aristotle's Masterpiece* in Eighteenth-Century England', in Robert P. Maccubbin (ed.), *'Tis Nature's Fault: Unauthorized Sexuality during the Enlightenment* (Cambridge: Cambridge University Press, 1988), 1–21.

Posner, Richard A., *Sex and Reason* (Cambridge, MA: Harvard University Press, 1992).

Potter, John, *Archaeologia Graeca*, vol. II (London: John Knapton et al., 1722).

Preus, Anthony, 'Galen's Criticism of Aristotle's Conception Theory', *Journal of the History of Biology*, 10 (1977): 65–85.

Pucci, Pietro, *Hesiod and the Language of Poetry* (Baltimore, MD: Johns Hopkins University Press, 1977).

Rademaker, Adriaan, '"Most Citizens Are *Euruprôktoi* Now": (Un)manliness in Aristophanes', in Ralph Rosen and Ineke Sluiter (eds), *Andreia: Studies in Manliness and Courage in Classical Antiquity* (Leiden: Brill, 2003), 115–26.

Read, Kirk D., 'Touching and Telling: Gendered Variations on a Gynaecological Theme', in Kathleen P. Long (ed.), *Gender and Scientific Discourse in Early Modern Culture* (Aldershot: Ashgate, 2010), 259–78.

— *Birthing Bodies in Early Modern France: Stories of Gender and Reproduction* (Aldershot: Ashgate, 2011).

Reardon, Bryan P., *Collected Ancient Greek Novels*, 2nd edition (London and Berkeley, CA: University of California Press, 2008).

Reeve, Michael D., 'Hyginus', in Leighton D. Reynolds (ed.), *Texts and Transmission: A Survey of the Latin Classics* (Oxford: Oxford University Press, 1983).

Reinach, Salomon, 'Le Rire rituel', in ibid., *Cultes, mythes et religions*, vol. IV (Paris: E. Leroux, 1912).

Resnick, Irven M., 'Medieval Roots of the Myth of Jewish Male Menses', *Harvard Theological Review*, 93 (2000): 241–63.

Rétat, Pierre, *Le Dictionnaire de Bayle et la lutte philosophique au XVIIIe siècle* (Paris: Imprimerie Audin, 1971).

Reynolds, Leighton D. (ed.), *Texts and Transmission: A Survey of the Latin Classics* (Oxford: Oxford University Press, 1983).

Ricci, James V., *Aetios of Amida: The Gynaecology and Obstetrics of the VIth Century A.D.* (Philadelphia, PA: Blakiston, 1950).

Richards, Penny, 'A Life in Writing: Elizabeth Cellier and Print Culture', *Women's Writing*, 7 (2000): 411–25.

Riolan, Jean, *Discours sur les Hermaphrodits* (Paris: Pierre Ramier, 1614).

Robert, Louis, 'Femmes médecins' s.v. *Mousa Agathokleos iatreinê*, in Nezih Firatli and Louis Robert (eds), *Les Stèles funéraires de Byzance gréco-romaine* (Paris: Adrien Maisonneuve, 1964), 175–8.

Roodenburg, Herman W., 'The Maternal Imagination: The Fears of Pregnant Women in Seventeenth-Century Holland', *Journal of Social History*, 21 (1988): 701–16.

Rooks, Judith, *Midwifery and Childbirth in America* (Philadelphia, PA: Temple University Press, 1999).

Rose, H.J., 'An Unrecognized Fragment of Hyginus, *Fabvlae*', *Classical Quarterly*, 23 (1929): 96–9.

— *Hygini Fabulae* (Leiden: A.W. Sijthoff, 1936).

— 'Second Thoughts on Hyginus', *Mnemosyne*, 11 (1958): 42–8.

Rose, Valentin, *Theodori Prisciani, Euporiston libri III* (Leipzig: Teubner, 1894).

Rouget, François, 'De la sage-femme à la femme sage: réflexion et réflexivité dans les *Observations* de Louise Boursier', *Papers on French Seventeenth-Century Literature*, 25 (1998): 483–96.

Rouyer, Jules, *Études médicales sur l'ancienne Rome* (Paris: Adrien Delahaye, 1859).

Rueff, Jakob, *De conceptu et generatione hominis* (Zurich, 1554).

— *The Expert Midwife, or An Excellent and Most Necesary Treatise of the Generation and Birth of Man* (London: printed by E. G[riffin] for S. B[urton], 1637).

Rütten, Thomas, *Demokrit – lachender Philosoph und sanguinischer Melancholiker. Eine pseudohippokratische Geschichte* (Leiden: Brill, 1992).

Sacombe, Jean-François, *La Luciniade ou l'art des accouchements, poème didactique* (Paris: chez Courcier, 1792).

Sadler, John, *Sick Woman's Private Looking-Glass* (London: Anne Griffith, for Philemon Stephens and Christopher Meridith, 1636).

Sama, Catherine M. (ed. and tr.), *Elisabetta Caminer Turra: Selected Writings of an Eighteenth-Century Venetian Woman of Letters* (Chicago, IL: University of Chicago Press, 2003).

Sankovitch, Tilde A., *French Women Writers and the Book: Myths of Access and Desire* (Syracuse, NY: Syracuse University Press, 1988).

Sawday, Jonathan, *The Body Emblazoned: Dissection and the Human Body in Renaissance Culture* (London and New York: Routledge, 1995).

Scarborough, John, 'Galen *Redivivus*: An Essay Review', *Journal of the History of Medicine and Allied Sciences*, 43 (1988): 313–21.

The Scarlet Beast Stripped Naked, Being the Mistery of the Meal-Tub The Second Time Unravelled (London: D. Mallet, 1680).

Schacher, Polycarpus F. and Joannes H. Schmidius, *Dissertatio historico-critica de feminis ex arte medica claris* (Leipzig: ex officina Langenhemiana, 1737).

Schaps, David M., 'The Woman Least Mentioned: Etiquette and Women's Names', *Classical Quarterly*, 27 (1977): 323–30.

Schenck von Grafenburg, Johannes, *Observationes Medicae Rarae, Novae, Admirabiles et Monstrosae* (Frankfurt: Becker, 1596).

Schiebinger, Londa, 'Skeletons in the Closet: The First Illustrations of the Female Skeleton in Eighteenth-Century Anatomy', *Representations*, 14 (1986): 42–82.

— 'Skelletestreit', *Isis*, 94 (2003): 307–13.

Schleiner, Winfried, 'Early Modern Controversies about the One-Sex Model', *Renaissance Quarterly*, 53 (2000): 180–91.

Schmidt, Moritz, *Hygini Fabulae* (Jena: Dufft, 1872).

Schochow, Maximilian, *Die Ordnung der Hermaphroditen-Geschlechter: eine Genealogie des Geschlechtsbegriffs* (Berlin: Akademie Verlag, 2009).

Schott, Gaspar, *Physica curiosa* (Würzberg: Michael and Johann Friedrich Endter, 1667).

Screech, Timon, *Sex and the Floating World: Erotic Images in Japan, 1700–1820* (London: Reaktion, 1999).

Sebesta, Judith Lynn, 'Women's Costume and Feminine Civic Morality in Augustan Rome', in Maria Wyke (ed.), *Gender and the Body in the Ancient Mediterranean* (Oxford: Blackwell, 1998), 105–17.

Semonin, Paul, 'Monsters in the Marketplace: The Exhibition of Human Oddities in Early Modern England', in Rosemarie Garland Thomson (ed.) *Freakery. Cultural Spectacles of the Extraordinary Body* (New York: New York University Press, 2006), 69–81.

Sermon, William, *The Ladies Companion or the English Midwife* (London: Edward Thomas, 1671).

Sharp, Jane, *The Midwives Book, Or, the Whole Art of Midwifry Discovered* (London: Simon Miller, 1671); modern edition, Elaine Hobby (ed.), *The Midwives Book* (New York and Oxford: Oxford University Press, 1999).

Sheridan, Bridgette, 'Whither Childbearing: Gender, Status, and the Professionalization of Medicine in Early Modern France', in Kathleen Long (ed.), *Gender and Scientific Discourse in Early Modern Culture* (Aldershot: Ashgate, 2010), 239–58.

Shuttleworth, Sally, 'Review of Thomas Laqueur, *Making Sex*', *Journal of the History of Sexuality*, 3 (1993): 633–4.

Siena, Kevin, 'The "Foul Disease" and Privacy: The Effects of Venereal Disease and Patient Demand on the Medical Marketplace in Early Modern London', *Bulletin of the History of Medicine*, 75 (2001): 199–224.

Simili, Alessandro, *Gerolamo Mercuriale lettore e medico a Bologna* (Bologna: Azzoguidi–Società Tipografica Editoriale, 1966).

Simons, Patricia, *The Sex of Men in Premodern Europe: A Cultural History* (Cambridge: Cambridge University Press, 2011).

Simpson, James Young, 'Hermaphroditism', in Robert B. Todd (ed.), *The Cyclopaedia of Anatomy and Physiology*, vol. 2, DIA–INS (London: Longman, Brown, Green, Longmans and Roberts, 1839).

Singer, Peter N., (tr.) *Galen: Selected Works* (Oxford: Oxford University Press, 1977).

Siraisi, Nancy G., 'Vesalius and Human Diversity in *De humani corporis fabrica*', *Journal of the Warburg and Courtauld Institutes*, 57 (1994): 60–88.

— 'Vesalius and the Reading of Galen's Teleology', *Renaissance Quarterly*, 50 (1997): 1–37.

— 'History, Antiquarianism, and Medicine: The Case of Girolamo Mercuriale', *History of Ideas*, 64 (2003): 231–51.

— *History, Medicine, and the Traditions of Renaissance Learning* (Ann Arbor, MI: University of Michigan Press, 2007).

'Sketch of Henry Carrington Bolton', *Popular Science Monthly*, 43 Sept. (1893): 688–95.

Smellie, William, *A Treatise on the Theory and Practice of Midwifery*, 2nd edition, corrected (London: D. Wilson, 1752).

Smit, Christopher R., 'A Collaborative Aesthetic: Levinas's Idea of Responsibility and the Photographs of Charles Eisenmann and the Late Nineteenth-Century Freak-Performer', in Marlene Tromp (ed.), *Victorian Freaks. The Social Context of Freakery in Britain* (Columbus, OH: Ohio State University Press, 2008), 283–311.

Smith, Lisa, 'Imagining Women's Fertility before Technology', *Journal of Medical Humanities*, 31 (2010): 69–79.

Smith, R. Scott and Stephen Trzaskoma, *Apollodorus' Library and Hyginus' Fabulae* (Indianapolis, IN: Hackett Publishing, 2007).

Smith, Wesley D., *The Hippocratic Tradition* (Ithaca, NY: Cornell University Press, 1979); revised edition, 2002, <http://www.biusante.parisdescartes.fr/medicina/Hippo2.pdf>.

— 'Introduction' to Loeb Classical Library, *Hippocrates* VII (Cambridge, MA and London: Harvard University Press, 1994), 1–15.

Smyth, Adam, *'Profit and Delight': Printed Miscellanies in England, 1640–1682* (Detroit: Wayne State University Press, 2004).

Soranus: Soranus d'Éphèse, *Maladies des Femmes*, Paul Burgière, Danielle Gourevitch and Yves Malinas (eds), tr. and comm. (Budé editions, Paris: Les Belles Lettres, 1988–2000).

Spach, Israel, *Gynaeciorum sive de Mulierum tum communibus, tum gravidarum, parientium et puerperarum affectibus et morbis libri Graecorum, Arabum, Latinorum veterum et recentium quotquot extant, partim nunc primum editi, partim vero denuo recogniti, emendati* (Strasbourg: Zetsner, 1597).

Sprague, James S., 'Agnodice', *Dominion Monthly and Ontario Medical Journal*, 38 (1912): 13–17.

Stafford, Emma, 'Masculine Values, Feminine Forms: On the Gender of Personified Abstractions', in Lin Foxhall and John Salmon (eds), *Thinking Men: Masculinity and its Self-Representation in the Classical Tradition* (London and New York: Routledge, 1988), 43–56.

Starnes, DeWitt T. and Ernest William Talbert, *Classical Myth and Legend in Renaissance Dictionaries: A Study of Renaissance Dictionaries in their Relation to the Classical Learning of Contemporary English Writers* (Chapel Hill, NC: University of North Carolina Press, 1955).

Stepan, Nancy Ley, 'Race and Gender: The Role of Analogy in Science', *Isis*, 77 (1986): 261–77.

Stephanson, Raymond, 'Review of Karen Harvey, *Reading Sex in the Eighteenth Century*', *Eighteenth-Century Fiction*, 19 (2006): 222–4.

Stephens, Elizabeth, *Anatomy as Spectacle: Public Exhibitions of the Body from 1700 to the Present* (Liverpool: Liverpool University Press, 2011).

Stern, Rebecca, 'Our Bear Women, Ourselves. Affiliating with Julia Pastrana', in Marlene Tromp (ed.), *Victorian Freaks. The Social Context of Freakery in Britain* (Columbus, OH: Ohio State University Press, 2008), 200–233.

Stolberg, Michael, 'A Woman Down to her Bones. The Anatomy of Sexual Difference in the Sixteenth and Early Seventeenth Centuries', *Isis*, 94 (2003): 274–99.

Stramaglia, Antonio (ed.), *Phlegon Trallianus, Opuscula de rebus mirabilibus et de longaevis. Bibliotheca scriptorum Graecorum et Romanorum Teubneriana* (Berlin and New York: Walter de Gruyter, 2011).

Suzuki, Mihoko, (ed.) *The Early Modern Englishwoman: A Facsimile Library of Essential Works*, Series II, *Printed Writings, 1641–1700: Part 3*, Volume 5 (Aldershot: Ashgate, 2006).

Swain, Simon (ed.), *Seeing the Face, Seeing the Soul: Philemon's Physiognomy from Classical Antiquity to Medieval Islam* (Oxford: Oxford University Press, 2007).

Swedberg, Richard, *The Max Weber Dictionary: Key Words and Central Concepts* (Stanford, CA: Stanford University Press, 2005).

Sylvius, Jacobus, *In Hippocratis et Galeni physiologiae partem anatomicam Isagoge* (Paris: apud Joannem Hulpeau, 1555).

Tarte, Kendall B., *Writing Places: Sixteenth-Century City Culture and the Des Roches Salon* (Newark, DE: University of Delaware Press, 2007).

Taruffi, Cesare, *Hermaphrodismus und Zeugungsunfähigkeit. Eine systematische Darstellung der Missbildungen der menschlichen Geschlectsorgane* (Berlin: Verlag von Hermann Barsdorf, 1903).

[Thicknesse, Philip] *Man-Midwifery Analysed: and the Tendency of that Practice Detected and Exposed* (London: R. Davis, 1764).

Thivel, Antoine, *Cnide et Cos? Essai sur les doctrines médicales dans la Collection Hippocratique* (Paris: Les Belles Lettres, 1981).

Thomas Dangerfield's Answer to a Certain Scandalous Lying Pamphlet, Entituled, Malice Defeated (London: printed for the Author, 1680).

Tiraqueau, André (Andreas Tiraquellus), *De nobilitate, et de iure primigeniorum*, 5th edition (Basel: Froben, 1561; first edition 1549).

— *De legibus connubialibus* (Venice, 1576; first edition 1513).

To the Praise of Mrs. Cellier the Popish Midwife: On her Incomparable Book (London: Walter Davis, 1680).

Tone, Andrea (ed.), *Controlling Reproduction: An American History* (Wilmington, DE: Scholarly Resources Books, 1997).

Torquemada, Antonio de, *Jardin de floras curiosas* (En Enveres: En casa de Iuan Corderio, 1575).

— *The Spanish Mandeuile of miracles. Or The garden of curious flowers* (London: printed by J.R. for Edmund Matts, 1600).

— *Histoires en forme de Dialogue sérieux* (Rouen: Jean Roger, 1625).

Torrentinus, Hermannus, *Elucidarius carminum et historiarum seu Vocabularius poeticus* (Paris: ex officina Roberti Stephani, 1550).

Tortelli, Giovanni, *De orthographia dictionum e Graecis tractarum* (1449; first printed Rome: Gallus, 1471).

Totelin, Laurence, *Hippocratic Recipes. Oral and Written Transmission of Pharmacological Knowledge in Fifth- and Fourth-Century Greece* (Leiden: Brill, 2009).

— 'Old Recipes, New Practice? The Latin Adaptations of the Hippocratic Gynaecological Treatises', *Social History of Medicine*, 24 (2011): 74–91.

Tougher, Shaun, 'Byzantine Eunuchs: An Overview, with Special Reference to their Creation and Origin', in Liz James (ed.), *Women, Men and Eunuchs: Gender in Byzantium* (London and New York: Routledge, 1997), 168–84.

Toulalan, Sarah, 'Introduction', in Sarah Toulalan and Kate Fisher (eds), *Bodies, Sex and Desire from the Renaissance to the Present* (Basingstoke: Palgrave Macmillan, 2011), 1–24.

Towler, Jean and Joan Bramall, *Midwives in History and Society* (Beckenham: Croom Helm, 1986).

Traub, Valerie, 'The Psychomorphology of the Clitoris, or, The Reemergence of the *Tribade* in English Culture', in Valeria Finucci and Kevin Brownlee (eds), *Generation and Degeneration: Tropes of Reproduction in Literature and History from Antiquity to Early Modern Europe* (Durham, NC and London: Duke University Press, 2001), 153–86.

Treadgold, Warren T., *The Nature of the Bibliotheca of Photius* (Washington, DC: Dumbarton Oaks Center for Byzantine Studies, 1980).

The Tryal and Sentence of Elizabeth Cellier; for Writing, Printing, and Publishing, a Scandalous Libel, called Malice Defeated (London: Thomas Collins, 1680).

Tuccille, Jerome, *Trump: The Saga of America's Most Powerful Real Estate Baron* (Washington, DC: Beard Books, 1985).

Velasco, Sherry, '*Marimachos, hombrunas, barbudas*: The Masculine Woman in Cervantes', *Cervantes*, 29 (2000): 69–78.

Venuti, Lawrence, *The Translator's Invisibility* (London and New York: Routledge, 1995).

Vergil, Polydore, *De rerum inventoribus* (Venice: Christophorus de Pensis, 1499).

Vernant, Jean-Pierre, 'À la table des hommes: Mythe de fondation du sacrifice chez Hésiode', in Marcel Detienne and Jean-Pierre Vernant, *La Cuisine du sacrifice en pays grec* (Paris: Gallimard, 1979), 37–132.

Vesalius, Andreas, *De humani corporis fabrica* (Basel: Joannes Oporinus, 1543).

— *De humani corporis fabrica* (Basel: Joannes Oporinus, 1555).

— William Frank Richardson and John Burd Carman, *On the Fabric of the Human Body: A Translation of De Humani Corporis Fabrica libri septem*, Book V, *The Organs of Nutrition and Generation* (San Francisco, CA: Norman Publishing, 2007).

von Staden, Heinrich, *Herophilus. The Art of Medicine in Early Alexandria* (Cambridge: Cambridge University Press, 1989).

— '"In a Pure and Holy Way": Personal and Professional Conduct in the Hippocratic Oath?', *Journal of the History of Medicine and Allied Sciences*, 51 (1996): 404–37.

Voss, Heinz-Jürgen, *Making Sex Revisited. Dekonstruktion des Geschlechts aus biologisch-medizinischer Perspektive* (Bielefeld: transcript, 2010).

Wahrman, Dror, 'Change and the Corporeal in Seventeenth- and Eighteenth-Century Gender History: Or, Can Cultural History Be Rigorous?', *Gender and History*, 20 (2008): 584–602.

Walker, Richard, *Memoirs of Medicine, Including a Sketch of Medical History*, Book 1 (London: J. Johnson, 1799).

Walker, Susan, 'Women and Housing in Classical Greece: The Archaeological Evidence', in Averil Cameron and Amélie Kuhrt (eds), *Images of Women in Antiquity*, 2nd edition (London: Routledge, 1993), 81–91.

Ward, James, *An Essay Written in Defence of the Beard* (n.d., probably 1854; reprinted London: Lion and Unicorn Press, 1954).

Wear, Andrew, *Knowledge and Practice in English Medicine, 1550–1680* (Cambridge: Cambridge University Press, 2000).

Weber, Max, *The Methodology of the Social Sciences* (eds and tr. Edward A. Shils and Henry A. Finch) (New York: The Free Press, 1959).

Weil, Rachel, '"If I did say so, I lyed": Elizabeth Cellier and the Construction of Credibility in the Popish Plot Crisis', in Susan D. Amussen and Mark A. Kishlansky (eds), *Political Culture and Cultural Politics in Early Modern England: Essays Presented to David Underdown* (Manchester: Manchester University Press, 1995), 189–209.

— *Political Passions: Gender, the Family and Political Argument in England 1680–1714* (Manchester: Manchester University Press, 1999).

Wertz, Richard and Dorothy, *Lying In: A History of Childbirth in America* (New York: Free Press, 1977).

West-Pavlov, Russell, *Bodies and their Spaces: System, Crisis and Transformation in Early Modern Theatre* (Amsterdam: Rodopi, 2006).

Whatley, E. Gordon, 'More than a Female Joseph: The Sources of the Late-Fifth-Century *Passio Sanctae Eugeniae*', in Stuart McWilliams (ed.), *Saints and*

Scholars. New Perspectives on Anglo-Saxon Literature and Culture in Honour of Hugh Magennis (Suffolk: Boydell and Brewer, 2012), 87–111.

Whitmarsh, Tim (ed.), *The Cambridge Companion to the Greek and Roman Novel* (Cambridge: Cambridge University Press, 2008).

Whittington, Karl, 'The Cruciform Womb: Process, Symbol and Salvation in Bodleian Library MS. Ashmole 399', *Different Visions: A Journal of New Perspectives on Medieval Art*, 1 (2008): 1–24; <http://www.differentvisions.org/issue1PDFs/Whittington.pdf> accessed 20 June 2012.

Wier, Jacob, *De praestigiis daemonum, et incantationibus ac veneficiis libri sex* (Basle: Joannes Oporinus, 1564).

— *Cinq livres de l'imposture et tromperie des diables* (tr. Jacques Grevin) (Paris: Jacques de Puys, 1567).

— *Opera omnia* (Amsterdam: Petrus vanden Berge, 1660).

Wiesner-Hanks, Merry, *The Marvellous Hairy Girls* (New Haven, CT and London: Yale University Press, 2009).

Williams, Craig A., *Roman Homosexuality: Ideologies of Masculinity in Classical Antiquity* (New York and Oxford: Oxford University Press, 1999).

Willughby, Percival, *Observations in Midwifery*, ed. Henry Blenkinsop (Warwick: Cooke, 1863).

Wilson, Adrian, *The Making of Man-Midwifery. Childbirth in England, 1660–1770* (Cambridge, MA: Harvard University Press, 1995).

— 'Midwifery in the "Medical Marketplace"', in Mark Jenner and Patrick Wallis (eds), *Medicine and the Market in England and its Colonies, c.1450–c.1850* (Basingstoke: Palgrave Macmillan, 2007), 153–74.

Wilson, Nigel G., *From Byzantium to Italy: Greek Studies in the Italian Renaissance* (London: Duckworth, 1992).

Winkler, John, J., 'Laying Down the Law: The Oversight of Men's Sexual Behavior in Classical Athens', in David M. Halperin, John J. Winkler and Froma I. Zeitlin (eds), *Before Sexuality: The Construction of Erotic Experience in the Ancient Greek World* (Princeton, NJ: Princeton University Press, 1990), 171–210.

Winn, Colette H., 'De sage (-) femme à sage (-) fille: Louise Boursier, *Instructions à ma fille* 1626)', *Papers on French Seventeenth-Century Literature*, 24 (1997): 61–83.

Wirth, Gerhard, *Diodorus. Griechische Weltgeschichte Fragmente Buch XXI–XL*, vol. 1 (Stuttgart: Anton Hiersemann, 2008).

Withers, Maurine, 'Agnodike. The First Midwife/Obstetrician', *Journal of Nurse-Midwifery*, 24 (1979): 4.

Witkowski, Gustav Joseph, *Accoucheurs et sages-femmes célèbres: esquisses biographiques* (Paris: Steinheil, 1891).

Witty, Francis J., 'The *Pinakes* of Callimachus', *Library Quarterly*, 28 (1958): 132–7.

The Works of Aristotle, in Four Parts, Containing His Complete Master Piece ... His Experienced Midwife ... His Book of Problems ... His Last Legacy (London, 1777).

The Works of Aristotle, in Four Parts, Containing His Complete Master Piece ... His Experienced Midwife ... His Book of Problems ... His Last Legacy (London, 1791).

The Works of Aristotle, the Famous Philosopher, in Four Parts. Containing His Complete Master Piece ... His experienced Midwife ... His Book of Problems ... His Last Legacy (Philadelphia, 1799).

Zanker, Paul, *The Mask of Socrates: The Image of the Intellectual in Antiquity* (Berkeley, CA: University of California Press, 1995).

Zeitlin, Froma, 'The Poetics of *Eros*: Nature, Art, and Imitation in Longus' *Daphnis and Chloe*', in David M. Halperin, John J. Winkler and Froma I. Zeitlin (eds), *Before Sexuality: The Construction of Erotic Experience in the Ancient Greek World* (Princeton, NJ: Princeton University Press, 1990), 417–64.

Zervos, Skevos, *Aetii sermo sextidecimus et ultimus* (Leipzig: Mangkos, 1901).

Index